Operative Techniques
in Epilepsy Surgery

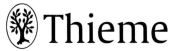

Operative Techniques in Epilepsy Surgery

Gordon Baltuch, MD, PhD, FRCS(C)
Associate Professor
Department of Neurosurgery
University of Pennsylvania
Philadelphia, Pennsylvania

Jean-Guy Villemure, MD, FRCS(C)
Professor and Chairman
Department of Neurosurgery
University of Montreal
Montreal, Quebec, Canada

Thieme
New York • Stuttgart

Thieme Medical Publishers, Inc.
333 Seventh Ave.
New York, NY 10001

Associate Editor: Ivy Ip
Executive Editor: Kalen Conerly
Vice President, Production and Electronic Publishing: Anne T. Vinnicombe
Production Editor: Kenneth L. Chumbley, Publication Services
Vice President, International Marketing and Sales: Cornelia Schulze
Chief Financial Officer: Peter van Woerden
President: Brian D. Scanlan
Compositor: Manila Typesetting Company
Printer: Everbest Printing Company, Ltd.

Library of Congress Cataloging-in-Publication Data

Operative techniques in epilepsy surgery / [edited by] Gordon Baltuch, Jean-Guy Villemure.
    p. ; cm.
  Includes bibliographical references and index.
  ISBN 978-1-60406-030-0 (alk. paper)
  1. Epilepsy--Surgery. 2. Brain--Surgery. I. Baltuch, Gordon H. II. Villemure, Jean-Guy.
  [DNLM: 1. Epilepsy--surgery. 2. Neurosurgical Procedures. WL 385 O61 2009]
  RD594.O64 2009
  617.4'81--dc22
                    2008017403

Important note: Medical knowledge is ever-changing. As new research and clinical experience broaden our knowledge, changes in treatment and drug therapy may be required. The authors and editors of the material herein have consulted sources believed to be reliable in their efforts to provide information that is complete and in accord with the standards accepted at the time of publication. However, in view of the possibility of human error by the authors, editors, or publisher of the work herein or changes in medical knowledge, neither the authors, editors, nor publisher, nor any other party who has been involved in the preparation of this work, warrants that the information contained herein is in every respect accurate or complete, and they are not responsible for any errors or omissions or for the results obtained from use of such information. Readers are encouraged to confirm the information contained herein with other sources. For example, readers are advised to check the product information sheet included in the package of each drug they plan to administer to be certain that the information contained in this publication is accurate and that changes have not been made in the recommended dose or in the contraindications for administration. This recommendation is of particular importance in connection with new or infrequently used drugs. Some of the product names, patents, and registered designs referred to in this book are in fact registered trademarks or proprietary names even though specific reference to this fact is not always made in the text. Therefore, the appearance of a name without designation as proprietary is not to be construed as a representation by the publisher that it is in the public domain.

Printed in China

5 4 3 2 1

ISBN: 978-1-60406-030-0

To our patients and their families who inspired us with their courage, trust, and support.

Gordon H. Baltuch
Jean-Guy Villemure

Contents

Preface

Epilepsy is an important illness with a high prevalence (5 per 1000). It is the second most common cause of mental health disability, particularly among young adults, but it affects individuals of all ages, races, and socioeconomic backgrounds. Recent advances in neuroimaging and surgical technique have improved the surgical treatment of epilepsy to such an extent that some experts now suggest that physicians should offer surgery early to patients with surgically remediable epileptic syndromes, instead of waiting years until multiple anticonvulsants have failed. This interest in surgical strategies has also been powered by a renaissance in neuromodulatory approaches to the brain, which have revolutionized functional neurosurgery over the last 15 years.

While there are classic texts in the field that describe in detail indications, outcomes, and controversies in epilepsy surgery, we endeavored to contribute a *techniques* text that would be readable by neurosurgeons and neurosurgeons in training, who want to learn how to perform the classic resective procedures of epilepsy surgery and some of the more recent and investigational neuromodulatory approaches. We sought out contributors whom we felt reflected a modern and innovative surgical approach in this field. We believe this text will also be of interest to those practicing in neurology and neuroradiology as well as to those working in clinical and cognitive neuroscience, who are curious as to what transpires once the operating theater doors are closed.

Acknowledgments

We would like to acknowledge Brian Scanlan, Kalen Conerly, Ivy Ip, and Elsie Starbecker at Thieme Publishers, as well as Kenny Chumbley, for their tremendous efforts in making this text a reality. Their assistance has been invaluable and is highly appreciated.

Gordon H. Baltuch
Jean-Guy Villemure

Contributors

Jeffrey D. Atkinson, MD, FRCS(C)
Assistant Professor
Department of Neurosurgery
McGill University
Montreal Children's Hospital
Montreal, Quebec, Canada

Gordon H. Baltuch, MD, PhD, FRCS(C)
Associate Professor
Department of Neurosurgery
University of Pennsylvania
Philadelphia, Pennsylvania

Fabrice Bartolomei, MD, PhD
Service de Neurophysiologie Clinique
Marseille, France

Joel A. Bauman, MD
Department of Neurosurgery
University of Pennsylvania
Philadelphia, Pennsylvania

Warren W. Boling, MD, FRCS(C)
Associate Professor
Department of Neurosurgery
West Virginia University
Morgantown, West Virginia

Patrick Chauvel, MD
Department of Stereotactic and Functional Neurosurgery
Timone University Hospital
Marseille, France

Patrick J. Connolly, MD
Assistant Professor
Department of Neurosurgery
Temple University
Philadelphia, Pennsylvania

G. Rees Cosgrove, MD
Professor
Department of Neurosurgery
Lahey Clinic Medical Center
Tufts University School of Medicine
Burlington, Massachusetts

Roy Thomas Daniel, MCh
Professor
Department of Neurological Sciences
Christian Medical College
Vellore, India

Jean-Pierre Farmer, MD, FRCS
Professor
Department of Neurosurgery
McGill University
Montreal Children's Hospital
Montreal, Quebec, Canada

Casey Halpern, MD
Department of Neurosurgery
University of Pennsylvania
Philadelphia, Pennsylvania

Gregory G. Heuer, MD, PhD
Department of Neurosurgery
University of Pennsylvania
Philadelphia, Pennsylvania

Jurg L. Jaggi, PhD
Department of Neurosurgery
University of Pennsylvania
Philadelphia, Pennsylvania

Barbara C. Jobst, MD
Assistant Professor
Department of Medicine
Section of Neurology
Dartmouth Medical School
Lebanon, New Hampshire

Padmaja Kandula, MD
Assistant Professor
Department of Neurology and Neuroscience
Weill Cornell Medical College
New York Presbyterian Hospital
New York, New York

Brian Litt, MD
Department of Neurology
University of Pennyslvania
Philadelphia, Pennyslvania

Ram Mani, MD
Department of Neurology
University of Pennsylvania
Philadelphia, Pennsylvania

Christopher R. Mascott, MD, FRCS(C)
Department of Neuroscience
Beacon Epilepsy Institute
Beacon Hospital
Dublin, Ireland

Douglas Maus, MD, PhD
Department of Neurology
University of Pennsylvania
Philadelphia, Pennsylvania

Sandeep Mittal, MD, FRCS(C)
Assistant Professor
Department of Neurosurgery
Wayne State University
Detroit, Michigan

José-Luis Montes, MD
Professor
Department of Neurosurgery
McGill University
Montreal Children's Hospital
Montreal, Quebec, Canada

Dimitris G. Placantonakis, MD, PhD
Department of Neurological Surgery
Weill Cornell Medical College
New York Presbyterian Hospital
New York, New York

Claudio Pollo, MD
Department of Neurosurgery
Centre Hospitalier Universitaire Vaudois
Lausanne, Switzerland

Jean Régis, MD
Professor
Department of Stereotactic and Functional Neurosurgery
Timone University Hospital
Marseille, France

David W. Roberts, MD
Professor
Department of Medicine
Section of Neurosurgery
Dartmouth Medical School
Lebanon, New Hampshire

Abdulrahman J. Sabbagh, MD
Neurosurgery Residency Program Director
Department of Neurosurgery
King Fahd Medical City
Riyadh, Saudi Arabia

Uzma Samadani, MD, PhD
Assistant Professor
Department of Neurosurgery
New York University
New York, New York

James Schuster, MD, PhD
Assistant Professor
Department of Neurosurgery
University of Pennsylvania
Philadelphia, Pennsylvania

Theodore H. Schwartz, MD
Associate Professor
Department of Neurological Surgery, Neurology, Neuroscience, and Otolaryngology
Weill Cornell Medical College
New York Presbyterian Hospital
New York, New York

Phillip B. Storm, MD
Assistant Professor
Department of Neurosurgery
University of Pennsylvania
Philadelphia, Pennsylvania

Albert E. Telfeian, MD, PhD
Neurosurgical Associates, LLP
Lubbock, Texas

Jean-Guy Villemure, MD, FRCS(C)
Professor and Chairman
Department of Neurosurgery
University of Montreal
Montreal, Quebec, Canada

Robert E. Wharen Jr., MD
Professor
Department of Neurosurgery
Mayo Clinic College of Medicine
Jacksonville, Florida

Surgical Planning

1 Image Guidance and Epilepsy Surgery

Christopher R. Mascott

Navigational systems have gained widespread acceptance in the neurosurgical community over the past decade. There is hardly a contemporary neurosurgery center that does not have one or several image-guided surgery (IGS) systems in the operating room. However, the utilization of these systems still does vary from institution to institution and from one surgeon to the next.[1] For the most part, epilepsy surgeons embraced computer-guidance technology early on because stereotaxis already was an integral component of techniques needed and employed by most epilepsy surgeons.[2–6]

Development of IGS

Stereotaxis

Although stereotactic frames were used in animals in the 19th century and early prototypes for human use have been reported,[7,8] the first use in humans is generally attributed to Spiegel and Wycis initially in the context of treating psychiatric disorders, then for pain and movement disorder surgery.[9] The application of frames for the stereotactic placement of depth electrodes to study epilepsy was reported in the 1950s by Bancaud and Talairach.[10] At the time, centers already performing surgery for epilepsy on the basis of scalp and intraoperative electroencephalogram (EEG) recordings, seizure semiology, and to a limited degree imaging studies (pneumoencephalography, angiography) gradually adopted stereotactic methodology for the investigation of subsets of patients. Renewed interest in epilepsy surgery in the 1980s, along with the advent of computed tomography (CT)-based and magnetic resonance imaging (MRI)-based stereotaxis, led to more extensive use of frame-based stereotaxis for invasive EEG studies.[11–13]

CT/MRI

Discussion of the enormous impact of computer-based neuroimaging modalities of CT and especially MRI on epilepsy surgery is beyond the scope of this chapter. With regard to stereotaxis, these imaging modalities were used to supplement or replace atlas-based strategies that relied on ventriculography, stereotactic angiography, or both. Stereotactic angiography is still employed in some centers as an adjunct to avoid vascular injury during electrode placement and possibly to increase accuracy.[12] The improvement of CT and MRI, the possibility of acquiring "volumetric" imaging datasets, and the increase of computer power used to correlate these datasets to stereotactic space paved the way for image-guided technology. Patrick Kelly was one of the pioneers in the correlating of three-dimensonally (3-D)-defined image datasets with surgical stereotactic space as defined by a stereotactic frame.[14–16]

Early IGS in the 1990s

When image datasets are acquired as a volume, the head can be reconstructed in 3-D in image space and the surfaces can be "rendered." In this manner the surface of the skin and (when using CT) the skull can be used to reference the location of targets in the brain instead of a stereotactic frame. Thus the concept of *frameless stereotaxis* was born.[17–21] To match target points of the image dataset with surgical targets in the operating room, the surface of the imaging-rendered volume must be correlated point for point with the surface of the patient's head at surgery. This process is known as *registration* and is of considerable importance with regard to the ensuing accuracy and reliability of image guidance at surgery.[22] Registration is dependant on a tracking system that can determine the position of points in space with regard to a fixed reference at the time of surgery. The earliest forms of frameless registration used ultrasound or mechanical arms for tracking, and these were applied to epilepsy surgery.[3,6,23] Most currently available image-guidance systems have moved to optical tracking where the position of a pointer and reference are triangulated by pole-mounted cameras, or to magnetic tracking where the head and instrument positions are defined within the reference of a generated magnetic field.[1,24–26]

Is IGS Necessary for Epilepsy Surgery?

It cannot be overstressed that technology cannot be a substitute for anatomical knowledge or medical and surgical knowledge and experience. Any surgeon undertaking surgery for epilepsy should have the appropriate medical and surgical background and training. Knowledge of neuroanatomy and concepts of functional neuroanatomy and localization of function are more critical to epilepsy surgery than any other area of neurosurgery. Within these parameters, the author has found image guidance to be a remarkable adjunctive tool in epilepsy surgery strategies. Although epilepsy surgeons should be able to plan and perform surgery without reliance on image-guidance technology, the author hopes to highlight the multifaceted usefulness of image-guidance technology in the contemporary approach to surgery for epilepsy.

IG for Preoperative Assessment and Planning

Image guidance is not restricted to use in the operating theater. For general neurosurgery, the planning of cranial procedures can be instructional in assessing a variety of approaches and surgery strategies on a virtual basis using the IGS planning station. This preoperative role can be greatly expanded in the epilepsy context.

Because of the overwhelming importance of a variety of imaging modalities to the contemporary investigation of epilepsy, an IGS workstation can be used as a tool to bring these imaging modalities together for analysis and discussion, even in patients that end up not being candidates for surgery.

Preoperative Analysis

Many of the software options incorporated into current generation IGS systems can be used to great effect for image analysis and correlation in epilepsy, quite independently of surgical guidance issues. Although similar analysis can be performed on imaging workstations not related to IGS, not all medical centers have all of these options at their disposal. More important, image processing and quantification can be quite labor-intensive and dedicated personnel may not be available. A neurosurgeon familiar with the more sophisticated aspects of IGS workstations can contribute valuable analysis options to a multidisciplinary team involved in epilepsy surgery workups.

Quantitative MRI

With the advent of MRI, previously recognized epilepsy-related physiopathological entities such as mesiotemporal sclerosis (MTS) became visible on preoperative imaging studies.[27,28] This has simplified surgical decision making for clearly visualized MTS with congruent electrophysiological and neuropsychological findings.[29] On the other hand, when imaging findings have been less clear-cut in both temporal and extratemporal epilepsy, many epilepsy centers have resorted to the quantification of structure volumes on MRI with the hope of gaining additional localizing information in epilepsy investigations.[30,31] This can be performed on volumetrically acquired MRI data on an imaging workstation, and more recently on a regular PC or laptop with the installation of the appropriate software. In several different centers, the author has taken advantage of the fact that MRI volumetric acquisition appropriate for epilepsy-imaging protocols was also appropriate for subsequent image guidance at surgery. In this manner, imaging protocols can be designed for both analysis and surgery, a cost-effective strategy to avoid repeat imaging. With this dual role of imaging in mind, **Table 1.1** lists the author's basic, routine imaging sequences for epilepsy/epilepsy surgery with discussion of add-on sequences for specific indications.

There is a wealth of literature on volumetric studies that quantify MRI volumes of hippocampus, amygdala, entorhinal cortex, other cortical areas, total temporal, frontal lobe or whole brain, thalamic nucleus, etc.[32-35] The motivation behind these strategies and the anatomical knowledge of the structural boundaries involved are beyond the scope of this chapter. The following brief discussion will be restricted to practical consideration for using an IGS workstation to perform volume analysis. This is predicated on the fact that most IGS systems will give a readout of volume estimation of any model that is built on the workstation. For research purposes, absolute volumes as given by IGS workstations need to be validated against other volumetric measurement strategies such as non-IGS workstation segmentation and stereology.[36]

Most of the author's experience in volumetric assessment using an IGS workstation has been with the StealthStation (Medtronic IGN, Louisville, CO). Each IGS manufacturer limits

Table 1.1 MRI Imaging Protocol

MRI Sequence	Slice Thickness	Orientation	Advantage	Comment	Routine or Additional
SPGR (GE) MPRAGE (Siemens) with contrast	1.3–1.5 mm (volumetric, no gap)	Axial	Volumetric acquisition. Optimized accuracy for IGS	Contrast mainly for cortical vein rendering	Routine
FLAIR	1–3 mm, no gap	Coronal	High sensitivity for low-grade tumors, dysplasia, gliosis, etc.		Routine
Inversion recovery	1–1.5 mm	Coronal	High resolution. Gray white definition, dysplasia	Particularly good for quantitative MRI (volumetrics)	Additional or routine if available
T2-weighted	1–3 mm	Coronal	Sensitive		Additional
DTI			Fiber tracking	DSI even more interesting	Additional

Abbreviations: SPGR MPRAGE, spoiled gradient echo-magnetization prepared rapid gradient echo; FLAIR, fluid attenuated inversion recovery; DTI, diffusion tensor imaging.

the number of volumes that can be defined. On most recent systems, whole brain volume can be segmented relatively automatically, and an appropriate menu will provide the volume readout for this. For other structures, such as the hippocampus, the author has relied on mainly manual segmentation (**Fig. 1.1**). This means that the structure of interest must be manually outlined on a sequential slice-by-slice basis, usually on coronal planes at higher magnification. It is usually useful in correctly identifying the structure of interest to set the screen view to simultaneously show axial and sagittal reformats. It is important to define the outlines of the structure of interest in only one plane as you progress through the volume. Once the volume has been defined on the last slice of the MRI, it is crucial to save the volume because acquisition is quite time-consuming and if one fails a "save" instruction, everything will be lost. As soon as the volume is saved, a readout of the measured volume becomes available on most systems. Because IGS workstations are designed for general neurosurgeons, not epilepsy surgeons, right and left hippocampal volumes may have to be designated as "skull" and "ventricles," respectively (for example). Color coding of volumes is usually available to help clarify matters somewhat.

Image Fusion

In the overall investigation of possibly surgically treatable epilepsy, the correlation of different imaging sequences and modalities is very useful. Here again, most contemporary IGS systems incorporate algorithms for image correlation or "fusion." Of available "routine" MRI sequences, the author has used fluid-attenuated inversion recovery (FLAIR) sequences the most frequently to help define areas of potential cortical dysplasia, gliosis, or low-grade tumor.[37] It is helpful to acquire any image sequence intended for routine importation into an image-guidance system in as "volumetric" an acquisition as possible (i.e., thin sequential cuts with no gap).

Current "image fusion" software in IGS systems will compensate for suboptimally acquired secondary imaging datasets to some degree. This will be at the expense of image quality in the reformatted planes. Most IGS systems now have software that "automatically" performs image fusion between different datasets based on mutual shared information algorithms. This works very well in most cases. Manual fusion is still available when automatic fusion seems suboptimal. From a practical standpoint, manual image correlation is performed by selecting matching anatomical points on the two sequences to be correlated.[22] If fiducial markers (either adhesive or skull-implanted) are present, they can be used for this. Otherwise, the author recommends the pituitary stalk, optic chiasm, anterior and posterior commisures, and vascular bifurcations (carotids, basilar tip, vertebrobasilar junction, some cortical veins). The same landmarks can be examined to assess the reliability of an automatically performed image fusion. Newer anatomical MR imaging sequences of interest in epilepsy include diffusion tensor imaging (DTI)[38,39] and higher field MRI inversion recovery sequences. In most cases, these image sequences need to be correlated or "fused" to a primary volumetric dataset for 3-D localization and image-guidance purposes.

Multimodal Correlation

In addition to the correlation of different MRI anatomical imaging sequences, the co-registration of other non-MRI modalities can be facilitated by IGS station software. This includes source localization from EEG, magnetoencephalography (MEG), positron emission tomography (PET), and ictal single photon emission tomography (SPECT) to name just a few (**Fig. 1.2**).[25,40–43] The main goal is to provide 3-D–defined brain localization for functional or metabolic data. This can then be presented at multidisciplinary meetings for discussion and interpretation (**Fig. 1.3**).

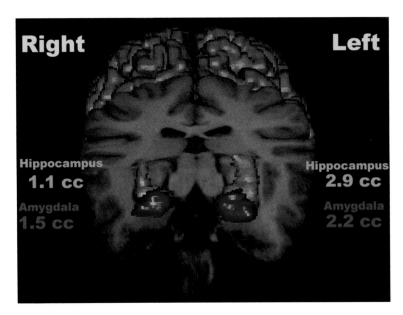

Fig. 1.1 This is an illustration of a 3-D model built on an IGS workstation (StealthStation, Medronic, Colorado). The right and left amygdalar (red) and hippocampal (models) were segmented slice by slice on coronal images. The individual models give a volume readout when built. From a practical standpoint, it is important to save the individual models frequently as they are being built to not lose the work in progress.

Functional Correlation

Functional imaging modalities can involve activation studies in functional MRI (fMRI) or in some of the modalities mentioned above (PET, MEG, magnetic resonance spectroscopic imaging [MRSI], EEG, etc.). As previously mentioned, it is useful to attempt localization of the modality being tested to a cortical area, if possible. In this manner it can be possible to compare localization of function to that of epileptic activity and anatomical landmarks. Frequently, cortical vein modeling provides useful landmarks to help localize target areas in the brain (**Figs. 1.2 and 1.3**).

Risk versus Benefit Assessment

The overall goal of epilepsy investigations in view of possible surgery is the same as that when considering any medical treatment: an assessment of the risks of a particular procedure compared with the likelihood and degree of benefit.

In this context, an IGS workstation used to correlate and present multiple investigations can be a powerful tool. Discussing possible vascular risks, functional risks, and surgical challenges is best done when looking at a workstation multimodal display.

Application Accuracy

In patients who are thought to be suitable candidates for epilepsy surgery, image guidance can be helpful for actual neuronavigation. If a variety of imaging modalities have already been correlated using the image-guidance workstation, these datasets can be used during surgery with relatively little further refinement. It remains essential, however, to highlight that for most common surgical procedures for epilepsy, surgeons should have an intimate knowledge of neuroanatomy, the literature regarding functional localization, and the neuropsychological risks related to resective or disconnective procedure variants. As with any technology, neuronaviga-

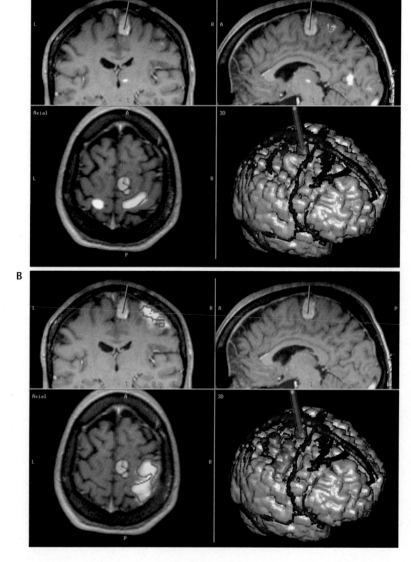

Fig. 1.2 This patient with longstanding epilepsy had new hemorrhage in the right central area (in green on the brain renderings in **[A,B]**). She had very brief "reflex"-type motor seizures. **(A)** Fusion of ictal SPECT data with a volumetric MRI sequence. The area of activation in the right hemisphere has been rendered in red on the 3-D model and with activity predominantly within the posterior bank of the central sulcus. Note that there is also some mirror-image activation in the left hemisphere, which has not been rendered. **(B)** Functional MRI data fused with the same volumetric MRI sequence. The fMRI in this illustration was performed with motor activation of the left hand, and this is rendered in blue on the 3-D model.

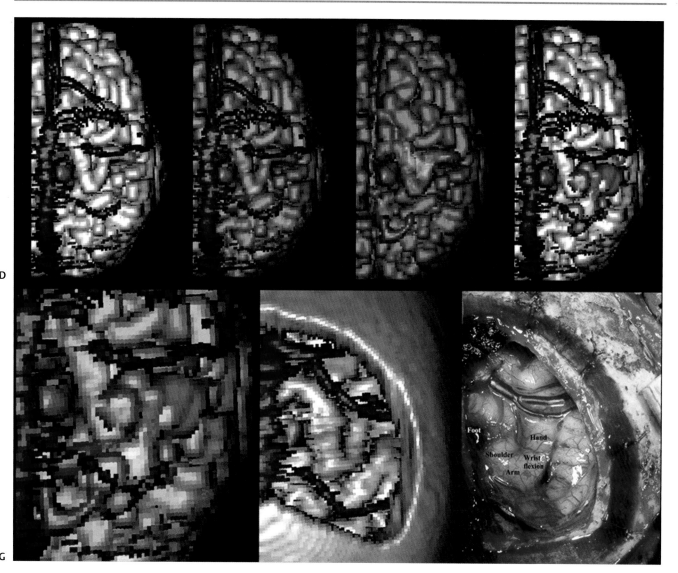

Fig. 1.3 This is a further example of multimodal image fusion from the same patient as in **Fig. 1.2**. **(A)** A 3-D–rendered brain from MRI with contrast as viewed from above. Note the rendered sagittal sinus and cortical veins. The area of hemorrhage is again rendered in green. **(B)** This image illustrates the rendered SPECT activation (in red) shown in **Fig. 1.2A** as seen from this angle. **(C)** Left leg motor activation fMRI data (in purple on 3-D model) fused with the same volumetric sequence. **(D)** This image illustrates the rendered left hand motor activation fMRI data (blue) shown in **Fig. 1.2A**, as seen from this angle. **(E)** The simultaneous 3-D renderings of **(A–D)**. **(F)** The craniotomy exposure at surgery. This image was obtained by fusing the preoperative MRI brain volume with a postoperative volumetric CT and building a skull model of the craniotomy exposure. **(G)** The surgical exposure. The hemorrhagic lesion has been excised after stimulation motor mapping. Electrocorticography showed active spiking in the postcentral gyrus, which has undergone subpial transection including down into the posterior bank of the central sulcus.

tion should be an adjunct to refine treatment, as opposed to a crutch. In more demanding situations that require a heavier reliance on image guidance, it becomes essential to be aware of how reliable and accurate this technology may be during surgery. Most contemporary imaging protocols that have evolved for use with image guidance have been streamlined to introduce relatively minimal error into the procedure. There remain, however, many other sources of localization error of neuronavigation during surgery. The final error of localizing targets during surgery is the cumulative result of all the possible sources of error when correlating targets on the IGS workstation (in "image space") with corresponding targets at surgery (in "surgical space"). The term *application accuracy* has been introduced to refer to this cumulative error.[22,44–46] Application accuracy will vary from case to case. There are methods that can lead to higher levels of accuracy, which can be crucial in some situations but unnecessary in others.

With the assumption that imaging protocols used are optimized for IGS, and that the mechanical accuracy of the various IGS systems has also been optimized, two main sources of localization error at surgery need to be considered here, registration and brain shift.[47]

- *Registration* is the process by which the anatomy on the images (of the IGS system) is correlated with the surgical anatomy of the patient. This is done by matching defined points or surfaces in image space with their counterparts in surgical space after defining the latter within a frame of reference (e.g., by means of optical, magnetic, or mechanical triangulation).[1,22] There is an overall consensus among most investigators that the calculated accuracy displayed by IGS systems can be a poor indicator of the real surgical (application) accuracy. This author has found that most common methods of registration using point matching with anatomical landmarks (i.e., tragus, bridge of the nose, etc.) or adhesive scalp fiducials, or surface matching (using 45 or 100 points) result in similar application accuracies in the 4 mm ± 2 mm range. (Note: in an individual case, observed accuracy could be 2 mm, and in another case it could be 8 mm.)[22] This may be reasonable accuracy for many common procedures in epilepsy surgery. There has been, however, a highly statistically significant accuracy advantage in registrations using skull-implanted fiducial markers, with accuracies of 1.7 ± 0.9 mm. This is slightly more invasive and warrants consideration in cases where higher accuracy and reliability are necessary (**Fig. 1.4**). A stereotactic frame is also an alternative in these situations.[48] The author's protocol for fiducial screw placement is given in **Table 1.2**.

- *Brain shift* occurs at the time of surgery when cerebrospinal fluid (CSF) is lost or when a resection creates shift of adjacent brain areas. Because IGS employs preoperative imaging information, dynamic changes during surgery are not taken into account and the new postshift location of an intracranial structure will no longer correlate with its presurgical images. Shift must be kept in mind as a source of localization error at surgery. It is wise to address any critical IGS dependant targets early during surgery prior to shift effects or to consider updating imaging information during surgery by intraoperative imaging when available (ultrasound, CT, or MRI).[49-52] In the author's experience, prioritizing critical areas for image guidance has minimized the need for intraoperative imaging.

IGS for Investigative Epilepsy Surgery

When information for suitability for resective surgery is insufficient or when there is conflicting information between EEG, imaging and/or neuropsychology testing, invasive EEG studies may be indicated. When placing intracranial electrodes, IGS systems can be useful in targeting anatomical or pathological areas on imaging studies.

Depth Electrodes

Traditionally, penetrating depth electrodes (DE) have been placed stereotactically by means of stereotactic frames.[10,12] Some institutions have used frameless IGS strategies for DE placement.[3,53,54] To optimize the accuracy and reliability of DE placement, the author strongly recommends using implanted screw fiducials for subsequent imaging and registration. This is a perfect example of the need for optimized application accuracy.

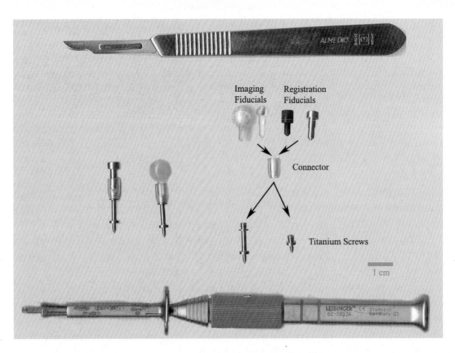

Fig. 1.4 Titanium fiducial bone screw markers (Stryker Leibinger, Inc., Kalamazoo, MI). The screwdriver is used to place the self-drilling screws following local anesthesia and a stab incision. Via the plastic connector, imaging fiducials are attached to the screws and serve as landmarks on MRI or CT. Just the screws are left in place until surgery. At surgery, registration fiducials are attached to the screws, so that the registration probe touches these in a manner that corresponds to the center of the imaging fiducials.

Table 1.2 Skull Fiducial Screw Placement

Procedure	Time Course	Objective	Comment
EMLA cream to 4–5 scalp locations	1 hour before screw placement	Decreases burning of local anesthetic	Not essential but more comfortable for patients. Prior to EMLA, we used sublingual lorazepam for patient comfort.
Local infiltration of lidocaine with epinephrine	Prior to screw placement	Local anesthesia; epinephrine for hemostasis	
After sterile prep, no. 15 blade scalpel stab incision. Periosteum is displaced with tip of blade.	Prior to screw placement	Incision just wide enough for screw	Supplemental local with epinephrine for hemostasis; rarely a stitch
Self-drilling titanium screws inserted	Screw can be placed 0–10 days before surgery. Average for the author is 3–5 days.	Base for localizing markers	Screws are usually placed fairly high. Lower screws tend to loosen and cause more pain and irritation.
Connectors and markers attached to screws	Prior to imaging (CT, MRI, or both)	These are the markers visualized on images for registration.	
IGS protocol imaging	Any time after marker attachment	Volumetric dataset for image guidance	The markers can also be used for manual image fusion.
Removal of connectors and markers leaving screws in place	Prior to discharge home	More discreet appearance and decreased chance of screw loosening	Screw location has been selected to avoid planned craniotomy incisions. Thin areas of skull are also avoided.
Surgical planning	Anytime between image acquisition and surgery	Surgical planning, cortical rendering, image fusion, and image registration	"Decoupling" of imaging and planning from the day of surgery is one of the advantages of "frameless" over frame-based stereotaxis.
Surgery: replacement of connectors to screws along with registration cup; removal at the end of surgery	In the OR after positioning and head immobilization	Registration for IGS	Nonsterile connectors and cups can be replaced by sterile ones attached to the screws through the drapes if intraoperative re-registration is necessary.

Abbreviations: EMLA, brand name: Astra Zeneca; OR, operating room.

The author's usual sequence for IGS DE placement is outlined in **Table 1.3**. Frequent targets for DEs include the mesiotemporal structures (amygdala and hippocampus). The mesiotemporal structures can be targeted via an orthogonal approach or from a posterior longitudinal approach. Using image guidance, the author has used both approaches (**Fig. 1.5**). When using a posterior approach, the author prefers to target the temporal horn of the ventricle for electrode placement to avoid bilateral longitudinal hippocampal penetrations. The IGS strategy to accomplish consistent temporal horn placement of electrodes involves targeting the atrium of the ventricle on each side from a high enough angle to let the electrode enter the temporal horn. The stylet of the electrode is then removed and the electrode advanced to allow it to follow the curvature of the temporal horn. The electrode is then immobilized at the level of the skull when the resistance of the tip of the temporal horn is encountered.[55]

In extratemporal DE explorations, these are usually placed in areas of suspected epileptogenesis on the basis of structural imaging (dysplasia, tumor, etc.), functional imaging (PET, SPECT, fMRI, MEG, etc.), or EEG and clinical information. For all DE placements described herein, skull-implanted fiducials were combined with volumetric MRI sequences (spoiled gradient echo [SPGR], magnetization prepared rapid gradient echo [MPRAGE]) with contrast. The addition of contrast allows the visualization of veins and arteries so that the DE trajectories can be planned to avoid vascular structures and thus decrease the risk of hemorrhage.

Table 1.3 IGS DE Placement

Procedure	Technique	Objective	Comment
Skull-implanted fiducial screw placement	See **Table 1.2.**	Optimizing registration and application accuracy	Electrode placement should be as accurate as possible.
Imaging	Volumetric MRI with contrast; formerly combined with CT but no accuracy advantage noted	MRI for 3-D brain rendering; contrast for vascular rendering	Other imaging modalities fused as needed
Planning	Electrode trajectories are planned by selecting a target and entry point for each electrode.	Once a trajectory has been defined, it is important to switch into trajectory view and probe's eye view on the workstation.	Running along the trajectory view, check for proximity of cortical veins and other vessels. Alter electrode trajectory to avoid vascular structures.
Registration at surgery using implanted screws	See **Table 1.2.**	Optimized application accuracy	
Depth electrode placement	The author prefers pediatric bur holes to twist drill holes for final verification of cortical vein avoidance.		
Electrode immobilization	Skull bolts are available for immobilization. The author prefers tunneling the electrodes to vertex.	Tunneling eliminates CSF leaks and facilitates bedside removal. Fixation is via a skull-mounted silicone clamp or silicone sheet on scalp.	

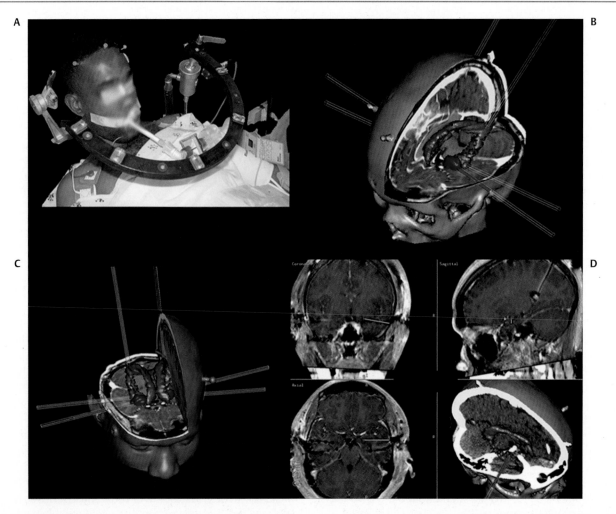

Fig. 1.5 **(A–D)** Frameless image-guided depth electrode placement. Trajectory planning on a fused CT-MRI dataset is shown on the models in **(B)** the upper right and **(C)**. Note the presence of skull-implanted fiducial markers throughout. Position at surgery with the reference arc and imaging fiducial in place is shown in **(A)**. A fusion of immediate postoperative volumetric MRI with preoperative planned trajectories on CT and MRI is shown in **(C)**. This has been used to assess actual electrode position versus intended electrode position.[26] CT and MRI shown in **(D)**.

Grids and Strips

When subdural electrodes are placed for the investigation of epilepsy either in isolation or combined with DEs, image guidance can be useful. This is particularly true when the individual electrode contacts are localized at the time of electrode (grid or strip) placement or at removal and when these localizations are superimposed on a 3-D brain rendering.[56] To aid in the localization of specific brain areas, building a model of cortical veins provides a particularly helpful landmark as previously mentioned.

IGS for Resective Surgery

Neuronavigation can be used in all resective epilepsy surgery. Overall, lesional epilepsy cases should be distinguished from nonlesional cases. In the latter, cortical areas are the target for surgical resection as opposed to a distinct "lesion." There can be some confusion in the definition of a lesion because some authors refer to all imaging abnormalities including volume loss and signal change in brain structures (i.e., hippocampal sclerosis) as a lesion. In this chapter, *lesional* will refer to distinct abnormalities thought to be more than cortical alterations.

Lesional IGS Epilepsy Surgery

In surgical approaches to lesions associated with epilepsy, it is important to highlight that some of these may be small, deep, and challenging to locate. Conversely, larger lesions may be in difficult locations (i.e., insula, cingulate gyrus, etc.) or may be hard to visually differentiate from normal cortex at surgery (i.e., low-grade gliomas, cortical dysplasias, etc.). For this reason, it may again be advisable to increase the application accuracy in some of these cases by using skull-implanted fiducials along with taking advantage of fused datasets that optimize lesion identification (i.e., fused FLAIR or T2 sequences, etc.) (**Fig. 1.6**). It is also possible to salvage poor accuracy at the time of surgery by rendering cortical veins on the IGS workstation and using these as visual landmarks to define lesion location in cases where image guidance is thought to be inaccurate (**Fig. 1.7**).

Nonlesional IGS Epilepsy Surgery

When select cortical or subcortical structures are targeted for resection, neuronavigation can be employed to improve the overall procedure so that the desired resection is predictably performed. Also, intraoperative stimulation mapping and electrocorticography (ECoG) can be localized on a 3-D–rendered brain and correlated with preoperative anatomical and physiological information.

Temporal Lobe Epilepsy

The temporal lobe is the most common target for resective surgery in adult epilepsy. There is great variability from center to center as to what procedures are performed in nonlesional temporal lobe epilepsy. Some institutions perform

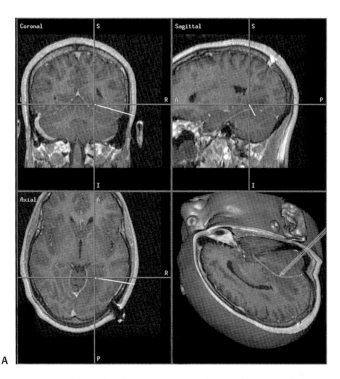

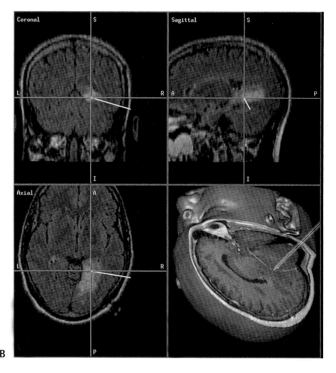

Fig. 1.6 A lesional epilepsy case in which a grade II mixed oligoastrocytoma with surrounding gliotic changes (as determined by histology of resection and multiple biopsies) was best visualized on the FLAIR sequence in **(B)**. **(A)** A volumetric (SPGR) sequence to which the FLAIR sequence in **(B)** was fused for assessment and surgical guidance.

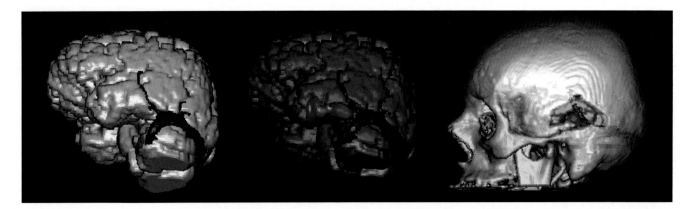

Fig. 1.7 This patient with longstanding epilepsy had a cavernous angioma (purple) in the fusiform gyrus of the left temporal lobe. The vein of Labbé served as an anatomical landmark for finding the lesion. Planning the surgery also took into account that endangering the vein of Labbé would carry the risk of venous infarction with a danger of speech disturbance because this was the dominant temporal lobe (sodium amytal test proven). A low craniotomy with a small neocorticectomy and no retraction on the vein of Labbé was performed. Intraoperative electrocorticography showed no epileptiform activity in the radiologically normal hippocampus (green) and amygdala (red), but it did lead to an extension of fusiform gyrus resection where spikes were observed. The image on the right shows a fusion of the preoperative MRI brain model with a postoperative volumetric CT. The actually performed craniotomy is illustrated.

surgery awake with stimulation mapping and ECoG, others asleep with or without ECoG.[57,58] Resections can be tailored according to the aforementioned physiological studies or standardized as an anterior temporal lobectomy (ATL),[59] anteromesial resection,[60] selective amygdalohippocampectomy (selAH)[61] or hippocampectomy, or other variants and combinations. Functional temporal lobe disconnections have also been described.[62,63] Discussion of these surgical variants is beyond the scope of this chapter. How image guidance can be useful for some of these procedures will now be addressed.

On a basic level, image guidance can assist the novice or trainee so that the craniotomy for surgical exposure of the temporal lobe or part thereof is optimized (**Figs. 1.3 and 1.7**). On a more advanced level, the temporal lobe can be measured on an MRI-rendered model before surgery, and the extent of resection can be planned and related to cortical veins such as the vein of Labbé. Intraoperative stimulation mapping and ECoG can be related to the same model. More interestingly, acute DEs can be placed with image guidance into deep mesiotemporal structures at the time of surgery to supplement ECoG (**Fig. 1.8**). As previously mentioned, neuronavigation should not substitute for anatomical knowledge or ability to perform a procedure. The author has found the following specific elements of surgery to benefit from image guidance:

1. If a radical removal of the amygdalar complex is intended, the superomedial aspect of this structure has no discernable boundary and is continuous with the basal ganglia. If radical amygdalectomy is desired, it is best to define a superomedial plane with the help of neuronavigation early in the mesiotemporal removal before more extensive brain shift, and before opening the temporal horn of the ventricle (**Fig. 1.9**).

2. Image guidance can assist in locating the temporal horn when performing a selective amygdalo-hippocampectomy. The temporal horn is the key anatomical landmark when locating the hippocampus. It is relatively easy to find the temporal horn when performing an ATL by sectioning the temporal stem in a coronal plane. When performing a selAH, however, the approach to the temporal horn is in a parallel rather than a perpendicular plane, whether the approach is transsylvian, transcortical, or transsulcal. It can be disconcerting not to find the temporal horn during these approaches, and image guidance is helpful in reorienting the angle of approach to find this crucial landmark.

3. Neuronavigation can also be used to confirm the extent of resection along the hippocampus (**Fig. 1.8**), entorhinal cortex, or other areas.

Extratemporal Epilepsy

Extratemporal resections within the frontal, occipital, and parietal lobes present additional challenges when compared with temporal lobe surgery, in that there are fewer defined anatomical landmarks available (**Fig. 1.10**). For classic "lobectomy"-type approaches, this is of less consequence, but with a modern trend toward more selective "neocorticectomies," identification of specific cortical areas and avoidance of functionally eloquent areas are essential. It should be underscored that stimulation mapping at surgery remains the gold standard for identifying eloquent areas at surgery. Functional imaging information used in conjunction with image guidance can be very helpful but is not always reliable, at the time of this writing. Again, cortical veins are important landmarks. Areas of cortical dysplasia may be visualized on MRI, but not at surgery, leading to greater reliance on image guidance in this context.

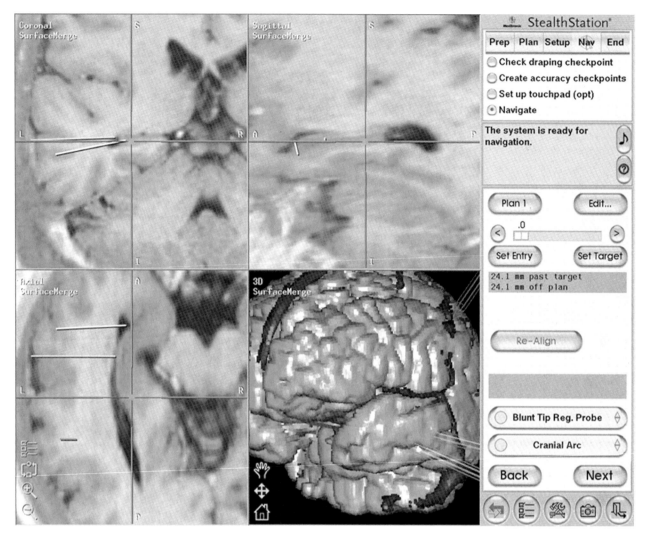

Fig. 1.8 Intraoperative screen capture during transsulcal selective hippocampectomy sparing amygdala. The two temporal trajectories illustrated represent intraoperative placement of acute depth electrodes during electrocorticography. The crosshairs of this screen capture denote the posterior resection margin of the hippocampus.

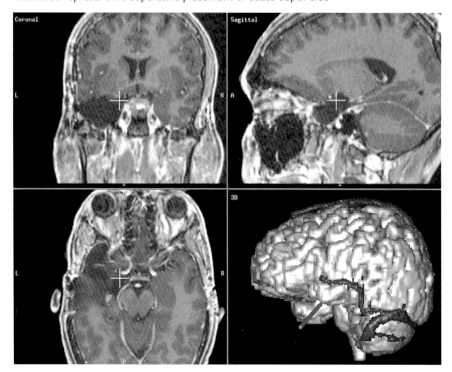

Fig. 1.9 IGS workstation reconstruction of a postoperative volumetric MRI following left anterior temporal lobe resection. In this case, a more radical amygdalar removal was intended (abdominal aura with fear, invasive monitoring with early amygdalar EEG involvement). Amygdalar resection was performed with image guidance for defining superomesial limits prior to opening the temporal horn of the ventricle.

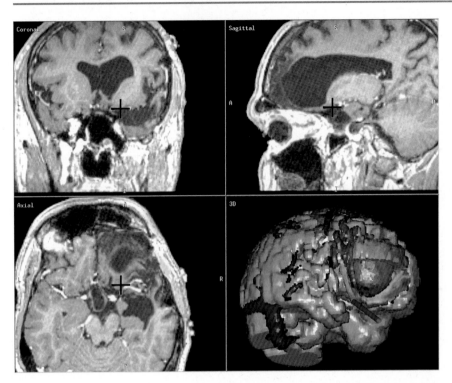

Fig. 1.10 This patient in his late 20s developed very intractable epilepsy following two craniotomies during childhood for a suprasellar craniopharyngioma. The case is also a good illustration for advocating avoidance of brain retraction, when possible. The right frontal and temporal encephalomalacia seen is secondary to surgical retraction at that time (no radiation therapy ever given). Seizures were predominantly frontal in semiology and on scalp EEG. Due to extensive gliosis, a functional disconnection of the frontal lobe was performed, as opposed to a resection. This was thought to be safer for preventing vascular injuries. The cross on the screen capture illustrates the posterior extent of orbitofrontal disconnection.

IGS for Disconnective Epilepsy Surgery

In addition to resective surgical options, some surgical treatment for epilepsy involves disconnection of cortical and subcortical areas. Disconnection can be a stand-alone procedure as with corpus callosotomy[64] or may be combined with resection to various degrees. It should be kept in mind that many classic "resective" operations have a corollary disconnective component. For example, a selAH also disconnects neocortical areas by temporal stem disruption during the surgical approach and by anterior commisure disruption at the time of amygdalectomy. On the other hand, functional hemispherectomy variants, in which disconnection predominate, lead to near-complete functional isolation of a cerebral hemisphere, which is the functional equivalent to complete removal.

Corpus Callosotomy

There are good anatomical surgical landmarks for callosotomy (interhemispheric fissure, pericallosal artery, etc.). The author would like to highlight a few select points where image guidance can fine-tune this surgical approach.

1. Preoperative identification of bridging veins to the sagittal sinus that may impede the interhemispheric approach. The approach can be varied to avoid the sacrifice of significant veins.
2. Guidance at the level of the rostrum of the corpus callosum, which can be difficult to visualize at surgery and is often found to be intact on postcallosotomy imaging.
3. Verification of the posterior extent of disconnection.

Functional Hemispherectomy

Hemispherectomy for intractable epilepsy is a remarkably effective option in a select population of patients with extensive pathological changes in one cerebral hemisphere leading to loss of function along with uncontrollable seizures originating in that hemisphere. Because of the long-term complications associated with complete removal of a cerebral hemisphere, several "functional" surgical variants have developed that disconnect the hemisphere while leaving it in situ. The author is most familiar with the periinsular hemispherotomy variant of functional hemispherectomy, and this shall be used to illustrate IGS application in hemispheric disconnection.[65]

1. Image-guided craniotomy for optimized exposure of perisylvian area.
2. After opercular resection, IGS can be used for entry into the circular sulcus around the insula, thus disconnecting the corona radiata by targeting the lateral ventricle circumferentially. If the ventricle is small, IGS is particularly helpful in minimizing resection.
3. Amygdalar resection: The same parameters apply to the superomedial extent of resection as previously described in temporal lobe surgery.
4. A verification of level posterior disconnection of hippocampus and fimbria-fornix is performed.
5. Parasagittal callosotomy performed by incising the medial roof of the body of the lateral ventricle to locate the pericallosal artery (**Fig. 1.11A**). This can then be followed by subpial aspiration. Posteriorly, this landmark is lost when the disconnection progresses more laterally toward the posterior choroidal fissure again with IGS.

6. Frontobasal disconnection: This is performed in a subpial plane down to the floor of the anterior fossa in a coronal plane. Neuronavigation is used to determine how far back to make this cut and for feedback with regard to progression toward the midline (**Fig. 1.11B**).

Subpial Transection

Subpial transection is a technique of disconnection reserved for functionally eloquent cortical areas. The principle is to make superficial cuts perpendicular to the cortical surface to disrupt tangential seizure spread while maintaining the integrity of cortical columns and therefore function.[66] There is some controversy as to whether the histological outcome of the transections corresponds to the intended disconnection, and the efficacy of the procedure is also debated.[67,68] The usefulness of image guidance in this context consists in the identification and anatomical correlation of eloquent cortex targeted for transection (**Fig. 1.3**). Again, it must be stressed that stimulation mapping remains the gold standard for the determination of cortical function. The author has used image guidance in combination with stimulation mapping when performing subpial transections. In some cases under general anesthesia, epileptiform activity on ECoG may be seen in cortex that may be involved in speech function, such as more posterior dominant temporal neocortex. In this context, where general anesthesia precludes speech mapping,

image guidance can confirm the location of posterior spiking and subpial transection can be substituted for resection in areas with a higher risk for speech representation by their anatomical location.

Other Disconnective Epilepsy Surgical Procedures

Experience with the disconnective aspects of functional hemispherectomy has led to some disconnective lobar procedures. These will probably not gain widespread acceptance because the disconnected cortex continues to have epileptic discharges. If residual or recurrent seizures occur from a nondisconnected area of cortex, the epileptic activity in the disconnected lobe would confound the localization of the area in need of additional surgery. This being said, there can be some advantages to functional lobar disconnection as opposed to resection, especially in the presence of scarring or adhesions that would increase the vascular risk of a resection (**Fig. 1.10**).

IG for Neurostimulation and Radiosurgery

Neurostimulation and radiosurgery are under active investigation for the treatment of epilepsy. The image-guidance aspects of these potential treatments shall briefly be reviewed.

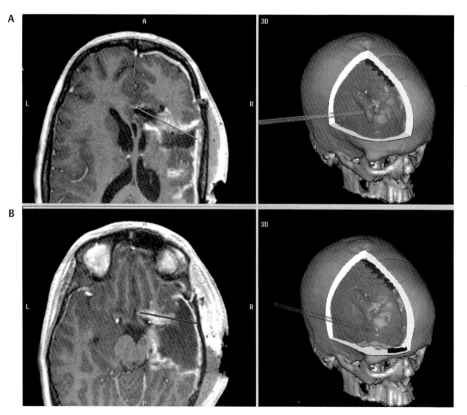

Fig. 1.11 This is a postoperative MRI of a functional hemispherectomy variant (fused to preoperative CT). The MRI study was performed with contrast 10 days after surgery so that postsurgical contrast enhancement would highlight the areas of disconnection. The operative trajectory for the anterior aspect of the parasagittal callosotomy component is superimposed on the resultant disconnection in **(A).** The trajectory of frontobasal disconnection is superimposed on the surgical result in **(B).** Note that unlike a typical periinsular hemispherotomy, there is a full temporal lobe resection. This was because a more posterior disconnection was not performed due to the desire to preserve intact visual fields.

DBS, Cortical Stimulation, and Closed-Loop Strategies

Several neurostimulation strategies are being investigated for epilepsy. These include continuous or intermittent stimulation of deep brain targets such as the thalamus or the subthalamic nucleus or the hippocampus.[69–75] There are also stimulation protocols of superficial cortical targets. Some protocols use a closed-loop strategy in which a recording electrode in or on the brain records a seizure onset that activates a stimulator to activate an electrode in an attempt to abort the seizure. At present, DEs for deep brain stimulation (DBS) are placed by means of a stereotactic frame by most investigators. There is recent evidence that frameless image-guided electrode placement is at least as accurate as frame placement provided that care is taken to optimize application accuracy (implanted skull fiducials).[26,44]

Radiosurgery

Radiosurgery will be dealt with in a separate chapter. It should be mentioned that radiosurgery is essentially computer-guided stereotactic radiation. Therefore, many of the aspects of imaging, image fusion, and surgical planning for image guidance in epilepsy surgery can be extrapolated to radiosurgery.[76–78]

IG for Postoperative Assessment

The utility of image guidance extends beyond surgery to postoperative assessment. The author has taken care to ob-

tain postoperative imaging sequences to match those obtained preoperatively for image guidance. In this way, the result of surgery can be assessed in a quantitative manner (**Figs. 1.3, 1.5, 1.7, 1.9, 1.11, 1.12**).

Intraoperative Imaging

Immediate postresection imaging can be performed during surgery prior to closure if intraoperative imaging systems (ultrasound, CT, or MRI) are available.[50,79] Because there are no absolute criteria that define what extent of surgical resection is necessary or desirable, the author feels that this is of limited value at present outside of lesional cases (i.e., brain tumors). This may change as we learn more about epilepsy and epileptogenesis.

Feedback for Improvement

Postoperative imaging (predominantly MRI) acquired 6 months or more after surgery can be loaded on an IGS workstation, compared with preoperative studies, and analyzed with regard to resultant seizure control. Lessons learned in this way can be applied to IGS planning of future patients.[80]

Future Use for IG in Treatment of Epilepsy

For many years now, the author has been convinced that surgically treated epilepsy should be viewed in terms of the disruption of an epileptogenic network as opposed to the resection of an epileptic "focus" or "zone." With the assump-

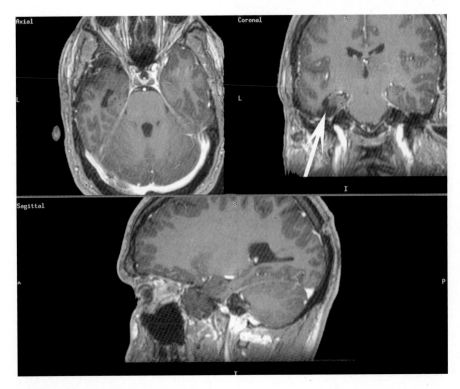

Fig. 1.12 This was an unusual case of temporal lobe epilepsy with a small hippocampus on the right but predominant seizure activity on the left (temporopolar and temporobasal on invasive monitoring with depth electrodes and subdural strips). Left temporopolar cortex and posterior entorhinal cortex were resected (*arrow*) sparing amygdala, anterior entorhinal cortex, and hippocampus (for fear of impairing memory). We expected the surgery to be palliative. The patient has been seizure and aura free for more than 4 years.

tion that no two networks or patients are exactly the same, there may come a time when it will be possible to determine an individualized surgical strategy for each patient that is as minimal as possible, and that nevertheless will result in seizure freedom. Strategies may include resection, disconnection, neurostimulation, radiosurgery, cell therapy, or gene therapy. Targets may be as small as a thalamic nucleus or as a subdivision of the entorhinal cortex. Image guidance will be essential to accurately access these targets.

Case Examples

1. This patient (**Fig. 1.2**) had a 20-year history of "reflex"-type epilepsy with predominantly motor features and falls. Sudden-onset left-sided weakness led to an MRI that demonstrated a hemorrhage in the right central area suggestive of an underlying cavernous angioma. Review of previous MRIs was unremarkable. In view of the surgical indication to prevent future hemorrhage, the patient was also reinvestigated with video EEG. Ictal events were brought on by cigarette smoking and were very short. Ictal EEG changes were minimal, but an ictal SPECT showed uptake in the central sulcus and postcentral gyrus, not immediately adjacent to the area of hemorrhage. Activation fMRI studies were performed for arm and leg motor functions. All these datasets were fused on the IGS workstation. At surgery, this information was used for guidance. ECoG confirmed spiking in the postcentral gyrus. Motor stimulation mapping confirmed the location of the motor strip. The lesion was resected. Epileptiform activity was confined to the postcentral gyrus (at a distance from the lesion) where a subpial transection was performed. The patient had a brief transient sensory deficit after surgery. Seizures decreased on follow-up, but mild motor seizures still occur occasionally. This is probably due to the underlying more "generalized" nature of the reflex epilepsy. IGS uses include multimodal preoperative fusion of MRI, fMRI, and ictal SPECT and intraoperative correlation with ECoG and stimulation mapping. Image guidance did not have optimal accuracy in this case, but the cortical veins and gyral anatomy could be used for correlation between image space and surgical space.
2. This patient (**Fig. 1.6**) presented with an 18-month history of simple partial seizures with visual semiology (flashing lights, left hemifield). The patient underwent a frame-based stereotactic biopsy in another institution, which was nondiagnostic. The MRI shows a subtle lesion in the right posterior parahippocampal and occipital area. The

lesion is much more evident on a FLAIR sequence. Preoperative formal visual fields were remarkable for a moderate homonymous field defect. A subtemporal approach was used to approach the lesion using the FLAIR sequence fused to the SPGR for guidance and skull-implanted fiducials for registration. The tumor was a low-grade oligoastrocytoma. Serial biopsies showed that the posterior aspect of the FLAIR-bright lesion was consistent with gliosis and not tumor (confirmed on permanent section). The posterior aspect of the FLAIR abnormality was not resected to avoid worsening the visual defect. The patient was seizure free at last follow-up 3 years after surgery. IGS uses include SPGR-FLAIR sequence fusion for lesion identification, image-guided biopsies of posterior FLAIR-bright area for assessment of gliosis versus tumor in view of risk to visual fields, and IGS resection of tumor.
3. This patient (**Fig. 1.8**) had a 35-year history of seizures. Seizure onset was characterized by right upper extremity sensory-motor phenomena including dystonic posturing. There was no autonomic semiology. Imaging showed a small left hippocampus. Hippocampal and amygdala models were constructed on the IGS workstation confirming marked left hippocampal volume loss but symmetrical amygdalar volumes. The seizure semiology was thought to represent suprasylvian spread from a left hippocampal onset. There was no autonomic semiology to suggest amygdaloinsular involvement. The surgical plan was to perform just a left selective hippocampectomy, sparing amygdala and anterior entorhinal cortex. At surgery, a subdural electrode strip was slipped toward the motor strip with image guidance from the superior aspect of the craniotomy to rule out any independent central epileptiform activity that might have accounted for the sensory-motor semiology. No epileptiform activity was identified. Electrodes placed along the hippocampus at surgery showed active spiking. An acute DE placed in the amygdala with image guidance did not demonstrate epileptic activity. A selective hippocampectomy was performed, and the patient has been seizure (and aura) free since surgery (4 years). IGS uses include volumetrics/localization of acute EEG electrodes at surgery and IGS for resection.

Conclusion

The potential uses for image-guidance should expand in parallel to the evolution of imaging in epilepsy, but may also expand as our understanding of the underlying mechanisms of epilepsy improves.

References

1. Mascott CR. Comparison of magnetic tracking and optical tracking by simultaneous use of two independent frameless stereotactic systems. Neurosurgery 2005;57(4, Suppl)295–301, discussion 295–301

2. Tanaka T, Olivier A, Hashizume K, et al. Image-guided epilepsy surgery. Neurol Med Chir (Tokyo) 1999;39(13):895–900
3. Olivier A, Germano IM, Cukiert A, et al. Frameless stereotaxy for surgery of the epilepsies: preliminary experience. Technical note. J Neurosurg 1994;81(4):629–633

4. Murphy M, O'Brien TJ, Morris K, et al. Multimodality image-guided epilepsy surgery. J Clin Neurosci 2001;8(6):534–538

5. Van Roost D, Schaller C, Meyer B, et al. Can neuronavigation contribute to standardization of selective amygdalohippocampectomy? Stereotact Funct Neurosurg 1997;69(1–4, Pt 2):239–242

6. Olivier A, Alonso-Vanegas M, Comeau R, et al. Image-guided surgery of epilepsy. Neurosurg Clin N Am 1996;7(2):229–243

7. Jensen RL, Stone JL, Hayne R. Use of the Horsley-Clarke stereotactic frame in humans. Stereotact Funct Neurosurg 1995;65(1–4):194–197

8. Olivier A, Bertrand G, Picard C. Discovery of the first human stereotactic instrument. Appl Neurophysiol 1983;46(1–4):84–91

9. Gildenberg PL. Spiegel and Wycis—the early years. Stereotact Funct Neurosurg 2001;77(1–4):11–16

10. Talairach J, Szikla G. Application of stereotactic concepts to the surgery of epilepsy. Acta Neurochir Suppl (Wien) 1980;30:35–54

11. Motti ED, Marossero F. Head-holder interfacing computed tomography with Talairach stereotactic frame. J Neurosurg Sci 1983;27(3):219–223

12. Olivier A, Bertrand G, Peters T. Stereotactic systems and procedures for depth electrode placement: technical aspects. Appl Neurophysiol 1983;46(1–4):37–40

13. Peters TM, Olivier A. C.T. aided stereotaxy for depth electrode implantation and biopsy. Can J Neurol Sci 1983;10(3):166–169

14. Kelly PJ, Sharbrough FW, Kall BA, et al. Magnetic resonance imaging-based computer-assisted stereotactic resection of the hippocampus and amygdala in patients with temporal lobe epilepsy. Mayo Clin Proc 1987;62(2):103–108

15. Kelly PJ. State of the art and future directions of minimally invasive stereotactic neurosurgery. Cancer Control 1995;2(4):287–292

16. Kelly PJ. Computer-assisted stereotaxis: new approaches for the management of intracranial intra-axial tumors. Neurology 1986;36(4):535–541

17. Bucholz RD, McDurmont L. From discovery to design: image-guided surgery. Clin Neurosurg 2003;50:13–25

18. Roberts DW, Strohbehn JW, Hatch JF, et al. A frameless stereotaxic integration of computerized tomographic imaging and the operating microscope. J Neurosurg 1986;65(4):545–549

19. Watanabe E, Watanabe T, Manaka S, et al. Three-dimensional digitizer (neuronavigator): new equipment for computed tomography-guided stereotaxic surgery. Surg Neurol 1987;27(6):543–547

20. Reinhardt H, Meyer H, Amrein E. A computer-assisted device for the intraoperative CT-correlated localization of brain tumors. Eur Surg Res 1988;20(1):51–58

21. Barnett GH, Kormos DW, Steiner CP, et al. Use of a frameless, armless stereotactic wand for brain tumor localization with two-dimensional and three-dimensional neuroimaging. Neurosurgery 1993;33(4):674–678

22. Mascott CR, Jean-Christophe S, Bousquet P, et al. Quantification of true in vivo (application) accuracy in cranial image-guided surgery: influence of mode of patient registration. Neurosurgery 2006;59(1, Suppl 1)ONS146–ONS156

23. Mascott CR, et al. Frameless stereotactic placement of depth electrodes for investigation of epilepsy. Meeting of the American Association of Neurological Surgeons, 1995

24. Gumprecht HK, Widenka DC, Lumenta CB. BrainLab VectorVision Neuronavigation System: technology and clinical experiences in 131 cases. Neurosurgery 1999;44(1):97–104, discussion 104–105

25. Hogan RE, Lowe VJ, Bucholz RD. Triple-technique (MR imaging, single-photon emission CT, and CT) coregistration for image-guided surgical evaluation of patients with intractable epilepsy. AJNR Am J Neuroradiol 1999;20(6):1054–1058

26. Mascott CR. In vivo accuracy of image guidance performed using optical tracking and optimized registration. J Neurosurg 2006;105(4):561–567

27. Cascino GD. Clinical correlations with hippocampal atrophy. Magn Reson Imaging 1995;13(8):1133–1136

28. Cendes F, Andermann F, Dubeau F, et al. Early childhood prolonged febrile convulsions, atrophy and sclerosis of mesial structures, and temporal lobe epilepsy: an MRI volumetric study. Neurology 1993;43(6):1083–1087

29. Diehl B, Luders HO. Temporal lobe epilepsy: when are invasive recordings needed? Epilepsia 2000;41(Suppl 3):S61–S74

30. Luby M, Spencer DD, Kim JH, et al. Hippocampal MRI volumetrics and temporal lobe substrates in medial temporal lobe epilepsy. Magn Reson Imaging 1995;13(8):1065–1071

31. Oppenheim C, Dormont D, Hasboun D, et al. Bilateral mesial temporal sclerosis: MRI with high-resolution fast spin-echo and fluid-attenuated inversion-recovery sequences. Neuroradiology 1999;41(7):471–479

32. Van Paesschen W, Sisodiya S, Connelly A, et al. Quantitative hippocampal MRI and intractable temporal lobe epilepsy. Neurology 1995;45(12):2233–2240

33. Cendes F, Leproux F, Melanson D, et al. MRI of amygdala and hippocampus in temporal lobe epilepsy. J Comput Assist Tomogr 1993;17(2):206–210

34. Bernasconi N, Bernasconi A, Andermann F, et al. Entorhinal cortex in temporal lobe epilepsy: a quantitative MRI study. Neurology 1999;52(9):1870–1876

35. Salmenpera T, Kalviainen R, Partanen K, et al. Quantitative MRI volumetry of the entorhinal cortex in temporal lobe epilepsy. Seizure 2000;9(3):208–215

36. Doherty CP, Fitzsimons M, Meredith G, et al. Rapid stereological quantitation of temporal neocortex in TLE. Magn Reson Imaging 2003;21(5):511–518

37. Mahvash M, König R, Urbach H, et al. FLAIR-/T1-/T2-co-registration for image-guided diagnostic and resective epilepsy surgery. Neurosurgery 2006;58(1, Suppl)ONS69–ONS75

38. Concha L, Gross DW, Wheatley BM, et al. Diffusion tensor imaging of time-dependent axonal and myelin degradation after corpus callosotomy in epilepsy patients. Neuroimage 2006;32(3):1090–1099

39. Briellmann RS, Pell GS, Wellard RM, et al. MR imaging of epilepsy: state of the art at 1.5 T and potential of 3 T. Epileptic Disord 2003;5(1):3–20

40. Levesque MF, Zhang JX, Wilson CL, et al. Stereotactic investigation of limbic epilepsy using a multimodal image analysis system. Technical note. J Neurosurg 1990;73(5):792–797

41. Murphy MA, O'Brien TJ, Morris K, et al. Multimodality image-guided surgery for the treatment of medically refractory epilepsy. J Neurosurg 2004;100(3):452–462

42. Gaillard WD, Bhatia S, Bookheimer SY, et al. FDG-PET and volumetric MRI in the evaluation of patients with partial epilepsy. Neurology 1995;45(1):123–126

43. Duffner F, Freudenstein D, Schiffbauer H, et al. Combining MEG and MRI with neuronavigation for treatment of an epileptiform spike focus in the precentral region: a technical case report. Surg Neurol 2003;59(1):40–46

44. Holloway KL, Gaede SE, Starr PA, et al. Frameless stereotaxy using bone fiducial markers for deep brain stimulation. J Neurosurg 2005;103(3):404–413

45. Henderson JM, Holloway KL, Gaede SE, et al. The application accuracy of a skull-mounted trajectory guide system for image-guided functional neurosurgery. Comput Aided Surg 2004;9(4):155–160

46. Maciunas RJ, Galloway RL Jr, Latimer JW. The application accuracy of stereotactic frames. Neurosurgery 1994;35(4):682–694, discussion 694–695

47. Maurer CRJ, Rohlfing T, Dean D, et al. Sources of error in image registration for cranial image-guided neurosurgery. In: Germano, IM, ed. *Advanced Techniques in Image-Guided Brain and Spine Surgery*. New York and Stuttgart: Thieme; 2002:10–36

48. Maurer CR Jr, Fitzpatrick JM, Wang MY, et al. Registration of head volume images using implantable fiducial markers. IEEE Trans Med Imaging 1997;16(4):447–462

49. Nimsky C, Ganslandt O, Fahlbusch R. 1.5 T: intraoperative imaging beyond standard anatomic imaging. Neurosurg Clin N Am 2005;16(1):185–200, vii

50. Nimsky C, Ganslandt O, Fahlbusch R. Functional neuronavigation and intraoperative MRI. Adv Tech Stand Neurosurg 2004;29:229–263

51. Buchfelder M, Ganslandt O, Fahlbusch R, et al. Intraoperative magnetic resonance imaging in epilepsy surgery. J Magn Reson Imaging 2000;12(4):547–555

52. Schwartz TH, Marks D, Pak J, et al. Standardization of amygdalohippocampectomy with intraoperative magnetic resonance imaging: preliminary experience. Epilepsia 2002;43(4):430–436

53. Murphy MA, O'Brien TJ, Cook MJ. Insertion of depth electrodes with or without subdural grids using frameless stereotactic guidance systems–technique and outcome. Br J Neurosurg 2002;16(2):119–125

54. Mehta AD, Labar D, Dean A, et al. Frameless stereotactic placement of depth electrodes in epilepsy surgery. J Neurosurg 2005;102(6):1040–1045

55. Song JK, Abou-Khalil B, Konrad PE. Intraventricular monitoring for temporal lobe epilepsy: report on technique and initial results in eight patients. J Neurol Neurosurg Psychiatry 2003;74(5):561–565

56. Winkler PA, Vollmar C, Krishnan KG, et al. Usefulness of 3-D reconstructed images of the human cerebral cortex for localization of subdural electrodes in epilepsy surgery. Epilepsy Res 2000;41(2):169–178

57. Karatas A, Erdem A, Sava A, et al. Identification and removal of an epileptogenic lesion using Ictal-EEG, functional-neuronavigation and electrocorticography. J Clin Neurosci 2004;11(3):343–346

58. Wennberg R, Quesney F, Olivier A, et al. Mesial temporal versus lateral temporal interictal epileptiform activity: comparison of chronic and acute intracranial recordings. Electroencephalogr Clin Neurophysiol 1997;102(6):486–494

59. Polkey CE. Effects of anterior temporal lobectomy apart from the relief of seizures: a study of 40 patients. J R Soc Med 1983;76(5):354–358

60. Spencer DD, Spencer SS, Mattson RH, et al. Access to the posterior medial temporal lobe structures in the surgical treatment of temporal lobe epilepsy. Neurosurgery 1984;15(5):667–671

61. Wieser HG, Yasargil MG. Selective amygdalohippocampectomy as a surgical treatment of mesiobasal limbic epilepsy. Surg Neurol 1982;17(6):445–457

62. Chabardes S, Minotti L, Hoffmann D, et al. Temporal disconnection for intractable temporal lobe epilepsy: results of a series of 45 consecutive patients. Acta Neurochir (Wien) 2006;148(10):8–9

63. Cossu M, et al. Disconnective surgery for drug-resistant focal epilepsy. Acta Neurochir (Wien) 2006;148(10):27–28

64. Hodaie M, Musharbash A, Otsubo H, et al. Image-guided, frameless stereotactic sectioning of the corpus callosum in children with intractable epilepsy. Pediatr Neurosurg 2001;34(6):286–294

65. Villemure JG, Mascott CR. Peri-insular hemispherotomy: surgical principles and anatomy. Neurosurgery 1995;37(5):975–981

66. Morrell F, Whisler WW, Bleck TP. Multiple subpial transection: a new approach to the surgical treatment of focal epilepsy. J Neurosurg 1989;70(2):231–239

67. Kaufmann WE, Krauss G, Uematsu S, et al. Treatment of epilepsy with multiple subpial transections: an acute histologic analysis in human subjects. Epilepsia 1996;37(4):342–352

68. Whisler WW. Treatment of epilepsy with multiple subpial transection: an acute histological analysis in human subjects. Epilepsia 1997;38(2):258–259

69. Kerrigan JF, Litt B, Fisher RS, et al. Electrical stimulation of the anterior nucleus of the thalamus for the treatment of intractable epilepsy. Epilepsia 2004;45(4):346–354

70. Andrade DM, Zumsteg D, Hamani C, et al. Long-term follow-up of patients with thalamic deep brain stimulation for epilepsy. Neurology 2006;66(10):1571–1573

71. Osorio I, Frei MG, Manly BF, et al. An introduction to contingent (closed-loop) brain electrical stimulation for seizure blockage, to ultra-short-term clinical trials, and to multidimensional statistical analysis of therapeutic efficacy. J Clin Neurophysiol 2001;18(6):533–544

72. Vonck K, Boon P, Claeys P, et al. Long-term deep brain stimulation for refractory temporal lobe epilepsy. Epilepsia 2005;46(Suppl 5):98–99

73. Velasco AL, Velasco F, Jiménez F, et al. Neuromodulation of the centromedian thalamic nuclei in the treatment of generalized seizures and the improvement of the quality of life in patients with Lennox-Gastaut syndrome. Epilepsia 2006;47(7):1203–1212

74. Fountas KN, Smith JR, Murro AM, et al. Implantation of a closed-loop stimulation in the management of medically refractory focal epilepsy: a technical note. Stereotact Funct Neurosurg 2005;83(4):153–158

75. Morrell M. Brain stimulation for epilepsy: can scheduled or responsive neurostimulation stop seizures? Curr Opin Neurol 2006;19(2):164–168

76. Regis J, Bartolomei F, Hayashi M, et al. Gamma Knife surgery, a neuromodulation therapy in epilepsy surgery! Acta Neurochir Suppl (Wien) 2002;84:37–47

77. Mathieu D, Kondziolka D, Niranjan A, et al. Gamma knife radiosurgery for refractory epilepsy caused by hypothalamic hamartomas. Stereotact Funct Neurosurg 2006;84(2–3):82–87

78. Eder HG, Feichtinger M, Pieper T, et al. Gamma knife radiosurgery for callosotomy in children with drug-resistant epilepsy. Childs Nerv Syst 2006;22(8):1012–1017

79. Kelly JJ, Hader WJ, Myles ST, et al. Epilepsy surgery with intraoperative MRI at 1.5 T. Neurosurg Clin N Am 2005;16(1):173–183

80. Siegel AM, Wieser HG, Wichmann W, et al. Relationships between MR-imaged total amount of tissue removed, resection scores of specific mediobasal limbic subcompartments and clinical outcome following selective amygdalohippocampectomy. Epilepsy Res 1990;6(1):56–65

2 Invasive EEG Studies: Peg, Strip, and Grid Implantation

Gregory G. Heuer, Joel Bauman, Phillip B. Storm, and Gordon H. Baltuch

Epilepsy is a very common neurological disorder with a prevalence of 5 to 10 per 1000 in the population in North America.[1,2] About 20 to 30% of patients are not adequately controlled by medical treatment alone.[3,4] At least 12% of patients are candidates for surgical treatment, although this number may be larger with the development of new imaging and diagnostic technologies.[5] A randomized, controlled trial demonstrated that surgery is superior to medical therapy.[6] The goal of surgery is to remove the portion of brain that is responsible for the generation of seizure activity, a region known as the epileptogenic zone.

Prior to consideration for surgery, patients require a comprehensive evaluation. The purpose of presurgical evaluation of epilepsy patients is to localize the epileptogenic zone responsible for the patient's intractable seizures and determine if it is amenable to resection. Surgical treatment of epilepsy requires the precise location of the seizure focus to maximize the potential for surgical cure and minimize disruption of normal cortical function. The most common cause for failure in the surgical treatment of intractable epilepsy is incomplete surgical resection of the epileptogenic zone.[7]

Initial methods for localization of the epileptogenic zone involve noninvasive techniques such as external scalp electroencephalogram (EEG) monitoring, magnetoencephalography (MEG), interictal or ictal single-photon emission tomography (SPECT), positron emission tomography (PET), and various other neuroimaging techniques such as magnetic resonance imaging (MRI). Although helpful, these methods do not always provide sufficient information to guide resection.

Some criteria used by the surgeon to consider the use of invasive techniques instead of relying on noninvasive technologies are lack of lateralization or localization of the epileptogenic zone, discordant information on noninvasive studies, presence of the epileptogenic zone near eloquent cortex, and the need to define the relationship of the zone to a lesion present on neuroimaging.[8]

When noninvasive techniques are insufficient, there are several options for detection of the epileptogenic zone using invasive methods, or electrocorticography (ECoG), including epidural electrodes, subdural grids, strip electrodes, and depth electrodes. Unlike scalp EEG that has a significant amount of tissue between the recorded cells and the electrode, electrodes placed by invasive methods localize the electrode on or near the cell that is being recorded. This results in less attenuation of the signal. The amplitude of the potentials recorded from the cortex is typically 2 to 58 times greater than scalp recordings.[9]

Additionally, invasive monitoring can be used for intra-operative recordings only. Indications for intra-operative mapping include mapping of eloquent cortex such as motor or speech. Also, intra-operative monitoring is used in tailored resections of the epileptogenic zone, localizing epileptic spikes.

History

The first reported case of intracranial EEG monitoring to guide surgical resection was performed by Wilder Penfield and Herbert Jasper at the Montreal Neurological Institute in 1939.[10,11] The patient had recurrent refractory seizure activity since a head injury in 1937. Scalp EEG performed on the patient demonstrated bilateral temporal epileptiform discharges. The patient underwent invasive EEG monitoring in an attempt to lateralize the focus. Epidural electrodes were placed via bur holes bilaterally, and the patient was monitored for 3 days revealing abnormal activity on the left side. The patient was taken to the operating room where an awake left temporal craniotomy reveled a posterior temporal meningocerebral scar that was then resected.

Electrode Types

There are several types of surface electrodes that differ in their location in the cranial space, as well as their configuration. The choice of invasive monitoring depends on patient characteristics including the site of disease, the age of the patient, and results of preoperative testing.

Peg electrodes are mushroom-shaped electrodes consisting of a steel or platinum disk with a Silastic cover. These electrodes are normally placed via twist drill into the epidural space. The main clinical indication for peg electrodes is lateralization of seizure focus. These electrodes are used in patients for which scalp EEG is not possible because of anatomical reasons (e.g., bone defects) or in patients in which scalp EEG failed to lateralize the seizure activity.[12,13] Peg electrodes do not record directly on the cortical surface; therefore, they have limited ability to spatially define the epileptogenic zone. Also, because of their shape and configuration, they cannot be used to monitor subfrontal or subtemporal regions. However, modified peg electrodes with cylindrical forms have been used successfully in these regions.[14] Because the dura is left intact, these electrodes are believed to have a reduced rate of complications such as hematoma and infection.

Strip electrodes consist of a linear array of platinum or stainless steel contacts embedded into a silicon strip (**Fig. 2.1A**). These constructs normally consist of four to eight contacts spaced 10 mm apart. These electrodes are placed into the subdural space either through a bur hole or under the edge of a bone flap. This type of electrode is used both for intraoperative monitoring during tumor resections and for postoperative monitoring in seizure cases. These electrodes have some advantage over larger grid electrodes. Because of their narrow size they can be passed under bone edges considerable distances to monitor more distance sites. For example, this type of electrode is often passed around the temporal lobe to monitor mesial temporal structures.

Subdural grids consist of a square array of contacts embedded in silicon (**Fig. 2.1B**). These constructs normally consist of four to 64 contacts; however, custom-designed grid patterns are available. These grids are placed on the cortical surface after a large craniotomy. An additional advantage to strip and grid electrodes is that these electrodes, unlike peg or other epidural electrodes, can be used for stimulation studies.

Operative Technique

Strip electrodes are used over the cortical surface for recordings. These electrodes are passed in the subdural space through a bur hole or under the edge of a craniotomy. A Penfield dissector is used to create room to pass the strip in the subdural space and to direct the strip in the appropriate direction. Constant irrigation is used to reduce any friction as the strip is passed and to monitor for any subdural bleeding. Due to the risk of damaging cortical veins, extreme care must be taken if they are passed into the interhemispheric fissure, near large cortical veins such as the vein of Labbé, or near venous sinuses. Placement of strip electrodes can be aided by frameless stereotaxy.

Strip electrode placement is often used in suspected cases of temporal lobe epilepsy (TLE). The electrodes are placed in such a fashion as to cover the temporal lobe.[15,16] In standard placement, a temporal bur hole is placed 2 cm anterior to tragus and superior to zygoma. Through this bur hole, two four-contact strip electrodes are passed and directed medially toward the parahippocampus and posterior to middle and inferior temporal gyrus. Next, through a frontal bur hole 4 cm anterior to the coronal suture and 2 cm lateral to midline, two electrodes are passed. A four-contact strip is passed along the interhemispheric fissure to cover the cingulate gyrus and one eight-contact strip is passed toward the ipsilateral globe. An alternative to the classic method is placement of an anteromedial strip electrode. This strip is passed around the temporal pole and underneath the lesser wing of the sphenoid electrode to monitor the medial temporal lobe.[17] The end of the electrode is then passed through the dural defect and bur hole, and tunneled under the skin with a trocar. A nylon purse-string suture is placed around electrode, and a drain stitch is applied to secure the electrode. Each electrode has a unique color combination, and this color should be recorded along with the location of the electrode.

Subdural grids are placed over the lesion or region of interest with care taken to overlap any eloquent cortex that is

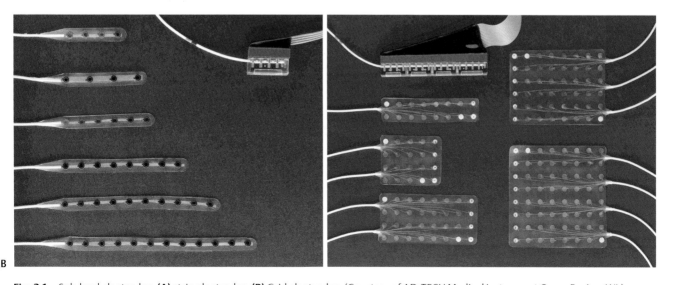

Fig. 2.1 Subdural electrodes. **(A)** strip electrodes. **(B)** Grid electrodes. (Courtesy of AD-TECH Medical Instrument Corp., Racine, WI.)

near. The placement of electrodes is affected by preoperative noninvasive studies. In patients with a suspected lesion present on preoperative imaging, grid placement is straightforward and can be aided by identification of the lesion with neuronavigation. In nonlesional cases, the electrodes are placed over the suspected epileptogenic focus based on scalp EEG recordings, MEG, ictal SPECT studies, or by semiology. Often a larger grid is used for nonlesional cases in an attempt to map the entire area.

A large craniotomy is performed, and a wide dural opening is made in a C-shaped fasion based on the sphenoid. Radial cuts are then made toward the sagittal sinus to visualize and avoid damaging bridging cortical veins. The grid is then placed over the cortical surface to cover the entire cortical surface in nonlesional cases (**Fig. 2.2A**) or to sufficiently cover the area around a suspected lesional seizure focus (**Fig. 2.2B**). Special attention is paid to the location and orientation of the grid with respect to the cortical surface and any lesion that may be present. An intraoperative photograph should be taken and a postimplantation volumetric computed tomography (CT) obtained to later aid the electrophysiologist in correlating the EEG information with the anatomical information. The color and position of each electrode is recorded prior to dural closure. It is important to assure that each electrode array has a unique color. The dura is closed if possible, or the dural closure is augmented with an onlay dural substitute such as DuraGen (Integra Lifesciences Corp., Plainsboro, NJ). The bone flap is loosely attached with

Tevdek sutures or cranial miniplates. The end of the electrode is passed out the bur hole and tunneled under the skin with a trocar. Leads are tunneled out the apex of the scalp to reduce the chance of cerebrospinal fluid (CSF) leaks. As with strip electrodes, the end is secured with a nylon purse-string and drain stitch. A subdural drain may be placed. Placement of a subdural drain may reduce the incidence of postoperative delayed subdural hematoma formation.[18]

Additionally, placement of the subdural grid can be guided by intraoperative cortical mapping using the Ojemann Cortical Stimulator (Integra Lifesciences Corp.), which can partially define the epileptogenic zone.[19] Such intraoperative mapping can be useful in resections in which the epileptogenic zone involves or is near the rolandic cortex and therefore greater surgical precision is required.[20] The stimulus, initially at a low setting such as 3 to 5 mA, 60 Hz 1-second pulse, is used, and the patient is carefully monitored for seizure activity. If a seizure does develop intraoperatively, this can be treated with irrigation with ice-cold saline or pharmacological methods.

Invasive monitoring can require repeat surgeries as recordings can occasionally fail to provide information to guide resection. There is some evidence that repositioning or adding electrodes can provide the information needed.[21,22] In one study of 183 patients, 18 patients underwent repositioning or implantation, 13 of these patients were found to have a new epileptogenic zone after repositioning. Also, reoperation with additional recordings has been shown to be

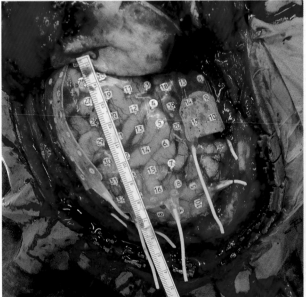 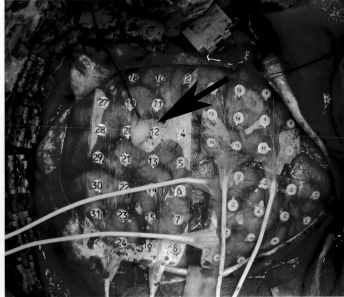

A,B

Fig. 2.2 Intraoperative grid placement (note: in both figures anterior is at the top and medial is at the left). **(A)** Wide grid placement across cerebral hemisphere in a nonlesional mapping case. **(B)** Grid placement around a lesion, indicated by the cotton ball (*large arrow*). Note the radial dural cuts made toward the sagittal sinus to avoid damaging bridging cortical veins.

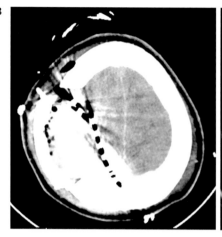
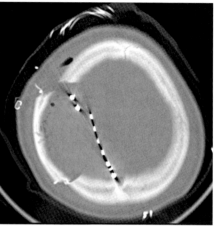

Fig. 2.3 Head CT in a patient with a symptomatic subdural collection that required evacuation. **(A)** Image windowed to view the parenchyma; note the significant artifact from the overlying grid. **(B)** Image windowed to view bone; note the deflection of the grid from the overlying subdural collection.

potentially beneficial in select patients with poor prognostic factors for surgical treatment.[23]

Postsurgical Monitoring

After placement of electrodes, the patient is monitored for several days and seizures are recorded from the electrodes. A reference electrode is placed at the vertex, and patients are additionally monitored with external EEG. Patients are monitored with video in a neurointensive care (NICU) setting or a specialized epilepsy monitoring unit (EMU). It is our practice to wait for at least five seizure episodes that localize the focus and are the typical seizure for the patient. Provocative measures are sometimes needed to induce seizures such as discontinuation of antiepileptic medicines, exercise, or sleep deprivation.

Normally perioperative and postoperative antibiotics are given. These antibiotics may be continued during the entire period of monitoring, a practice that may reduce the incidence of infection.[24] A short 1- to 3-day taper of steroids may be used to reduce cerebral swelling.[25] In the postoperative period special attention is paid to the development of any CSF leaks. When CSF leaks develop, they are managed with placement of purse-string sutures around the electrode and the head of the bed is elevated.

Postoperative imaging, including MRI and noncontrast CT is helpful to confirm the location of the electrode placement and to monitor for the development of any space-occupying collections.[26]

When sufficient information is obtained, the patient is brought into the operating room, where the electrodes are removed and the epileptogenic zone is resected. Some surgeons advocate culturing the subdural space and electrodes,[24] but this is not common practice at our institution.

Complications

With invasive monitoring, the overall rate of complications is between 13 and 19%, with a very low mortality rate (0 to 0.85%).[16,18,24,27–29] The complication rate is higher for patients with a greater number of electrodes and longer duration of monitoring.[28] Complications of chronic invasive monitoring include aseptic meningitis, infection (0 to 12.1%), and CSF leak (19 to 20%). Other complications include brain contusion/intracerebral hemorrhage (8%), epidural bleeds (2 to 2.5%), subdural bleeds (7 to 14%), and infarction (1.5%). The grid itself, even when not being stimulated, can lead to seizure activity that is not associated with the epileptogenic focus.[30]

Subdural collections are a common occurrence that can develop during monitoring due to the presence of the electrode in the subdural space. Although CT imaging can be useful in monitoring these lesions, clinical exam has been shown to be more useful in determining the need for surgical evacuation.[31] In our experience, analyzing CT scans that are windowed to view the brain can be misleading due to the substantial artifact of the subdural grid (**Fig. 2.3A**). For this reason, it is necessary to window the CT scan for bone. When viewed with these settings, the defection of the grid secondary to a subdural collection can be detected (**Fig. 2.3B**).

Conclusion

Invasive monitoring can be a useful and necessary technique for the surgical treatment of medically intractable epilepsy. Peg, strip, and grid electrodes can be used safely with a low complication rate. Often, these techniques are used in combination with each other or with depth electrodes to tailor surgical resections.

References

1. Hauser WA, Hesdorffer DC. Incidence and prevalence. In *Epilepsy: Frequency, Causes and Consequences.* Hauser WA, Hesdorffer DC, eds. New York: Demos: 1990:1–51

2. Wiebe S, Bellhouse DR, Fallahay C, et al. Burden of epilepsy: the Ontario Health Survey. Can J Neurol Sci 1999;26(4):263–270

3. Sander JW. Some aspects of prognosis in the epilepsies: a review. Epilepsia 1993;34(6):1007–1016

4. Kwan P, Brodie MJ. Early identification of refractory epilepsy. N Engl J Med 2000;342(5):314–319

5. Commission for the Control of Epilepsy and its Consequences. *Plan for Nationwide Action on Epilepsy.* Washington, DC: U.S. Government Printing Office; 1978. U.S. Dept. of Health, and Welfare. DHEW publication no. NIH 78–819

6. Wiebe S, Blume WT, Girvin JP, et al. A randomized, controlled trial of surgery for temporal-lobe epilepsy. N Engl J Med 2001;345(5):311–318

7. Wyler AR, Hermann BP, Richey ET. Results of reoperation for failed epilepsy surgery. J Neurosurg 1989;71(6):815–819

8. Dubeau F, McLachlan RS. Invasive electrographic recording techniques in temporal lobe epilepsy. Can J Neurol Sci 2000;27(Suppl 1): S29–S34

9. Fisch BJ. *Fisch and Spehlmann's EEG Primer.* New York: Elsevier; 1999

10. Penfield W. The epilepsies: with a note on radical therapy. N Engl J Med 1939;221:209–218

11. Almeida AN, Martinez V, Feindel W, et al. The first case of invasive EEG monitoring for the surgical treatment of epilepsy: historical significance and context. Epilepsia 2005;46(7):1082–1085

12. Barnett GH, Burgess RC, Awad IA, et al. Epidural peg electrodes for the presurgical evaluation of intractable epilepsy. Neurosurgery 1990;27(1):113–115

13. Awad IA, Assirati JA Jr, Burgess R, et al. A new class of electrodes of "intermediate invasiveness": preliminary experience with epidural pegs and foramen ovale electrodes in the mapping of seizure foci. Neurol Res 1991;13(3):177–183

14. Byrne RW, Smith M, Kanner A, et al. Presurgical intracranial monitoring with epidural cylindrical electrodes. Epilepsia 2000;41 (Suppl 7):79

15. Wyler AR, Ojemann GA, Lettich E, et al. Subdural strip electrodes for localizing epileptogenic foci. J Neurosurg 1984;60(6):1195–1200

16. Wyler AR, Walker G, Somes G, et al. The morbidity of long-term seizure monitoring using subdural strip electrodes. J Neurosurg 1991;74(5):734–737

17. Cohen-Gadol AA, Spencer DD. Use of an anteromedial subdural strip electrode in the evaluation of medial temporal lobe epilepsy. Technical note. J Neurosurg 2003;99(5):921–923

18. Lee WS, Lee JK, Lee SA, et al. Complications and results of subdural grid electrode implantation in epilepsy surgery. Surg Neurol 2000;54(5):346–351

19. Berger MS, Kincaid J, Ojemann GA, et al. Brain mapping techniques to maximize resection, safety, and seizure control in children with brain tumors. Neurosurgery 1989;25(5):786–792

20. Cohen-Gadol AA, Britton JW, Collignon FP, et al. Nonlesional central lobule seizures: use of awake cortical mapping and subdural grid monitoring for resection of seizure focus. J Neurosurg 2003; 98(6):1255–1262

21. Siegel AM, Roberts DW, Thadani VM, et al. The role of intracranial electrode reevaluation in epilepsy patients after failed initial invasive monitoring. Epilepsia 2000;41(5):571–580

22. Lee SK, Kim K-K, Nam H, et al. Adding or repositioning intracranial electrodes during presurgical assessment of neocortical epilepsy: electrographic seizure pattern and surgical outcome. J Neurosurg 2004;100(3):463–471

23. Bauman JA, Feoli E, Romanelli L, et al. Multistage epilepsy surgery: safety, efficacy, and utility of a novel approach in pediatric extratemporal epilepsy. Neurosurgery 2005;56(2):318–334

24. Wiggins GC, Elisevich K, Smith BJ, et al. Morbidity and infection in combined subdural grid and strip electrode investigation for intractable epilepsy. Epilepsy Res 1999;37(1):73–80

25. Araki T, Otsubo H, Makino Y, et al. Efficacy of dexamathasone on cerebral swelling and seizures during subdural grid EEG recording in children. Epilepsia 2006;47(1):176–180

26. Silberbusch MA, Rothman MI, Bergey GK, et al. Subdural grid implantation for intracranial EEG recording: CT and MR appearance. AJNR Am J Neuroradiol 1998;19(6):1089–1093

27. Swartz BE, Rich JR, Dwan PS, et al. The safety and efficacy of chronically implanted subdural electrodes: a prospective study. Surg Neurol 1996;46(1):87–93

28. Hamer HM, Morris HH, Mascha EJ, et al. Complications of invasive video-EEG monitoring with subdural grid electrodes. Neurology 2002;58(1):97–103

29. Onal C, Otsubo H, Araki T, et al. Complications of invasive subdural grid monitoring in children with epilepsy. J Neurosurg 2003;98(5):1017–1026

30. Wennberg R, Gross D, Quesney F, et al. Transient epileptic foci associated with intracranial hemorrhage in patients with subdural and epidural electrode placement. Clin Neurophysiol 1999;110(3):419–423

31. Mocco J, Komotar RJ, Ladouceur AK, et al. Radiographic characteristics fail to predict clinical course after subdural electrode placement. Neurosurgery 2006;58(1):120–125

3 Depth Electrodes in Invasive Epilepsy Monitoring

Dimitris G. Placantonakis, Padmaja Kandula, and Theodore H. Schwartz

Since the inception of electroencephalography (EEG) by Berger,[1] our understanding of the pathophysiological changes associated with neurological disorders has dramatically improved. EEG recordings have been particularly useful in helping clarify the electrophysiological basis of seizures. Seizures are abnormal neuronal discharges entrained by the synchronous and often oscillatory firing[2,3] of large neuronal ensembles.[4] Although theoretically many parts of the brain are capable of generating seizure-like discharges, the clinically relevant seizures are associated with the neocortex, the hippocampal archicortex, and corticothalamic networks.

Epilepsy is a disorder of abnormal neuronal excitability. Possible electrophysiological mechanisms accounting for epileptogenesis include abnormal synaptic inhibition,[4] aberrant ephaptic[5] or electrotonic[6,7] transmission, and deregulated ion channels.[8-11] At the clinical level, the etiology of seizure generation is broad and includes lesions such as tumors, infections, vascular malformations, and hemorrhages; structural abnormalities, including mesial temporal sclerosis, cortical dysplasia, and neuronal ectopias; and genetic mutations that produce specific seizure phenotypes.[8] In <30% of all cases, seizures cannot be attributed to a specific anatomical, functional, or genetic abnormality and are then considered idiopathic in origin.

The first line of treatment for nonlesional seizure disorders is medical management with antiepileptic agents. The pharmacological approach, however, is ineffective in many patients. In medically intractable cases of nonlesional epilepsy where a single focal origin is suspected, multiple diagnostic modalities are used to help identify the pathogenetic area: magnetic resonance imaging (MRI), functional MRI (fMRI), positron emission tomography (PET), subtraction ictal single-photon emission computed tomography (SPECT) coregistered to MRI (SISCOM), magnetoencephalography (MEG), and surface EEG. MRI, for example, is useful in identifying anatomical abnormalities such as mesial temporal sclerosis or neuronal ectopias, wheras PET and SISCOM can point to metabolically aberrant brain areas that may generate seizures.[12] MEG has been used in some centers to localize prominent synchrony and rhythmicity associated with epileptogenic foci.[13] In some cases, scalp EEG points out a focal origin of seizures. These diagnostic tools can direct the surgeon to a confined resectable locus, if they are concordant with the clinical semiology.

Scalp EEG electrodes, however, sit far from the underlying current sources and sinks, and their ability to localize ictal onset zones is limited by signal attenuation by the underlying skin and cerebrospinal fluid (CSF), as well as muscle artifact. For these reasons, scalp EEG often fails to identify the precise region of ictal onset. Invasive electrophysiological monitoring can help better localize ictal and interictal events, thus facilitating the identification of the epileptogenic focus and a possible therapeutic resection.[14] Simultaneous scalp and subdural recordings demonstrate the power of implanted electrodes to identify the precise origin and propagation patterns of seizures that cannot be localized with scalp recordings.[15] Invasive monitoring is achieved via placement of either subdural electrodes (e.g., strip and grid electrodes) or depth intraparenchymal electrodes.[14,16] In this chapter, we will focus on depth electrodes.

Indications for Depth Electrode Placement

Although subdural electrodes can provide high-quality recordings from a large number of neocortical sites, several deep structures that are considered highly epileptogenic and surgically treatable[17,18] can be monitored more efficiently with depth electrodes.[16] Such structures are found in the medial temporal lobe and include the hippocampus, amygdala, entorhinal cortex, and parahippocampal gyrus.[19] Although subtemporal strip electrodes can sample the mesial temporal lobe, they cannot always be placed reliably and can mislocalize the ictal onset zone compared with stereotactically placed depth electrodes.[20] Recordings from the cingulate gyrus, which is buried within the interhemispheric fissure, can be greatly facilitated by the use of depth electrodes. Likewise the insula is most easily sampled with depth electrodes.[21] Moreover, some institutions use depth electrodes to record from the depth of sulci or even from the neocortical layer.[22] It has been postulated that the use of depth electrodes in stereoelectroencephalography[22-24] can provide a three-dimensional map of the seizure focus and the spread of the discharge.[25] Finally, depth electrodes can be used to electrophysiologically monitor the activity of ectopic neuronal tissue located deep within the cerebral hemispheres such as periventricular heterotopias and hypothalamic hamartomas.[26]

Depth electrodes are typically of low impedance and, thus, record local field potentials (LFPs), the compound activity of neuronal ensembles.[14] However, there exist depth electrodes capable of capturing activity from single neurons. More recently, microdialysis probes have been inserted intraparenchymally to monitor simultaneously neurotransmitter levels and neuronal activity.[27]

Depth electrodes are used not only to record electrophysiological activity during ictal states and interictally; they can be used to functionally map the brain areas where they are inserted, which is of paramount importance when epileptogenic foci are adjacent to eloquent brain.[14] Moreover, single-unit recordings have been used to correlate neuronal activity to specific behavioral states, as well as to characterize oscillatory activity during seizure generation.[2,3,28]

Surgical Approach to Implantation of Depth Electrodes

Depth electrodes target deep structures that, by definition, are not visible to the surgeon. It is therefore essential to plan their trajectory using stereotaxy. The stereotactic placement of depth electrodes may be achieved by several means. An imaging modality, such as computed tomography (CT) or MRI, and the creation of stereotactic space, either frame-based or frameless, are essential components to a successful placement. In recent years, the advent of high-resolution gadolinium-enhanced MRI has rendered it the preferred imaging modality for surgical planning. Gadolinium-enhanced MRI has the advantage of not only differentiating well between gray and white matter, thus reliably delineating deep

structures such as the amygdala and hippocampus from the adjacent white matter, but also identifying vascular structures that may be encountered in the electrode trajectory.

The electrode path is carefully chosen so as to avoid injury to critical vascular structures, and, if possible, to not intersect the ventricular system. There are two main issues that arise from an intersection of the electrode trajectory and the ventricles, and the resulting CSF loss from the ventricle through the electrode track. First, an acute reduction in intraventricular volume can generate compensatory shifts in the topography of the brain parenchyma, which in turn may result in erroneous placement of the electrode away from its target. Second, if the depth electrodes are used for extended periods of time for invasive electrophysiological monitoring, a sustained CSF leak through the skin may predispose toward meningitis. It is thus preferred to plan trajectories that spare the ventricular system, although in certain cases this cannot be avoided. In fact, some authors recommend placement of the electrode within the ventricles to avoid damaging the hippocampus and potential "injury spikes."[29] We have not found this approach as reliable as intraparenchymal placement for providing reliable data.

Although stereotactic frames are still used in many institutions for depth electrode implantation, frameless stereotaxy can also be used with good accuracy and results. At our institution, we have exclusively used frameless stereotaxy for depth electrode placement in the context of epilepsy the past few years and have found it to be reliable and accurate (**Fig. 3.1**).[30]

A
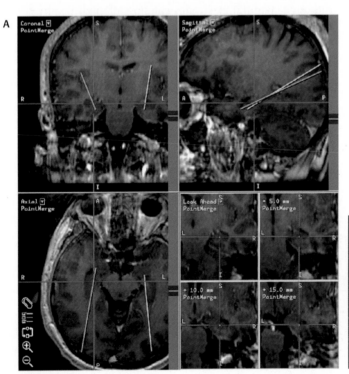

B
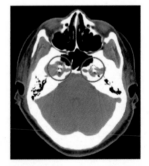
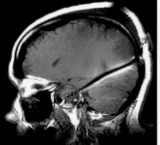
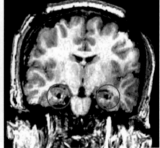

Fig. 3.1 Frameless stereotaxy for depth electrode implantation in the mesial temporal lobe. **(A)** Preoperative planning using a neuronavigation system for placement of a depth electrode into the mesial temporal lobe using an occipitotemporal approach. The planning was based on a brain MRI. **(B)** Postoperative imaging showing the depth electrodes on the axial (CT), sagittal (MRI), and coronal (MRI) planes. The electrode tips are circled.

The computer software that accompanies most commercially available frameless stereotaxy systems also allows for easy modification of the surgical plan and trajectory intraoperatively.

When depth electrodes are used to target the amygdala and hippocampus, the entry site can be either perpendicular to the temporal neocortex through the middle temporal gyrus, perpendicular to the frontal lobe through a precoronal trajectory, or through the occipitoparietal junction. The first two approaches are orthogonal to the long axis of the hippocampus and sample limited areas. Hence, multiple electrodes may be required to record from the entire amygdalohippocampal complex. In contrast, the occipitotemporal approach[19] passes through the long axis of the hippocampus and can sample the anterior and posterior hippocampus, as well as the amygdala, with one electrode. In our practice we use exclusively the temporal and occipitotemporal approaches (**Fig. 3.2**).

Recordings of ictal (**Fig. 3.3**) and interictal (**Fig. 3.4**) events from depth electrodes have been shown to facilitate the identification of epileptogenic foci and lead to surgical resection in up to 87% of cases.[23] Approximately 70% of those patients show substantial improvement in their seizure disorder (Engel classes I to II).[23] Importantly, depth electrodes are considered to be superior to subdural electrodes in identifying seizures originating from the deep structures of the mesial temporal lobe.[15,31]

Depth electrodes can be placed either in the context of a large craniotomy or through bur holes, depending on the clinical indications. We tend to use the temporal approach to sample the hippocampus and amygdala in conjunction with

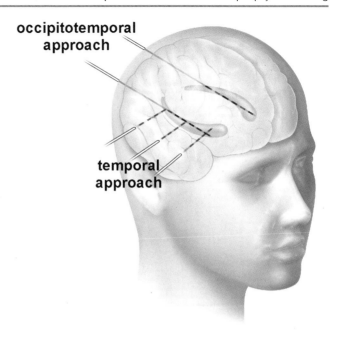

Fig. 3.2 Stereotactic placement of depth electrodes into the mesial temporal lobe. The hippocampal formation and amygdala of the mesial temporal lobe are the most frequent targets of depth electrodes for invasive epilepsy monitoring. Two different trajectories may be employed. First, the temporal route allows for stereotactic placement of electrodes into the target using a trajectory orthogonal to the long axis of the hippocampus. Second, the occipitotemporal approach utilizes a parietooccipital entry site and a trajectory parallel to the hippocampal long axis.

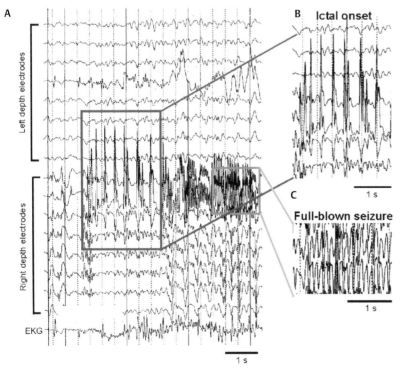

Fig. 3.3 Electrophysiological recording of a seizure using bilateral depth electrodes implanted into the mesial temporal lobes. **(A)** Recordings illustrating a full-blown seizure originating in the right mesial temporal lobe. Depth electrodes were implanted into both mesial temporal lobes in this patient using an occipitotemporal approach. Each electrode contained eight contacts. The bottom trace shows a concurrent electrocardiogram trace. Note the sudden onset of 3 Hz rhythmic discharges recorded from the right but not left depth electrode. These discharges are shown in higher sweep speed in **(B)**. The event subsequently evolves to recruit the entire right mesial temporal lobe, with a concomitant shift in the dominant frequency to 8 to 9 Hz at the origin **(C)**.

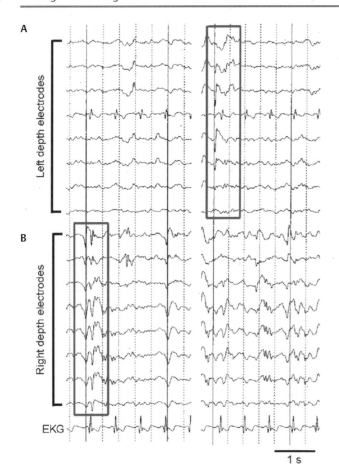

A

Left depth electrodes

B

Right depth electrodes

EKG

1 s

Fig. 3.4 Recordings of interictal spikes with bilateral depth electrodes. These traces represent recordings obtained with bilateral depth electrodes implanted into the mesial temporal lobes from the same patient as in **Fig. 3.2**. This patient suffered from seizures originating in the right mesial temporal lobe. However, interictal spikes arose independently from both temporal lobes. **(A)** Interictal spike originating in the right mesial temporal lobe with no involvement of the left temporal lobe. **(B)** A separate interictal spike now originates in the left mesial temporal lobe

a large craniotomy in which grids and strips are placed simultaneously because the temporal lobe is already exposed. The occipitotemporal approach is used when implanting bilateral depth electrodes in patients with preliminarily bitemporal epilepsy to determine the side of ictal onset. The electrode lead is eventually tunneled through the skin. The lead's path thus produces a potential corridor allowing communication of the intracranial space with the outside world via CSF leaks. To minimize the potential for CSF leak, we routinely place a purse-string suture around the lead's exit site on the skin. Moreover, we meticulously approximate the dura in the case of large craniotomies and subsequently use

Duraseal (Confluent Surgical, Waltham, MA) to help seal the dural edges. When bur holes are used for depth electrode placement, the hole is plugged with Gelfoam (Pfizer Inc., New York, NY) with subsequent application of Duraseal. Using this approach, we have not had any clinically significant CSF leaks through the leads' exit sites or associated infections, such as meningitis. To prevent accidental movement of the intracranial portion of the electrodes through accidental pulling, the leads are tethered to both the dura and the skin.

The perioperative care includes antibiotic administration before (single dose) and after (for a day) the procedure. Although the literature supports the use of perioperative antibiotics,[32,33] some centers avoid them while still maintaining low infection rates.[22] Steroids can be administered postoperatively to reduce the inflammation in the parenchyma from the electrode track. However, they should be tapered quickly as they have antiepileptic activity that may interfere with the electrophysiological monitoring.[34] By the same token, antiepileptic medications are titrated down to facilitate the monitoring. Although valproic acid has been shown to have some anticoagulant properties,[35] its use has not been shown to increase the risk of bleeding in prior studies of epilepsy surgery.[36] However, these studies were done during resections and not during electrode implantation. For this reason, we taper patients off valproic acid if possible prior to surgery. We prefer to place a head-wrap postoperatively to minimize the risk of the leads being pulled and to keep the incision and electrode exit sites clean. Finally, we avoid using subcutaneous heparin for deep venous thrombosis prophylaxis postoperatively while the depth electrodes are implanted. Instead, we rely on compression boots.

Complications

Major surgical complications from placement of depth electrodes include hemorrhage and infection. Such complications, however, are rare. A recent report[22] estimated the risk of hemorrhage to be 2.9% per hemisphere when multiple (four or more) electrodes were implanted in the frontal lobe. The incidence of intracranial abscess and meningitis in the same series was very rare, whereas 11% of the patients experienced psychiatric disturbances during the monitoring. Cossu et al[23] reported a 4.2% incidence of hemorrhagic complications. In the same series, the infection rate was 0.5%. Other complications included transient sensory deficits (0.5%) and fractured intraparenchymal electrodes requiring surgical removal (0.5%).[23] At our institution, we have not encountered clinically significant hemorrhagic or infectious complications from placement of depth electrodes.

Bilateral Depth Electrodes

The preliminary workup of epilepsy patients who are being considered for surgical treatment occasionally fails to reveal a focal origin, even when the clinician suspects a single epileptogenic focus based on clinical semiology. The reasons for the failure to obtain a diagnosis from scalp EEG or imaging studies include discordant diagnostic tests, where different tests suggest distinct foci; diagnostic results contradicting clinical semiology; and multiple foci being identified within the same diagnostic modality. In some patients, the uncertainty may involve hemispheric laterality. In such cases, bilateral hemispheric invasive monitoring may be employed to help identify the origin of the seizures.

At our institution, 45% of patients undergoing implantation of bilateral subdural recording electrodes also have depth electrodes placed into both mesial temporal lobes via the occipitotemporal route (**Fig. 3.5**). The depth electrode trajectories are preplanned with neuronavigation software and implemented with frameless stereotaxy. We have previously shown that frameless stereotaxy results in accurate placement of electrodes into the amygdala and hippocam-

pus with 98% of the electrodes providing informative recordings.[30] Bilateral bur holes are placed in the calvaria at the level of the lambda and ~4 cm from the midline as entry sites for such electrodes. This approach is facilitated by positioning the patient in a semi-sitting position with an appropriate amount of neck flexion. We have not encountered any complications with bilateral depth electrode placement.

Conclusion

Depth electrodes are of great value in the invasive electrophysiological monitoring of epilepsy patients. Such electrodes are routinely used to obtain recordings from the mesial temporal lobe and can also sample deep ictogenic structures such as subcortical heterotopias, cingulate gyrus, and the medial frontal lobe. Some centers also use multiple depth electrodes in the context of stereoelectroencephalography. Depth electrode implantation is associated with a low incidence of complications and is tolerated well by patients. The placement can be achieved reliably with either frame-based or frameless stereotaxy.

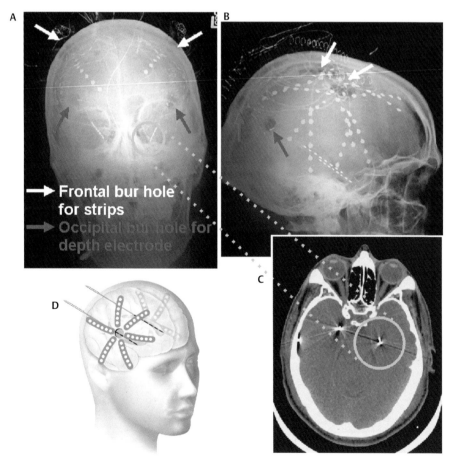

Fig. 3.5 Surgical approach in patients who require bilateral invasive monitoring. **(A,B)** Anteroposterior and lateral skull films showing the placement of bilateral subdural strip and depth electrodes. The depth electrodes are targeting the mesial temporal lobes. The *arrows* indicate the location of frontal (*white arrows*) and parietooccipital (*red arrows*) bur holes used as entry sites for the implantation of subdural and depth electrodes, respectively. **(C)** A slice from a noncontrast head CT from the same patient shows a portion of the left depth electrode in the left mesial temporal lobe. **(D)** Illustration summarizing our technique in patients whose hemispheric laterality is in question and who require implantation of bilateral electrodes. We typically use several subdural strip electrodes to monitor the neocortex, as well as depth electrodes into the mesial temporal lobe via the occipitotemporal approach in 45% of the cases.

References

1. Berger H. *On the Electroencephalogram of Man.* New York: Elsevier; 1969

2. Worrell GA, Parish L, Cranstoun SD, Jonas R, Baltuch G, Litt B. High-frequency oscillations and seizure generation in neocortical epilepsy. Brain 2004;127:1496–1506

3. Jirsch JD, Urrestarazu E, LeVan P, Olivier A, Dubeau F, Gotman J. High-frequency oscillations during human focal seizures. Brain 2006;129:1593–1608

4. McCormick DA, Contreras D. On the cellular and network bases of epileptic seizures. Annu Rev Physiol 2001;63:815–846

5. Ghai RS, Bikson M, Durand DM. Effects of applied electric fields on low-calcium epileptiform activity in the CA1 region of rat hippocampal slices. J Neurophysiol 2000;84:274–280

6. Nemani VM, Binder DK. Emerging role of gap junctions in epilepsy. Histol Histopathol 2005;20:253–259

7. Hempelmann A, Heils A, Sander T. Confirmatory evidence for an association of the connexin-36 gene with juvenile myoclonic epilepsy. Epilepsy Res 2006;71:223–228

8. Berkovic SF, Mulley JC, Scheffer IE, Petrou S. Human epilepsies: interaction of genetic and acquired factors. Trends Neurosci 2006;29:391–397

9. Graves TD. Ion channels and epilepsy. QJM 2006;99:201–217

10. Khosravani H, Zamponi GW. Voltage-gated calcium channels and idiopathic generalized epilepsies. Physiol Rev 2006;86:941–966

11. Vincent A, Lang B, Kleopa KA. Autoimmune channelopathies and related neurological disorders. Neuron 2006;52:123–138

12. Murphy MA, O'Brien TJ, Morris K, Cook MJ. Multimodality image-guided surgery for the treatment of medically refractory epilepsy. J Neurosurg 2004;100:452–462

13. Makela JP, Forss N, Jaaskelainen J, Kirveskari E, Korvenoja A, Paetau R. Magnetoencephalography in neurosurgery. Neurosurgery 2006;59:493–511

14. Engel AK, Moll CK, Fried I, Ojemann GA. Invasive recordings from the human brain: clinical insights and beyond. Nat Rev Neurosci 2005;6:35–47

15. Pacia SV, Ebersole JS. Intracranial EEG substrates of scalp ictal patterns from temporal lobe foci. Epilepsia 1997;38:642–654

16. Brekelmans GJ, van Emde Boas W, Velis DN, Lopes da Silva FH, van Rijen PC, van Veelen CW. Comparison of combined versus subdural or intracerebral electrodes alone in presurgical focus localization. Epilepsia 1998;39:1290–1301

17. Cohen-Gadol AA, Wilhelmi BG, Collignon F, et al. Long-term outcome of epilepsy surgery among 399 patients with nonlesional seizure foci including mesial temporal lobe sclerosis. J Neurosurg 2006;104:513–524

18. Sindou M, Guenot M, Isnard J, Ryvlin P, Fischer C, Mauguiere F. Temporo-mesial epilepsy surgery: outcome and complications in 100 consecutive adult patients. Acta Neurochir (Wien) 2006;148:39–45

19. Blatt DR, Roper SN, Friedman WA. Invasive monitoring of limbic epilepsy using stereotactic depth and subdural strip electrodes: surgical technique. Surg Neurol 1997;48:74–79

20. Eisenschenk S, Gilmore RL, Cibula JE, Roper SN. Lateralization of temporal lobe foci: depth versus subdural electrodes. Clin Neurophysiol 2001;112:836–844

21. Isnard J, Guenot M, Sindou M, Mauguiere F. Clinical manifestations of insular lobe seizures: a stereo-electroencephalographic study. Epilepsia 2004;45:1079–1090

22. de Almeida AN, Olivier A, Quesney F, Dubeau F, Savard G, Andermann F. Efficacy of and morbidity associated with stereoelectroencephalography using computerized tomography – or magnetic resonance imaging – guided electrode implantation. J Neurosurg 2006;104:483–487

23. Cossu M, Cardinale F, Castana L, et al. Stereoelectroencephalography in the presurgical evaluation of focal epilepsy: a retrospective analysis of 215 procedures. Neurosurgery 2005;57:706–718

24. Cossu M, Cardinale F, Colombo N, et al. Stereoelectroencephalography in the presurgical evaluation of children with drug-resistant focal epilepsy. J Neurosurg 2005;103:333–343

25. Gavaret M, Badier JM, Marquis P, et al. Electric source imaging in frontal lobe epilepsy. J Clin Neurophysiol 2006;23:358–370

26. Kahane P, Ryvlin P, Hoffmann D, Minotti L, Benabid AL. From hypothalamic hamartoma to cortex: what can be learnt from depth recordings and stimulation? Epileptic Disord 2003;5:205–217

27. Fried I, Wilson CL, Maidment NT, et al. Cerebral microdialysis combined with single-neuron and electroencephalographic recording in neurosurgical patients. Technical note. J Neurosurg 1999;91:697–705

28. Colder BW, Wilson CL, Frysinger RC, Chao LC, Harper RM, Engel J Jr. Neuronal synchrony in relation to burst discharge in epileptic human temporal lobes. J Neurophysiol 1996;75:2496–2508

29. Song JK, Abou-Khalil B, Konrad PE. Intraventricular monitoring for temporal lobe epilepsy: report on technique and initial results in eight patients. J Neurol Neurosurg Psychiatry 2003;74:561–565

30. Mehta AD, Labar D, Dean A, et al. Frameless stereotactic placement of depth electrodes in epilepsy surgery. J Neurosurg 2005;102:1040–1045

31. Alsaadi TM, Laxer KD, Barbaro NM, Marks WJ, Garcia PA. False lateralization by subdural electrodes in two patients with temporal lobe epilepsy. Neurology 2001;57:532–534

32. Barbaro NM. Stereoelectroencephalography using computerized tomography—or magnetic resonance imaging—guided electrode implantation. J Neurosurg 2006;104:480–482

33. Barker FG. Efficacy of prophylactic antibiotics for craniotomy: a meta-analysis. Neurosurgery 1994;35:484–492

34. Duport S, Stoppini L, Correges P. Electrophysiological approach of the antiepileptic effect of dexamethasone on hippocampal slice culture using a multirecording system: the Physiocard. Life Sci 1997;60:251–256

35. Pohlmann-Eden B, Peters CN, Wennberg R, Dempfle CE. Valproate induces reversible factor XIII deficiency with risk of perioperative bleeding. Acta Neurol Scand 2003;108:142–145

36. Anderson GD, Lin YX, Berge C, Ojemann GA. Absence of bleeding complications in patients undergoing cortical surgery while receiving valproate treatment. J Neurosurg 1997;87:252–256

II Cortical Resection

4 Temporal Lobectomy and Amygdalohippocampectomy

Patrick J. Connolly and Gordon H. Baltuch

Layout of the Operating Room and Positioning the Patient

A multidisciplinary team is required for epilepsy surgery and includes the anesthesiologist, circulating nurse, scrub nurse, surgical assistant or resident, neurophysiologist or neurologist, patient, and surgeon. The team utilizes several workstations that occupy floor space in the suite. They include the anesthesia machine, instrument tables, neurophysiology platform, navigational equipment, cautery machines, microscope, and operating table.

Walls support view boxes, suction canisters, and electricity. The ceiling delivers anesthesia gases, general and task lighting, and sometimes a microscope. Adequate space and thoughtful placement of these items are necessary to minimize clutter and to maintain a safe environment for patient and personnel. An example of an operating room arrangement in shown in **Fig. 4.1**. However, the arrangement ultimately depends on the location of electricity, plumbing, doors, lighting, and even the occasional window.

Surface Anatomy and Designing the Incision for Right Temporal Lobectomy

Place the patient in the supine position on the operating table, and secure him or her in the Mayfield headrest (Integra LifeSciences Corp., Plainsboro, NJ). There are two pinning options: (1) single pin in the forehead and two posteriorly; and (2) single pin at the root of the mastoid process, one pin in the forehead, and one just behind the hairline. The head is turned at least 45 degrees to the left. A shoulder roll may be necessary. Turn the bed as necessary to accommodate the various work zones. If surgical navigation is planned, attach the arm that holds the reference frame. It goes toward anesthesia, away from the operating field. Take care that the arm will not interfere with any retractor apparatus. Once this is done, then register the head into the surgical navigation software.

The temporal lobe is contained by the middle fossa. It is bounded above by sphenoid bone and sylvian fissure, below by the temporal bone and the tentorium. Anteriorly, it is bounded by lateral orbital wall. Posteriorly, it is bounded by the parietal lobe. Several surface landmarks reveal the location of the middle fossa (**Fig. 4.2**). A typical temporal skin incision accomplishes several tasks while providing exposure to the temporal lobe and associated structures. It is (1) mostly concealed by hair; (2) preserves blood supply to scalp and temporalis; (3) avoids the facial nerve; and (4) avoids the ear canal. Its boundaries are determined by the root of the zygoma, superior temporal line, and, on the face, the amount of anterior temporal exposure required.

For epilepsy surgery a fair amount of anterior exposure is necessary, so the scalp and temporalis are often dissected separately.

The incision is the form of a question mark, **Fig. 4.2**. With a marking pen, start just below the root of the zygoma, and just in front of the ear, curve posterior to the ear, then superiorly and anteriorly. Note that the incision may be different on the nondominant side, compared with the dominant side. In some dominant lobe resections, language mapping may be necessary, and this requires greater surface exposure. If you begin the incision more than 1 cm in front of the ear you are likely to encounter the facial nerve and the superficial temporal artery. The incision will show prominently as well. Try to follow the hairline to its most facial extent. Extend the mark onto the face by 1 to 2 cm in case extra exposure is needed. Prepare the skin and drape. Preplace the retractor clamps so that no extra time is spent once the dura is open. Infiltrate local anesthetic into the wound. Epinephrine helps with hemostasis. Do not inject the superficial temporal vessels.

Incision and Extracranial Dissection

Begin the incision rostrally, and open the scalp down to the bone until you reach the temporalis fascia. At that point, slide an elevator under the scalp to define a plane, then open sharply. Just open the skin for the last 2 cm of incision above the zygoma. Use Metzenbaum scissors to dissect in layers to the temporalis fascia, so that the superficial temporal vessels may be identified, secured with bipolar cautery, and cut. Cauterize any arteries in the scalp. Venous bleeding may be secured with Raney clips.

Once this is done, then separate the galea from the temporalis fascia by finger or sharp dissection or cautery. You will need to identify the frontal process of the zygoma. This marks the frontal extent of the craniotomy. The pterion is just behind it.

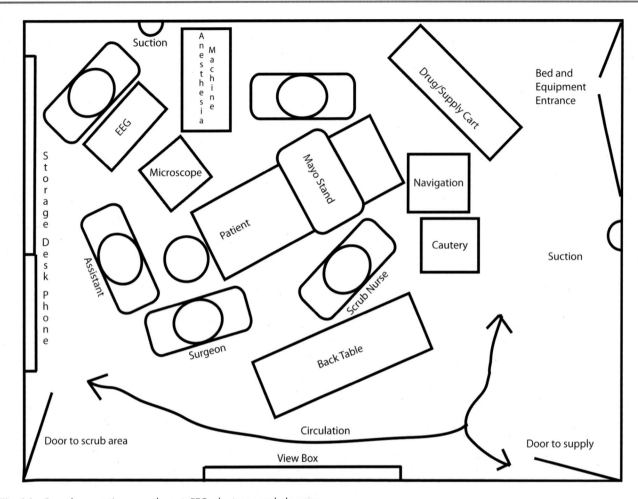

Fig. 4.1 Sample operating room layout. EEG, electroencephalogram.

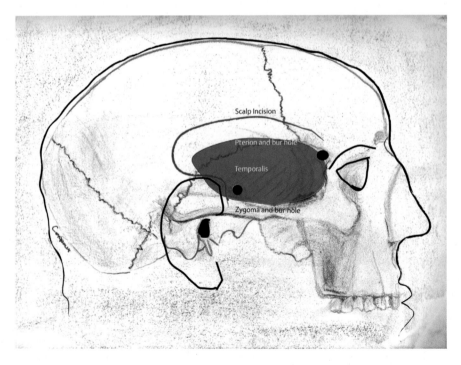

Fig. 4.2 Surface features demarcating the middle fossa. The zygoma outlines the anterior and inferior boundaries, the superior temporal line the superior boundary. The top of the tragus and external auditory meatus approximate the floor of the middle fossa. The position of the temporal lobe itself is estimated with red hatching within the temporalis. For brevity and clarity, the mandible is not drawn.

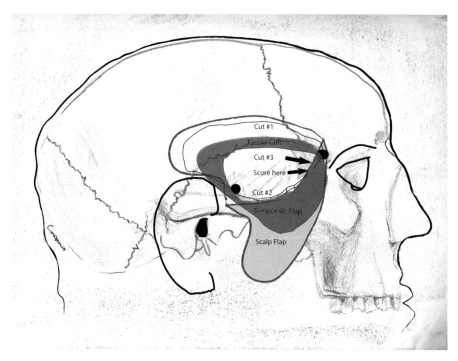

Fig. 4.3 Extracranial dissection. Temporalis and scalp are reflected separately for increased anterior exposure. Cover them with a damp sponge and place a rolled sponge under the scalp to prevent vascular kinking and ischemia. Leave a cuff of temporalis fascia to sew. Note craniotome cuts and suggested sequence. The craniotome will not cross the sphenoid wing. The sphenoid should be scored and cracked. Hatched area indicates rongeured bone. The exact amount will vary. Note again the red hatched area estimating the temporal lobe location.

Open the temporalis fascia sharply and curvilinearly from the frontal part of the zygoma to the root of the zygoma (**Fig. 4.3**). Leave a minimal 1 to 2 cm cuff of fascia to which to sew. Some surgeons prefer monopolar cautery to elevate the temporalis; others prefer to use periosteal elevators. Try to advance as anteriorly as possible along the lateral temporal bone.

Drill two bur holes (**Fig. 4.3**) with either an acorn bit or a perforator, one at the pterion, the other at the root of the zygoma. Use a no. 3 Penfield dissector or an Adson periosteal elevator to elevate the dura in the epidural space. You may drill a third at the posterior edge of the craniotomy, if desired.

Use a craniotome to make the long cuts first (**Fig. 4.3**). There will be two short cuts. First, advance anteriorly from the root of the zygoma along the middle fossa floor. Turn superiorly toward the pterional bur hole. The craniotome will be blocked by the wing of the sphenoid bone. Make a short cut (usually ~1 cm) from the pterion to the sphenoid wing. Score the remaining sphenoid segment with a craniotome bit without the footplate.

Use a no. 3 Penfield dissector to elevate the bone. The sphenoid part will crack. Carefully dissect the bone away from the dura with a periosteal elevator. Do not allow the bone to lever into the brain.

Obtain hemostasis. The middle meningeal artery may require attention at the sphenoid wing. There is often venous bleeding, which responds either to bone wax or to thrombin soaked Gelfoam powder (Pfizer Inc., New York, NY).

Continue the bony dissection by using a rongeur to remove 1 to 2 cm more of squamous temporal bone anteriorly and inferiorly toward the floor of the middle fossa (**Fig. 4.3**). Reserve the chips for closure. Note whether there are any opened mastoid air cells along the floor. Wax these thoroughly. It is often helpful to drill some of the sphenoid wing. You need not go to the superior orbital fissure. Once you obtain hemostasis, it is time to open the dura.

Durotomy and Surface Exposure

The dural flap should be based anteriorly. Make an apex posteriorly, then advance the durotomy medially and anteriorly. Then, advance it laterally and anteriorly, over the temporal lobe. Leave a 1-cm cuff of dura with which to close. Be careful about attached veins when reflecting the dura.

With a brain ribbon, verify that there are no veins between the craniotomy edge and the temporal tip. Measure 4 cm from the temporal tip to ensure that the craniotomy is satisfactory and to plan the lateral temporal lobectomy (**Fig. 4.4**).

Corticography is optional, depending on the case and preoperative mapping. It can be useful to record from the temporal and frontal areas with a subdural grid, either 4×4 or 4×5 contacts, particularly if subdural grids are not already present. A detailed discussion of electrocorticography can be found in Chapter 11. Once corticography has been performed, one can begin the resection (**Fig. 4.4**).

Lateral Lobectomy

Use a no. 7 Frazier suction and a bipolar cautery to make the initial pial incision ~4 cm posterior to the temporal tip, minding any large surface veins. The vein of Labbé has variable anatomy and is typically found over the posterior temporal lobe, but not always. Generally, the corticotomy can be made 3.5 to 4.5 cm from the temporal tip in the dominant

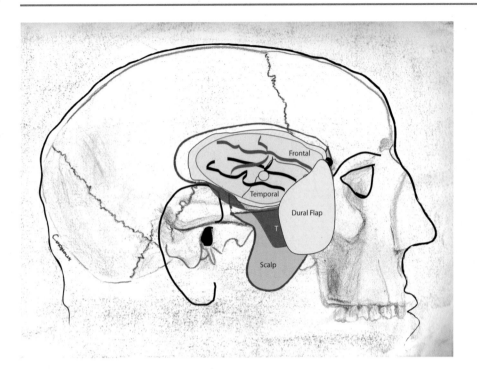

Fig. 4.4 Subdural exposure of temporal lobe. The thin black line denotes the corticotomy line 4 cm from the temporal tip and in the superior temporal gyrus. The resection is taken to, but not into, the sylvian fissure. The circle over the middle temporal gyrus estimates the location of the initial corticotomy used to find the ventricle. The ventricle is usually encountered ~3 cm below the surface (see **Fig. 4.5**). Veins are schematic, not anatomical. T, Temporalis flap.

hemisphere and 4 to 5 cm from the temporal tip in a nondominant hemisphere. Enter through the middle temporal gyrus and identify the ventricle. This will mark the medial extent of the lobectomy. Mark the ventricular opening with a cottonoid patty (**Fig. 4.5**). Work inferiorly along the posterior limb toward the floor of the middle fossa. For the rostral limb, some surgeons spare the superior temporal gyrus, others resect to the gray-white junction along the sylvian fissure, and still others resect all the way to the pia. It is neither necessary nor desirable to open the sylvian fissure.

The ventricle is in the same sagittal plane as the collateral sulcus, and it is identified during a lateral corticectomy by the collateral eminence, which is the lateral ventricular wall. Medial to the collateral sulcus is the mesial temporal lobe, specifically the parahippocampal gyrus, so do not yet resect there (**Fig. 4.6**). Work to connect the corticotomy incisions along the floor of the middle fossa. Use caution to control the temporal draining veins. They should be cauterized because they are somewhat of a nuisance if cut before doing so. Once you do this, the lateral lobectomy will be complete. Be careful not to resect any tissue posterosuperior to the tip of the temporal horn. This tissue may contain fibers of Meyer's loop and damaging them causes a contralateral superior temporal quadrantanopsia, the so-called pie in the sky field cut.[1] Additionally, excessive posterolateral resection or retraction can result in damage to the optic radiations.[2] Ready the retractor apparatus, either Greenberg (Codman & Shurtleff, Inc., Raynham, MA), Budde (Integra LifeSciences), or Leyla (Aesculap Inc., USA, Center Valley, PA) bar. Now it is time to bring in the microscope.

Microsurgical Resection of the Mesial Temporal Lobe

The hippocampus forms the medial surface of the temporal horn, and it is defined superolaterally by ependyma; medially by fimbria, choroidal fissure, and hippocampal sulcus; inferiorly by parahippocampal gyrus; and laterally by collateral eminence (**Fig. 4.6**).

Some surgeons use a low powered ultrasonic aspirator for subpial dissection and others use a bipolar cautery. One approach is to follow the pia from the collateral sulcus over the incisura and through the uncus, whereupon the hippocampal head and uncus will be resected by cautery or aspiration. The amygdala is partly removed during the lateral corticectomy because it forms an anterior cap over the temporal horn. The rest is removed with the uncus. Some surgeons use the inferior choroidal point as the posterior edge of the resection, a so-called pesectomy. The inferior choroidal point marks the posterior edge of the hippocampal head. Under the pia, you will also recognize the posterior cerebral artery, and the oculomotor nerve passing medial to it. The third nerve is quite fragile and can be easily traumatized, so it is particularly important to not violate this pial border. Beyond this is the ambient cistern. The advantages of the lesser approach are: (1) the choroidal fissure does not need to be opened, exposing the contents of the ambient and crural cisterns; and (2) the optic radiation is not at risk. The disadvantage is that the entire hippocampus is not removed, and this has implications for postoperative result.[3]

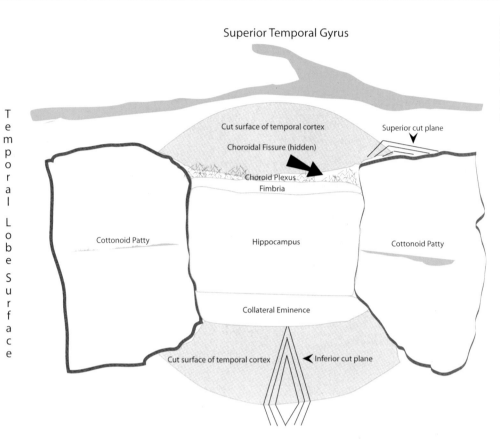

Fig. 4.5 Corticotomy through the middle temporal gyrus. This is an enlarged view of the circle in **Fig. 4.4**, and it is the entrance to the temporal horn. Anatomical landmarks are identified. Cut planes are indicated for the lateral temporal lobectomy.

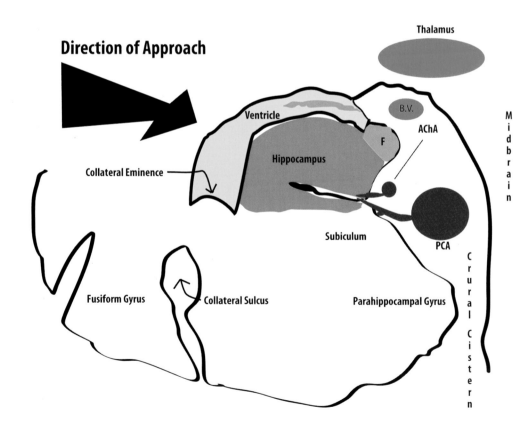

Fig. 4.6 Illustration depicting coronal section through mesial temporal lobe within the hippocampal body.[5] Note that the cut plane is behind the hippocampal head with the midbrain and crural cistern, so the oculomotor nerve is not represented. PCA, posterior cerebral artery; AChA, anterior choroidal artery and small hippocampal perforators; F, fimbria; B.V., basal vein of Rosenthal. The choroid plexus is drawn in green.

Fig. 4.7

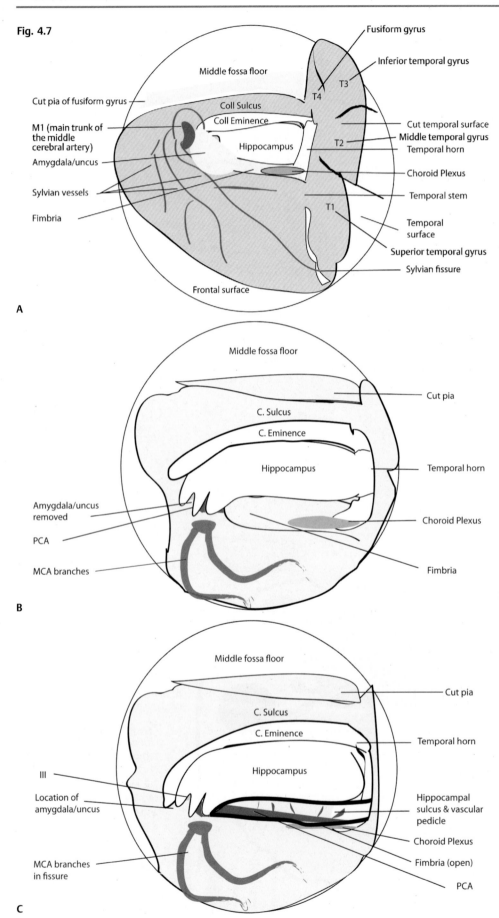

A

Middle fossa floor

Fusiform gyrus

Inferior temporal gyrus

T3

T4

Cut pia of fusiform gyrus

Coll Sulcus

Coll Eminence

M1 (main trunk of the middle cerebral artery)

Hippocampus

T2

Amygdala/uncus

Cut temporal surface

Middle temporal gyrus

Temporal horn

Choroid Plexus

Sylvian vessels

Temporal stem

Fimbria

T1

Temporal surface

Superior temporal gyrus

Sylvian fissure

Frontal surface

B

Middle fossa floor

Cut pia

C. Sulcus

C. Eminence

Hippocampus

Temporal horn

Amygdala/uncus removed

PCA

MCA branches

Choroid Plexus

Fimbria

C

Middle fossa floor

Cut pia

C. Sulcus

C. Eminence

Hippocampus

Temporal horn

III

Location of amygdala/uncus

Hippocampal sulcus & vascular pedicle

Choroid Plexus

Fimbria (open)

MCA branches in fissure

PCA

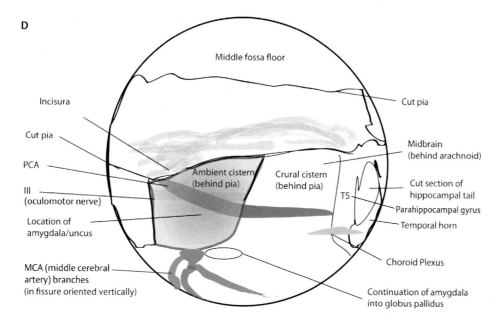

D

Middle fossa floor

Incisura

Cut pia

Cut pia

Midbrain
(behind arachnoid)

PCA

Ambient cistern
(behind pia)

Crural cistern
(behind pia)

Cut section of
hippocampal tail

III
(oculomotor nerve)

T5

Parahippocampal gyrus

Location of
amygdala/uncus

Temporal horn

MCA (middle cerebral
artery) branches
(in fissure oriented vertically)

Choroid Plexus

Continuation of amygdala
into globus pallidus

Fig. 4.7 (Continued) Sequence depicting hippocampectomy.[6] The illustration is highly schematized for clarity. **(A)** After the lateral lobectomy but before the mesial lobectomy. For clarity, the uncus is shown unresected, though it is partly removed with the lateral lobectomy. **(B)** The amygdala/uncus is removed. Do not enter the frontal lobe. The amygdala is continuous with the globus pallidus. The posterior cerebral artery (PCA) and III are now visible. **(C)** The entry line may be through the choroidal fissure or through the fimbria. Through the fimbria, the ambient and crural cisterns are traversed to the hippocampal sulcus. The PCA is visible behind the crural cistern arachnoid layer when the fimbria is opened. Use a bipolar cautery to secure the small hippocampal perforators on the surface of the hippocampal sulcus. Once the sulcus is open, dissect subpially to remove the subiculum and parahippocampus. **(D)** The hippocampus is amputated at the tail and removed with the parahippocampus. The brainstem is visible through the crural cistern. The oculomotor nerve exits behind the PCA. The ICA (internal carotid artery), MCA, and MCA divisions are visible through the sylvian arachnoid. The hippocampus condenses into a tail, marking the posterior extent of resection.

Removal of the hippocampal body is a larger resection. Additionally, a subpial dissection of the hippocampal head does not give an anatomical en bloc resection, which is desirable if a laboratory wants to use hippocampal slices. In that case, it is preferable to open the choroidal fissure and do a larger resection. A detailed description of this technique is given by Wen et al.[4] The inferior choroidal point is where the choroidal fissure begins. The anterior choroidal artery runs parallel, in the ambient, then the crural, cistern. The inferior choroidal point also demarcates the division between the hippocampal head anteriorly and body posteriorly.

You can place a 3/8' retractor lateral to the ventricle and another where needed, usually superiorly. As you near the choroidal point, you will find a tentlike pial structure underlying the hippocampus. This is the hippocampal sulcus, through which a small hippocampal branch of the anterior choroidal artery passes. Once the hippocampal head is removed subpially (the "anterior disconnection"), the body of the hippocampus can be removed by dissecting it from within the choroidal fissure along the arachnoid of the ambient and crural cisterns (medial disconnection). Cauterize the small hippocampal feeders along the pial surface. The posterior disconnection may be done by dividing the hippocampus at the desired point, and working laterally to the lateral cortical pia. A complete hippocampal resection enables you to see the contents of the ambient and crural cisterns as well as the cerebral peduncle, colliculi, and the pulvinar of the thalamus. You should also encounter choroid plexus and be able to see, if not encounter, the anterior choroidal artery in the crural cistern.

An alternative method for removing the hippocampal body is to dissect subpially along the hippocampal sulcus. This structure was initially identified during the resection of the hippocampal head. A bipolar or ultrasonic aspirator can be used to detach the body from the pia. This is almost en bloc, and it also spares the risk of opening the choroidal fissure and exposing ambient and crural cisternal structures. A similar method is to open the hippocampal sulcus through the fimbria, then cauterize hippocampal perforators and continue subpially along the subiculum and parahippocampus (**Figs. 4.6 and 4.7**).

Closure

Obtain hemostasis. Gelfoam powder, bipolar cautery, and Surgicel pieces are useful. Ascertain that the anesthesiologist was not using nitrous oxide, or has turned it off. Close the dura. Because the ventricle is open, a watertight closure is desirable. Backfill the resection cavity with irrigation before placing the final stitch. Pneumocephalus will often cause a severe headache. Replace the bone, close the temporalis fascia, and then close the galea aponeurotica and skin. The patient typically remains on the preoperative seizure medication regimen.

Conclusion

This chapter describes the technique for the classical temporal lobectomy and amygdalohippocampectomy. This is a workhorse procedure for all neurosurgeons. Its anatomy is relatively complex, but constant. Temporal lobectomy and amygdalohippocampectomy is an effective technique for refractory mesial temporal lobe epilepsy. Furthermore, the region is frequently entered in tumor surgery and traversed in vascular and skull base surgery.

Pearls

- Pin carefully and make sure you have enough space for the incision.
- Check the location of the navigation reference frame before registering.
- Use sharp dissection to isolate the superficial temporal artery.
- When making a bone flap, err on the larger side.
- Do as much as you can to expose the anterior part of the middle fossa.
- Carefully dissect any bridging dural veins.
- Identify the temporal horn during the lateral lobectomy.
- Make a watertight closure.
- Replace the rongeured bone. The large concavity may be cosmetically apparent.
- Close the wound well. Patients complain about combing across it if it is lumpy.

Pitfalls

- Removing too much hair
- Reflecting the temporalis without a fascial cuff
- Levering the bone into the brain when cracking the sphenoid
- Trying to do the lobectomy without adequate anterior exposure
- Resecting medial to the collateral sulcus during the lateral lobectomy
- Opening more of the lateral ventricular wall than necessary—optic radiations
- Resecting the roof of the temporal horn—Meyer's Loop
- Violating the uncal pia or resecting the uncus too superiorly—the rostral aspect of the amygdala merges with the globus pallidus.
- Opening the crural or ambient cistern arachnoid—it is not necessary.
- Forgetting to backfill the resection cavity with irrigation

---

References

1. Choi C, Rubino P, Fernandez-Miranda JC, et al. Meyer's Loop and the optic radiation in the transsylvian approach to the mediobasal temporal lobe. Neurosurgery 2006;59:228–236
2. Campero A, Trocolli G, Martins C, Fernandez-Miranda JC, Yasuda A, Rhoton AL Jr. Microsurgical approaches to the medial temporal region: an anatomical study. Neurosurgery 2006;59:279–308
3. Wyler A, Hermann BP, Somes G. Extent of medial temporal resection on outcome from anterior temporal lobectomy: a randomized prospective study. Neurosurgery 1995;37:982–991
4. Wen HT, Rhoton AL, de Oliveira E, et al. Microsurgical anatomy of the temporal lobe, Part 1: mesial temporal lobe anatomy and its vascular relationships as applied to amygdalohippocampectomy. Neurosurgery 1999;45(3):549–591
5. Duvernoy HM. *The Human Hippocampus: An Atlas of Applied Anatomy.* Munchen: JF Bergmann Verlag; 1988
6. Wyler A. Technique of temporal lobectomy. In: Rengachary SS, Wilkins RH, eds. *Neurosurgical Operative Atlas*, Vol 4. Rolling Meadows: AANS; 1995:131–138

5 Selective Amygdalohippocampectomy

Warren W. Boling

It is useful to categorize temporal lobe epilepsy into one of two types based on the anatomical site of seizure onset: neocortical (lateral temporal) or mesial temporal lobe epilepsy (MTLE). Although they share many features that may make diagnosis difficult in a single patient,[1,2] there are sufficient distinguishing characteristics for MTLE with hippocampal sclerosis to be considered a distinct syndromic entity.[3] In general, MTLE more commonly displays the typical temporal lobe seizure elements of an aura, staring, automatisms, and posturing.[4] MTLE is more related to childhood febrile convulsions, especially prolonged and complicated febrile convulsions.[5] The imaging hallmark of MTLE is mesiotemporal sclerosis (MTS).[6] Neocortical epilepsy may manifest signs related to perisylvian structures such as a simple auditory hallucination or, in the dominant hemisphere, postictal aphasia.[7,8]

Although localization of the temporal lobe seizure focus based on a noninvasive evaluation is often complex and may be unreliable,[9–11] when history, seizure semiology, electroencephalogram (EEG), and imaging findings point to MTLE, there can be a high degree of diagnostic certainty.[10,12] Intracranial electrode monitoring may be required in a subset of patients to confirm the site of seizure onset. Our approach at West Virginia University is to reserve invasive studies for patients in whom the diagnosis of temporal lobe epilepsy or lateralization of the seizure focus is in doubt.

In the 1950s, Paolo Niemeyer introduced the concept of selective amygdalohippocampectomy (SAH) **(Fig. 5.1)**.[13] His description of a small corridor through T2 to the temporal horn for the selective disconnection of the mesial temporal structures represented a dramatic shift from the temporal lobectomy popular at the time. In fact, as a result of research performed by Scoville and Milner[14] and Penfield and Milner[15] that stressed the important role of the hippocampus in memory, the trend at the time was to preserve the hippocampus. In the first published report of surgery for temporal lobe epilepsy, Penfield and Flanigin largely preserved the mesial temporal structures in the patients on which they operated.[16] Despite concerns of disrupting memory function, even in the early history of surgery for temporal lobe epilepsy, experimental evidence was mounting for the paramount role of the mesial structures in seizure genesis.[17–21] Much of this work was presented at the International Colloquium on Temporal Lobe in Marseille in 1954.[22] Penfield and Jasper showed that further removal of the hippocampus could convert a failed surgery into a success.[23] Removal of mesial temporal structures with the temporal lobectomy was shown to be successful with long-term follow-up by Morris in 1956.[24] Feindel and colleagues demonstrated the role of the amygdala in seizure generation and temporal lobe automatisms.[25,26]

More recently, considerable interest was raised for SAH after Yasargil et al developed an approach using the transsylvian route.[27] In Yasargil's technique, the arachnoid over the sylvian fissure is divided and the bottom of the circular sulcus exposed. An incision between two opercular temporal arteries exposes the ventricular horn allowing the hippocampal formation to be resected by an extrapial approach and the amygdala removed by subpial aspiration. More recently, Hori et al have described a subtemporal approach through the paraphippocampal gyrus.[28] Over many years now, a transcortical approach through the second temporal gyrus, similar to that demonstrated by Niemeyer, has been used at the Montreal Neurological Institute and now at West Virginia University.[29]

The SAH approach is based on the concepts first developed from Hughlings Jackson's description of a lesion in the uncus causing psychomotor seizures (Jackson called this a "dreamy state") and the role played by the mesial temporal structures in human epilepsy.[30] Subsequently, an abundance of experimental studies have pointed to a very important role of the mesial temporal structures in experimental and human epilepsies.[17,18,20,23,24,31,32] Results from many patients operated for MTLE with SAH confirms the overwhelming participation of the mesial temporal and limbic structures in temporal lobe epilepsy.[33–35] Furthermore, recently the International League Against Epilepsy determined that MTLE represents a sufficient cluster of signs and symptoms to comprise a specific epilepsy syndrome.[36]

The goal of SAH is to achieve the best possible results on the seizure tendency in the most selective manner, and to spare from resection those cerebral structures not involved in the seizure focus. At centers with experience in SAH, the results on seizure tendency clearly rival the results of corticoamygdalohippocampectomy (CAH) (see below).[27–29,32,35] Although the neuropsychological advantages of SAH have yet to be entirely proven,[37–39] the intuitive advantages are inescapable. Sparing brain tissue not involved with the seizure focus should be an important goal of epilepsy surgery.

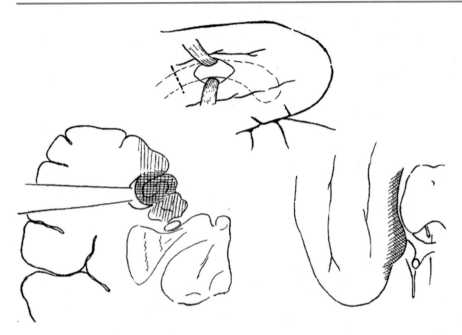

Fig. 5.1 Niemeyer's original description (1957) of the SAH.[13] A trans-T2, transventricular approach for selective removal of the mesial temporal structures. It is essentially the identical approach used today.

Surgical Anatomy of the Temporal Lobe with Emphasis on the Mesial Structures

Nineteenth-century neuroanatomists developed a numbering system for the gyri and sulci of the brain that today is still the preferred method of nomenclature.[40,41] It is a simple but useful system that emphasizes the concept of gyral ribbons interconnecting the convolutions of the brain.[41–43] There are five gyri running the length of the temporal lobe. The superior temporal gyrus is T1, middle temporal gyrus T2, inferior temporal gyrus T3, fusiform gyrus T4, parahippocampal gyrus T5, and the most medially located gyrus in the temporal lobe is the hippocampal complex (composed of the hippocampus proper and dentate gyrus) (**Fig. 5.2A**). Similarly, the temporal gyri are separated by four longitudinal sulci, which are: S1, S2, S3, and S4. The superior temporal gyrus (T1) is bounded above by the sylvian fissure. Below T1 the superior temporal sulcus (S1) is the deepest sulcus in the temporal lobe extending toward the temporal horn, and it is an important anatomical guide to localizing the ventricle. T4 is well demarcated from the parahippocampus (T5) by the constant and strong collateral fissure (S4) that produces an obvious bulge into the ventricle of the temporal horn called the collateral eminence (**Figs. 5.2B, 5.3, 5.4**).

The fifth temporal gyrus is better known as the parahippocampal gyrus because of its close relation to the hippocampus proper (**Fig. 5.2B**). The parahippocampus lies adjacent and inferolateral to the hippocampus. The parahippocampus is clearly delineated laterally by the collateral fissure (S4) and mesially by the hippocampal sulcus. Its anterior extent does not reach the temporal pole but ends ~2 cm behind it. Peter Gloor defines the entorhinal cortex in man to be the

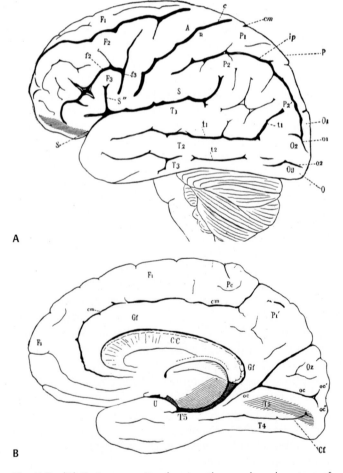

Fig. 5.2 **(A)** Brain convexity showing the numbered system of nomenclature. T1, T2, and T3 are visible on the lateral surface. **(B)** On the medial brain surface, T4, T5 (parahippocampus), and uncus (U) are plainly visible.

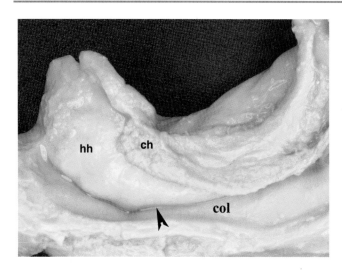

Fig. 5.3 Dissection of the left temporal lobe. The view is into the opened temporal horn. The arrowhead points to the lateral ventricular sulcus that is the entry into the parahippocampus. ch, choroid plexus; col, collateral emminance; hh, hippocampus head.

region of parahippocampus anterior to the most posterior limit of the uncus.[44] Posteriorly, the parahippocampal gyrus is divided into two branches by the anterior calcarine sulcus. The superior branch merges into the isthmus of the cingulate gyrus, and the inferior one becomes the lingual gyrus of the occipital lobe.

The uncus has a conical shape (**Fig. 5.5**). Its medial convex surface can be further subdivided into several small gyri including the semilunar gyrus superiorly, ambient gyrus, uncinate gyrus, band of Giacomini, and intralimbic gyrus that form its posterior apex. In fact, the rostral end of the hippocampus and dentate bends medialward to form most of the uncus. The anterosuperior uncus (semilunar gyrus) is occupied by the amygdala.

The hippocampus proper envelops the hippocampal sulcus (**Fig. 5.4**). Its two pial walls closely adhere to each other and contain the vascular supply of the hippocampus. The superomesial wall of the sulcus is formed by the dentate gyrus, whereas the subiculum and hippocampus proper form the inferolateral wall (**Fig. 5.4**). With the ventricle opened, the hippocampus appears as a distinct bulge on its inner surface covered by a white matter tract, the alveus, and a glistening ependymal layer (**Fig. 5.3**). The hippocampus lies just lateral to the cerebral peduncle. Its anterior portion, or head, is short and occupies the rostral extent of the temporal horn and curves mesially to form the bulk of the uncus. Its middle part (body) extends posteriorly into a narrower part called the "tail" that curves backward and upward to the trigone of the ventricle.

The fimbria is a white matter band that runs horizontally along the medial border of the hippocampus, just above the dentate gyrus, separated by the fimbriodentate sulcus. Its free aspect forms the inferolateral edge of the choroidal fissure. It ends anteriorly at the posterior gyrus of the uncus, the intralimbic gyrus (**Fig. 5.4**). Posteriorly, under the splenium, the fimbria becomes the fornix.

The choroid plexus partially covers the hippocampus as they both bulge into the temporal horn and is an important

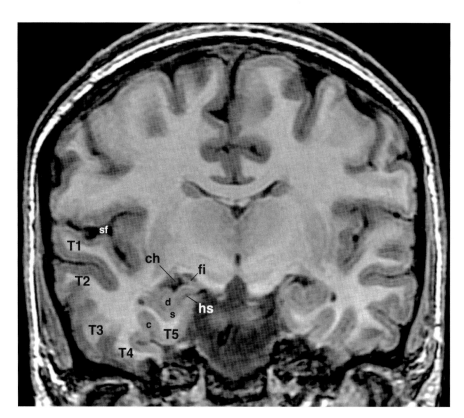

Fig. 5.4 Coronal T1 image at the level of the hippocampal body. T1 to T5 label the temporal gyri. c, collateral sulcus; ch, choroids plexus; d, dentate gyrus; fi, fimbria; hs, hippocampal sulcus; s, subiculum; sf, sylvian fissure.

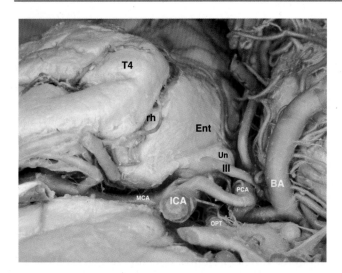

Fig. 5.5 Dissection of the left medial temporal lobe, ambient cistern, and related structures. BA, basilar artery; Ent, entorhinal cortex (anterior extension of parahippocampus); ICA, internal carotid artery; III, cranial nerve III; MCA, middle cerebral artery (M1 branch); OPT, optic tract; PCA, posterior cerebral artery; rh, rhinal sulcus; T4, fusiform gyrus; Un, uncus.

surgical landmark for orientation while working in the ventricle (**Fig. 5.3**). The choroid plexus arises from the tela choroidea, an ependymal and pial layer that fill the choroidal fissure. The tela choroidea spans the space between the fimbria and the stria terminalis, attached to the two white matter bundles (**Fig. 5.4**). The anterior choroidal artery enters the temporal horn at the inferior choroidal point to form the choroid plexus. Therefore, the choroid plexus can be reflected posteriorly to see the intralimbic gyrus. Tilting the choroid plexus laterally exposes the stria terminalis, and mesial retraction uncovers the fimbria and hippocampus.

The mesial temporal structures are defined as including the uncus, amygdala, hippocampal complex, fimbria, parahippocampus, and entorhinal cortex. The collateral sulcus and choroid plexus are important landmarks that define the mesial temporal area. The anatomical region of the mesial temporal area lies between the choroid plexus and collateral sulcus, also including the more anterior structures of the amygdala and uncus. Therefore, the lateral temporal region (often called iso- or neocortex to contrast with the archicortex named for the phylogenetically more primitive three-cortical-layered hippocampus) comprises the temporal lobe lateral to the collateral fissure. The parahippocampus (and especially the subiculum) is the transition between the six-layered neocortex and three-layered archicortex of the hippocampus.

Surgery for Temporal Lobe Epilepsy

Temporal Lobectomy

Temporal lobectomy consists of a removal of the entire temporal lobe including the mesial structures. This complete removal of the temporal lobe is rare today. Therefore,

to identify the typical anterior, lateral, and mesial structure resection, it is preferable to use the terms *anterior temporal resection* or *corticoamygdalohippocampectomy* to more accurately describe the extent of structures that have been removed.

Corticoamygdalohippocampectomy (CAH)

This is the standard temporal resection performed at most epilepsy centers. It essentially corresponds to an anterior temporal neocortical resection followed by a removal of the temporal mesial structures. Variations on this approach have been described including anatomically standardized resections[45,46] as well as a tailored type of operation.[47] Our approach to CAH is strictly image guided to localize anatomical landmarks that define the resection margins. Essentially, in the dominant hemisphere along T1 the resection extends no further posterior than the precentral sulcus (corresponding to ~3.5 to 4 cm), and in the nondominant hemisphere the posterior extent of the T1 removal is the central sulcus (corresponding to ~4 to 4.5 cm). The lateral cortex is removed en bloc as a specimen. The temporal horn is opened, and the mesial structures are disconnected exactly as is described below for the SAH.

Corticoamygdalectomy (CA)

As the name implies, CA consists of an anterior temporal cortical resection combined with an amygdalectomy, emptying of the uncus, and sparing of the hippocampal formation. The neocortical resection is limited as described for CAH. In the CA, the cortical resection is carried up to the collateral sulcus. The anterior temporal horn is opened for the purpose of identifying landmarks. The hippocampus and the adjacent parahippocampal gyrus are left undisturbed. The amygdala is resected as completely as possible, and the uncus is emptied in a subpial fashion. However, it is unavoidable to encroach on the anterior most part of the hippocampus that reflects back upon itself within the uncus. This surgical approach is used mainly in patients who have failed the ipsilateral sodium amytal test for memory and/or are at risk for a significant functional memory decline from a disconnection of the mesial temporal structures. CA has been shown to be useful for controlling the seizure tendency when the hippocampus retains significant memory function and cannot be included in the resection.[48,49]

Selective Amygdalohippocampectomy (SAH)

The SAH was introduced by Niemeyer to treat temporal lobe epilepsy arising from the mesial temporal structures (**Fig. 5.1**).[13] Subsequently, the overwhelming importance of MTLE in medically intractable temporal lobe epilepsy has been established. Building on the work of earlier investigators, modern reports of SAH have confirmed its utility for the treatment of mesial temporal structures.[29,32–34] To date, SAH has become the standard approach to treat pharmacoresistant MTLE at many epilepsy centers, including ours.

Surgical Technique of SAH

The scalp and bone exposure for SAH can range from a frontotemporal craniotomy to a keyhole approach. A larger craniotomy is required for electrocorticography (ECoG), and a keyhole approach is preferred if ECoG is not performed. All aspects of the SAH are enhanced with the use of image guidance, and in keyhole surgery image guidance is required.

The patient's head is immobilized in the three-pronged headholder. Anesthesia is general endotracheal. A roll is placed under the ipsilateral shoulder with the head turned toward the opposite shoulder. The vertex being lowered inferiorly allows the surgeon better access to the mesial structures, and when turned ~30 degrees from horizontal improves visualization of the structures more posterior in the ventricle.

The traditional frontotemporal craniotomy is exposed via a curvilinear question-mark–shaped scalp incision that starts at the zygoma, extends posterior just to the back of the ear, up to the superior temporal line, and anterior to the hair line. The scalp is reflected anterior with the temporalis muscle and retracted with hooks. The root of the zygoma must be visualized to confirm an adequate exposure to the floor of the middle fossa. A frontotemporal bone flap is elevated plus a craniectomy of the temporal bone is performed with a rongeur to the zygoma inferiorly and anterior to the apex of the middle fossa, if possible. An adequate bone opening is essential to allow a sufficient exposure of the temporal lobe and to fit the 16-channel ECoG, if required. The dura is reflected away from the temporal lobe. Once the brain is exposed, important sulcal and gyral landmarks are identified, namely the sylvian fissure, T1, T2, and the central sulcus.

A corticectomy measuring 2 to 3 cm is made along the upper border of the second temporal gyrus (T2) and just below the superior temporal sulcus (S1) (**Fig. 5.6**). The posterior extent of the corticectomy is the central sulcus on the nondominant side and the precentral sulcus in the dominant hemisphere. Image guidance is required to localize these sulcal landmarks that correspond to ~3.5 cm in the dominant hemisphere and 4.5 cm in the nondominant hemisphere from the temporal tip. If necessary, a small gyrectomy of T2 can be performed to facilitate maneuvers within the ventricle. Using an ultrasonic dissector at very low settings of suction and vibration, a corridor of ~3 to 4 cm in height is fashioned down to the ependymal lining that is opened (**Fig. 5.6**). The corridor is fashioned along and directed by the inferior wall of S1 that points to the temporal horn. A retractor is then inserted to provide an unobstructed view of the temporal horn and of the mesial temporal structures (**Fig. 5.7**). The ventricle is open completely from its anterior tip to the posterior limit of the corridor exposure.

Three ependymal-lined structures are now seen bulging into the ventricle. On the lateral surface is the collateral eminence and below is the hippocampus. Between them is the lateral ventricular sulcus (**Fig. 5.3**). Anterior to the choroid plexus and arising from the medial wall of the ventricle is the amygdala. The choroid plexus is an important intraventricular landmark that should be identified early. Often the hippocampus must be retracted laterally to see the choroid plexus, which is followed to its anterior origin in the choroidal fissure (inferior choroidal point) that marks the posterior limit of the uncus.

The entire mesial resection is endopial/subpial using the ultrasonic aspirator at its lowest settings of suction and vibration (using the CUSA (Integra Life Sciences, Plainsboro, NJ), suction and vibration are set at 10).The resection proper is begun by entering the lateral ventricular sulcus at the junction of the hippocampus with the collateral eminence (**Fig. 5.3**). This is the entry into the parahippocampal gyrus that is emptied subpially between the hippocampal sulcus and the collateral sulcus. This maneuver separates the hippocampus from its lateral connection and allows the hippocampus to be retracted laterally to facilitate subpial aspiration of the fimbria and disconnection mesially. The hippocampus is separated from the hippocampal tail posteriorly. Lifting the hippocampus off and separating it from its vascular pedicle, the hippocampal sulcus, completes the en bloc removal. The hippocampal vessels typically can be teased and separated from the hippocampus without coagulation and division. Additional hippocampus can be removed piecemeal posteriorly. The habitual posterior limit of the hippocampal formation resection corresponds to the midbrain tectum. These landmarks and the extent of hippocampal resection are readily identified with image guidance.

The anterior extent of the resection corresponds to the level of the rhinal sulcus that includes the entire uncus (**Fig. 5.5**). The uncus, normally herniated over the edge of the tentorium, should be completely emptied subpial. The third cranial nerve and posterior cerebral artery (P1) are expected to be seen in the cistern beneath the partially transparent uncal pia. The amygdala is removed piecemeal. Essentially, the structures found between the choroid plexus and collateral sulcus are removed entirely, taking care to keep the pial surface intact (**Figs. 5.6 and 5.7**). The posterior limit is the level of the midbrain tectum identified with image guidance (**Fig. 5.8**). Anterior to the choroid plexus the uncus is emptied completely. The mesial boundary of the amygdala resection is not precise. Essentially, medial to the level of the choroid plexus, the resection is only subpial aspiration of cortex.

Many of the pitfalls in SAH can be avoided by using image guidance, and image guidance provides useful corroboration for landmark identification. The extent of anterior temporal craniectomy and temporal lobe exposure is easily confirmed with image guidance. In the asleep patient, image guidance is required to identify the central and precentral sulci that mark the posterior limit of the T2 corticectomy. On occasion, the dominant draining vein is more related to S1 and does not take the expected course along the sylvian fissure, which must be recognized. Fashioning the corridor to the temporal horn is benefited by image guidance to help define and

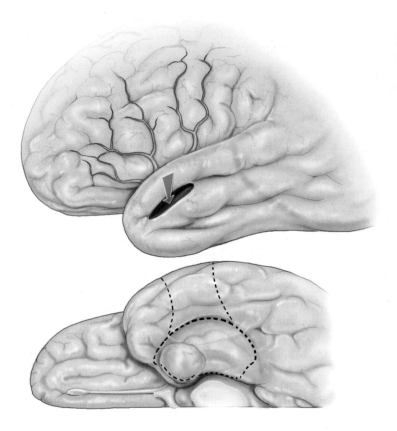

Fig. 5.6 SAH approach. Corticectomy through the upper portion of T2 and a corridor carried down to the ventricle that is opened. The mesial temporal structures are removed in a subpial fashion. The arrow points to the corticectomy. The dotted line outlines the corridor to the ventrical and structures included in the mesial temporal resection.

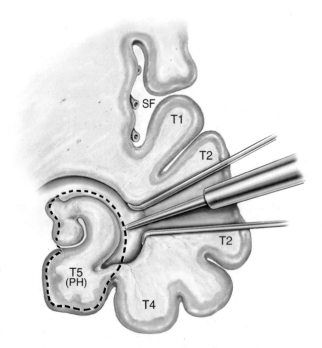

Fig. 5.7 Coronal view of the SAH approach. The retractors are within the T2 corticectomy and the ventricle is open. Dotted line outlines the mesial temporal structures that are removed in a subpial fashion. PH, parahippocampus; SF, sylvian fissure.

improve the trajectory to the target. Image guidance enhances the performance of SAH by confirming landmarks, aiding the fashioning of the corridor to the ventricle, and documenting the posterior limit of the hippocampal resection. Image guidance is utilized by the author in essentially all surgeries for epilepsy.

The resection of the mesial temporal structures is a strictly subpial dissection. The midbrain and contents of the ambient cistern lie adjacent to the mesial temporal lobe (**Fig. 5.5**). The posterior cerebral artery (P2) typically bulges into the parahippocampal pia, and the third cranial nerve is often adherent to the pia lining the uncus. The internal carotid artery and its bifurcation are closely related to the anteromedial uncus and amygdala (**Fig. 5.5**). The subpial technique provides additional safety while working around these critical structures. Our experience has been that using the ultrasonic aspirator at the lowest settings of suction and vibration enhances the subpial dissection technique.

Keyhole Approach in SAH

The rational of the SAH is to spare cerebral tissue not included in the seizure generator. The logical progression from a selective resection of the seizure focus is to minimize the scalp and bony opening to accomplish the SAH. In individuals with

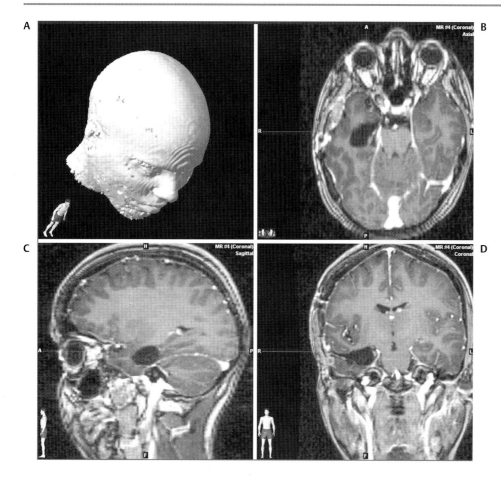

Fig. 5.8 T1-weighted axial, coronal, and sagittal MRI postoperative after right SAH. (**A**) 3D MRI reconstruction of the head. (**B–D**) T1 MRI showing completed right SAH in the axial, sagittal, and coronal planes, respectively.

clear-cut MTLE who are candidates for SAH, the keyhole approach can be considered. The caveats are that it is a strictly image-guided approach and ECoG cannot be performed adequately within the restricted keyhole exposure. Therefore, the surgeon must have sufficient confidence of MTLE prior to performing keyhole SAH. The evidence comes from congruent findings on the imaging, EEG, and semiology in the epilepsy investigation and/or from intracranial electrodes recording seizure onset in the mesial temporal structures.

SAH for temporal lobe epilepsy is performed when the data (neuroimaging, EEG, semiology) point to the mesial temporal structures as the seizure focus. The keyhole exposure lends itself especially well to an SAH approach. Although, ECoG cannot be accomplished with the keyhole approach due to the small cortical working space.[50,51] In the author's experience, most patients who have had the keyhole craniotomy approach did have intracranial electrode monitoring, although it has been used without intracranial electrodes in patients with the typical stigmata of MTLE (EEG, magnetic resonance imaging (MRI), and semiology congruent with MTLE).[48]

The keyhole approach is a strictly image-guided approach. The scalp incision is curvilinear starting at the zygoma (**Fig. 5.9**). The temporalis muscle is split and held open with

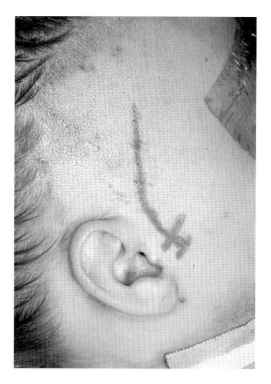

Fig. 5.9 Scalp incision for a keyhole approach to SAH.

hooks. The scalp opening is large enough to accommodate a bur hole and bone opening measuring ~3 cm in diameter, centered at the second temporal gyrus, and over the planned cortical incision. The SAH procedure is essentially identical to the nonkeyhole approach to SAH as described above. Image guidance confirms the corticectomy is positioned on the upper bank of T2 as well as anterior to the central sulcus in the nondominant hemisphere and anterior to the precentral sulcus on the dominant side (**Fig. 5.10**). The three-dimentional image-guided cortical reconstruction is especially useful for anatomical verification.

Electrocorticography for Temporal Lobe Epilepsy Surgery

The technique and role of ECoG in surgery for epilepsy is beyond the scope of this chapter. However, suffice it to say that ECoG is used routinely to guide the resection approach, but its utility in temporal lobe epilepsy surgery is somewhat controversial. At our center, the philosophy is that individuals who have not had chronic intracranial electrode recording from the mesial temporal structures will routinely undergo preresection ECoG. Sixteen channels of electrodes are positioned over the surface and two acute depth electrodes are inserted trans-T2 to the amygdala and hippocampus, directed with image guidance, and along the line of the SAH corticectomy.[50,52]

The ECoG recording is interictal and usually lasts at least 20 minutes. Inhalational anesthetic is stopped during the recording. Low-dose methohexital may be given to accentuate spiking activity in oligospikers. Enough spiking activity needs to be observed to localize the preponderance of epileptic potential, mesial versus lateral. A patient with temporal lobe epilepsy, the stigmata of MTLE, and strikingly more spiking activity in the mesial temporal structures on ECOG is a good candidate for SAH.

Results of SAH on Seizure Tendency

Underscoring the paramount role of the mesial temporal limbic structures in MTLE, excellent results reducing the seizure tendency have been found using diverse approaches to SAH, that is, the transsylvian,[53] subtemporal,[28] and trans-T2[29] described in this chapter.

In patients with temporal lobe epilepsy who underwent operation at West Virginia University in 2002 to 2004 with more than1 year postoperative follow-up,[48] 26 surgeries

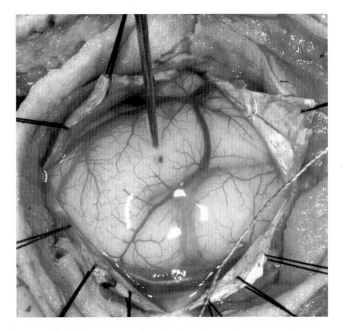

Fig. 5.10   Keyhole exposure of T2. This is a strictly image-guided approach that is required to confirm anatomical landmarks. After the cortex is exposed, the SAH is performed identically to the nonkeyhole approach.

(54%) were performed for SAH. CAH was performed in 15 individuals (31%). CA was performed in five (10%), one operation was lesionectomy only, and one was SAH later converted to CAH. Seizure freedom outcomes were similar in SAH and CAH groups (74% and 73%, respectively). Complications were one scalp infection that required removal of the bone flap and a cranial prosthesis placed later. One subject has had chronic atypical face and scalp pain since surgery. There were no neurological deficits or mortality from surgery.

Conclusion

SAH has become the standard approach in surgery for MTLE at many centers, including ours. The benefit to the patient is a selective disconnection and removal of the seizure focus with sparing of the cortical structures not primarily involved in epileptogenesis. In individuals with MTLE the results on seizure tendency have been excellent. The technique used is essentially the approach originally described by Niemeyer, which is a trans-T2 corridor to the temporal horn and then a subpial removal and emptying of the mesial temporal structures.

References

1. O'Brien TJ, Kilpatrick C, Murrie V, Vogrin S, Morris K, Cook MJ. Temporal lobe epilepsy caused by mesial temporal sclerosis and temporal neocortical lesions. A clinical and electroencephalographic study of 46 pathologically proven cases. Brain 1996;119(Pt 6):2133–2141

2. Burgerman RS, Sperling MR, French JA, Saykin AJ, O'Connor MJ. Comparison of mesial versus neocortical onset temporal lobe seizures: neurodiagnostic findings and surgical outcome. Epilepsia 1995;36: 662–670

3. Wieser HG. ILAE Commission Report. Mesial temporal lobe epilepsy with hippocampal sclerosis. Epilepsia 2004;45:695–714

4. Olivier A, Gloor P, Andermann F, Quesney LF. The place of stereotactic depth electrode recording in epilepsy. Appl Neurophysiol 1985; 48:395–399

5. Cendes F. Febrile seizures and mesial temporal sclerosis. Curr Opin Neurol 2004;17:161–164

6. Berkovic SF, Andermann F, Olivier A, et al. Hippocampal sclerosis in temporal lobe epilepsy demonstrated by magnetic resonance imaging. Ann Neurol 1991;29:175–182

7. Schramm J, Kral T, Grunwald T, Blumcke I. Surgical treatment for neocortical temporal lobe epilepsy: clinical and surgical aspects and seizure outcome. J Neurosurg 2001;94:33–42

8. Pacia SV, Devinsky O, Perrine K, et al. Clinical features of neocortical temporal lobe epilepsy. Ann Neurol 1996;40:724–730

9. Maillard L, Vignal JP, Gavaret M, et al. Semiologic and electrophysiologic correlations in temporal lobe seizure subtypes. Epilepsia 2004;45:1590–1599

10. Pfander M, Arnold S, Henkel A, et al. Clinical features and EEG findings differentiating mesial from neocortical temporal lobe epilepsy. Epileptic Disord 2002;4:189–195

11. Adam C, Clemenceau S, Semah F, et al. Variability of presentation in medial temporal lobe epilepsy: a study of 30 operated cases. Acta Neurol Scand 1996;94:1–11

12. Foldvary N, Lee N, Thwaites G, et al. Clinical and electrographic manifestations of lesional neocortical temporal lobe epilepsy. Neurology 1997;49:757–763

13. Niemeyer P. The transventricular amygdalo-hippocampectomy in temporal lobe epilepsy. In: Baldwin M, Bailey P, eds. *Temporal Lobe Epilepsy*. Springfield, IL: CC Thomas; 1958:461–482

14. Scoville WB, Milner B. Loss of recent memory after bilateral hippocampal lesions. J Neurol Neurosurg Psychiatry 1957;20:11–21

15. Penfield W, Milner B. Memory deficit produced by bilateral lesions in the hippocampal zone. Arch Neurol Psychiatry 1958;79:475–497

16. Penfield W, Flanigin H. Surgical therapy of temporal lobe seizures. Arch Neurol Psychiatry 1950;64:491–500

17. Kaada BR. Somatomotor, autonomic and electrographic responses to electrical stimulation of "rhinencephalic" and other structures in primates, cat and dog: a study of responses from limbic, subcallosal, orbito-insular, pyriform and temporal cortex, hippocampus, fornix and amygdala. Acta Physiol Scand Suppl 1951;83:1–285

18. Vigouroux R, Gastaut HR, Badier M. Provocation des principales manifestations cliniques de l'épilepsie dite temporale par stimulation des structures rhinencéphaliques chez le chat non-anaesthésié. Rev Neurol 1951;85:505–508

19. Gastaut H. So-called "psychomotor" and "temporal" epilepsy. Epilepsia 1953;2:59–76

20. Green JD, Shimamoto T. Hippocampal seizures and their propagation. Arch Neurol Psychiatry 1953;7:687–702

21. Sano K, Malamud N. Clinical significance of sclerosis of the cornu ammonis. Arch Neurol Psychiatry 1953;70:40–53

22. Morin G, Gastaut H, Colloquium concerning normal and pathological anatomical problems raised by epileptic discharges. Neurobiological Laboratory, Faculty of Medicine, Marseilles, France Nov. 15–18, 1954 (Reproduced by U.S. Department of Health, Education, and Welfare, Public Health Service, Washington, DC)

23. Penfield W, Jasper H. *Epilepsy and the Functional Anatomy of the Human Brain.* Boston: Little Brown; 1954:418, 468, 815, 816

24. Morris AA. Temporal lobectomy with removal of uncus, hippocampus and amygdala. Arch Neurol Psychiatry 1956;76:479–496

25. Feindel W, Penfield W. Localization of discharge in temporal lobe automatism. Arch Neurol Psychiatry 1954;72:605–630

26. Feindel W, Penfield W, Jasper H. Localization of epileptic discharge in temporal lobe automatism. Trans Am Neurol Assoc 1952;56:14–17

27. Yasargil MG, Teddy PJ, Roth P. Selective amygdalo-hippocampectomy: operative anatomy and surgical technique. In: Symon L, Brihaye J, Guidette B, eds. *Advances and Technical Standards in Neurosurgery,* Vol. 12. New York: Springler-Wien; 1985

28. Hori T, Tabuchi S, Kurosaki M, Kondo S, Takenobu A, Watanabe T. Subtemporal amygdalohippocampectomy for treating medially intractable temporal lobe epilepsy. Neurosurgery 1993;33(1): 50–56

29. Olivier A. Transcortical selective amygdalohippocampectomy in temporal lobe epilepsy. Can J Neurol Sci 2000;27(Suppl 1):S68–S76

30. Jackson JH, Colman WS. Case of epilepsy with tasting movements and "dreamy state" with very small patch of softening in the left uncinate gyrus. Brain 1898;21:580–590

31. Gastaut H, Vigouroux R, Naquet R. Lésions épileptogènes amygdalohippocampiques provoquées chez le chat par l'injection de crème d'albumine . Rev Neurol 1952;87:607–609

32. Wieser HG, Ortega M, Friedman A, Yonekawa Y. Long-term seizure outcomes following amygdalohippocampectomy. J Neurosurg 2003; 98:751–763

33. Olivier A. Relevance of removal of limbic structures in surgery for temporal lobe epilepsy. Can J Neurol Sci 1991;18(Suppl 4):628–635

34. Abosch A, Bernasconi N, Boling W, et al. Factors predictive of suboptimal seizure control following selective amygdalohippocampectomy. J Neurosurg 2002;97:1142–1151

35. Lutz MT, Clusmann H, Elger CE, Schramm J, Helmstaedter C. Neuropsychological outcome after selective amygdalohippocampectomy with transsylvian versus transcortical approach: a randomized prospective clinical trial of surgery for temporal lobe epilepsy. Epilepsia 2004;45:809–816

36. Wieser HG. ILAE Commission Report. Mesial temporal lobe epilepsy with hippocampal sclerosis. Epilepsia 2004;45:695–714

37. Jones-Gotman M, Zatorre RJ, Olivier A, et al. Learning and retention of words and designs following excision from medial or lateral temporal-lobe structures. Neuropsychologia 1997;35:963–973

38. Kessels RP, Hendriks M, Schouten J, Van Asselen M, Postma A. Spatial memory deficits in patients after unilateral selective amygdalohippocampectomy. J Int Neuropsychol Soc 2004;10:907–912

39. Gleissner U, Helmstaedter C, Schramm J, Elger CE. Memory outcome after selective amygdalohippocampectomy in patients with temporal lobe epilepsy: one-year follow-up. Epilepsia 2004;45:960–962

40. Broca P. *Mémoires sur le cerveau de l'homme et des primates.* Paris: C Reinwald; 1888

41. Ecker A. *Die Hirnwindungen des Menschen.* Braunschweig: Vieweg; 1883

42. Foville AL. *Traité complet de l'anatomie, de la physiologie et de la pathologie du système nerveux.* Paris: Fortin; 1884

43. Yasargil MG. *Microneurosurgery IVA CNS Tumors.* New York: Thieme Medical Publishers, Inc.; 1994

44. Gloor P. *The Temporal Lobe and Limbic System.* New York: Oxford University Press; 1997

45. Spencer DD, Spencer SS, Mattson RH, Williamson PD, Novelly RA. Access to the posterior medial temporal lobe structures in the surgical treatment of temporal lobe epilepsy. Neurosurgery 1984;15: 667–671

46. Olivier A. Temporal resections in the surgical treatment of epilepsy. Epilepsy Res Suppl 1992;5:175–188

47. Silbergeld DL, Ojemann GA. The tailored temporal lobectomy. Neurosurg Clin N Am 1993;4:273–281

48. Boling W, Longoni N, Palade A, Moran M, Brick J. Surgery for temporal lobe epilepsy. W V Med J 2006, Nov–Dec; 102(6):18–21

49. Kim HI, Olivier A, Jones-Gotman M, Primrose D, Andermann F. Corticoamygdalectomy in memory-impaired patients. Stereotact Funct Neurosurg 1992;58:162–167

50. Wennberg R, Quesney F, Olivier A, Dubeau F. Mesial temporal versus lateral temporal interictal epileptiform activity: comparison of chronic and acute intracranial recordings. Electroencephalogr Clin Neurophysiol 1997;102:486–494

51. Boling WW, Olivier A. Image Guided Keyhole Craniotomy for Selective Amygdalo-hippocampectomy. Epilepsia 2004;45(Suppl 7):333

52. Stefan H, Quesney LF, Abou-Khalil B, Olivier A. Electrocorticography in temporal lobe epilepsy surgery. Acta Neurol Scand 1991;83:65–72

53. Wieser HG. Selective amygdalo-hippocampectomy for temporal lobe epilepsy. Epilepsia 1988;29(Suppl 2):S100–S113

6 Cortical Resection in the Central Region

Ram Mani and G. Rees Cosgrove

The surgical treatment of epilepsy in the central region or rolandic cortex presents special challenges to neurosurgeons. Not only does the central region provide essential somatomotor and somatosensory control of the contralateral face and limbs, this region of the brain is highly epileptogenic. Lesions in this region often produce disabling and treatment refractory seizures, which can frequently result in episodes of focal status epilepticus. In this chapter, we will review the anatomy of the rolandic cortex, the seizure semiology, and the most appropriate presurgical evaluation as well as the various diagnostic and therapeutic surgical approaches in the management of intractable seizures of the central region.

Anatomical Considerations

The central or rolandic region is composed of the pre- and postcentral gyri. The precentral gyrus or motor strip is anatomically the most posterior portion of the frontal lobe, whereas the postcentral gyrus or sensory strip is the most anterior portion of the parietal lobe. The two central gyri are defined by the vertically oriented central sulcus, which runs from the region of the sylvian fissure superiorly and posteriorly toward the interhemispheric fissure. The central region is further defined by the pre- and postcentral sulci, which run roughly parallel to the central sulcus. The precentral sulcus is often discontinuous in its mid-portion (**Fig. 6.1**).

Whereas the pre- and postcentral gyri can be easily detected as the vertically oriented gyri in the central region of the brain on either an anatomical specimen or a three-dimensional (3-D) volumetric magnetic resonance imaging (MRI) rendering (**Fig. 6.1**), it is sometimes much more difficult to accurately define the central sulcus on standard sagittal, axial, or coronal MRI sections. Knowledge of sulcal anatomy and cerebral topography, however, can aid in the confident localization of the pre- and postcentral sulci even in the presence of local pathology. In the midsagittal plane, one can define the central sulcus by following the cingulate sulcus as it courses parallel to the corpus callosum to its marginal ramus that turns upward toward the vertex. The sulcus seen ~8 to 9 mm anterior to the end of the marginal ramus is the termination of the central sulcus (**Fig. 6.2A**). The marginal ramus of the cingulate sulcus defines the posterior border of the paracentral lobule, whereas the parasagittal portion of the precentral sulcus defines its anterior border. On an axial MRI scan near the vertex, one can also follow the superior frontal sulcus, which travels parallel to the interhemispheric fissure ~15 to 20 mm off the midline.

It typically terminates in a "T" intersection with the superior portion of the precentral sulcus. The two sulci running parallel and just posterior to the precentral sulcus are the central and postcentral sulci, respectively. The intraparietal sulcus is located on the lateral surface of the parietal lobe. It runs parallel to the interhemispheric fissure and often forms a T intersection anteriorly with the superior portion of the postcentral sulcus (**Fig. 6.2B**). In the axial MRI images near the vertex, it is also important to realize that the precentral gyrus or motor strip is actually wider and thicker than the postcentral gyrus. This is due to the fact that the gray matter in the precentral gyrus is on average 2.8 to 3.1 mm thick, whereas the gray matter cortical thickness in the sensory or postcentral gyrus is ~1.9 mm.[1] It is often possible to see an omega-shaped gyrus or knuckle, which represents the somatosensory localization of hand function.[2] One can also define the central region by its anatomical relationship to the sylvian fissure and the inferior frontal gyrus on a parasagittal MRI scan. In most cases, one is able to discern the horizontal and vertical rami in the inferior frontal gyrus dividing this gyrus into the pars opercularis, pars triangularis, and par orbitalis. The first sulcus immediately posterior to the pars opercularis and extending to the sylvian fissure is the precentral sulcus. The sulcus just posterior and running parallel to this but not reaching the sylvian fissure is the central sulcus (**Fig. 6.2C**).

The precentral gyrus or motor strip is composed of Brodmann's areas 4 and 6. Cytoarchitecturally, these areas are composed of a six-layer neocortex with giant pyramidal cells, an almost complete absence of granular cells, and numerous densely packed intracortical fibers, especially in the plexiform layer. The postcentral gyrus or sensory strip is composed of Brodmann's areas 3, 1, and 2. Cytoarchitecturally, this area contains granular cells and a modest number of pyramidal cells. It too has many intracortical connections along the postcentral gyrus and anteriorly into the precentral gyrus.[3] These connections are essential to normal sensorimotor function. The postcentral gyrus receives large numbers of afferents from the ventral posterior medial and lateral nuclei of the thalamus. The precentral gyrus gets most of its afferent information via the ventral lateral nucleus of the thalamus from the cerebellum. A supplementary sensory area (SM2) lies at the inferior portion of the postcentral gyrus along the insula and parietal operculum with extension on occasion into the precentral region.[4] There is some degree of somatotopy in this area, although it is much less distinct than in the primary somatosensory areas.

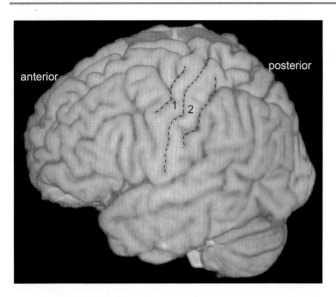

Fig. 6.1 Three-dimensional brain reconstruction. View of lateral surface. Precentral, central, and postcentral sulci are outlined with dashed line. 1, precentral gyrus; 2, indicates postcentral gyrus.

There are numerous thalamocortical and reciprocal connections in the central region. The primary efferent output of the central region is the corticospinal tract. This extends caudally from the central region, through the centrum semiovale, condensing as the pyramidal tract within the posterior limb of the internal capsule then distributing to their target motor nuclei either in the brainstem or spinal cord.

There is a distinct and important somatotopic arrangement to sensorimotor function in the central region. Penfield and Rasmussen classically described this somatotopic organization with the tongue and face represented in the inferior portion of the central region near the sylvian fissure.[5] The thumb, fingers, and hand are situated at the middle portion of the central region in the area of the omega gyrus with the upper extremity and trunk approaching the midline with parts of the lower extremity and foot in the paracentral lobule. The pharynx and oropharynx are typically localized along the operculum of the central region.

With functional MRI, we can now create accurate structural and functional models of individual patients' brains.[6] First, a 3-D volumetric acquisition and surface rendering is acquired, and then functional imaging data are obtained

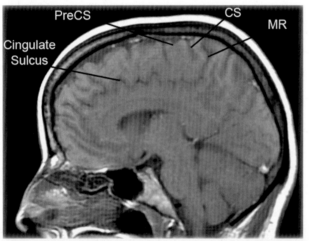

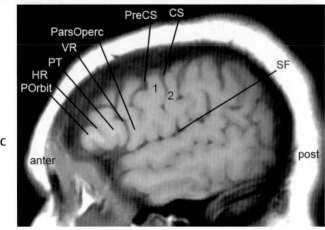

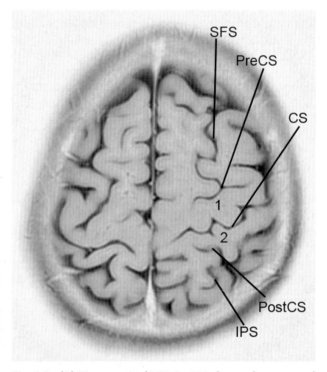

Fig. 6.2 **(A)** T1 parasagittal MRI. PreCS indicates the precentral sulcus. MR indicates the marginal ramus. CS indicates the central sulcus. **(B)** T2 high-axial MRI. SFS indicates the superior frontal sulcus. PreCS, indicates the precentral sulcus. IPS indicates the longitudinally running intraparietal sulcus. PostCS indicates the laterally running postcentral sulcus. 1 indicates the precentral gyrus. 2 indicates the postcentral gyrus. **(C)** T1 midsagittal MRI. Inferior frontal gyrus subdivided into pars orbitalis (POrbit), pars triangularis (PT), and pars opercularis (ParsOperc). The horizontal ramus (HR) and vertical ramus (VR) define the PT. The inferior portion of the PreCS defines the posterior portion of the ParsOperc. SF indicates the sylvian fissure.

while the subject performs a specific sensorimotor task. The areas of cortex activated during this task are then co-registered to the anatomical model thereby localizing the central sulcus. These images can be used preoperatively to define the location of the central region and plan surgical approaches (**Fig. 6.3**).

Seizures of the Central Region

The clinical semiology of seizures originating in the central region is much more stereotyped than focal epilepsy of the frontal, temporal, or parietal lobes. Seizures of the central region are rarely characterized by auras with subjective or emotional accompaniment. The majority of the attacks are heralded by primary somatomotor or somatosensory symptoms or signs. Seizures typically begin with clonic movements of the face, arm, or leg with no alteration of consciousness. The clonic movements may remain localized to the affected region or may spread and secondarily generalize. If the seizure spreads along the sensory or motor strip, the patient or clinician may observe progression of the clonic motor movements to involve more of the affected extremity or face and then spread to contiguous areas. This so-called Jacksonian march is the clinical accompaniment of the spread of epileptic discharges along the rolandic cortex.[7] The seizure may stop at this point or may go on to a secondary generalized tonic-clonic convulsion. If the seizures involve the inferior portion of the motor strip where face and tongue are represented, the patient often experiences a speech arrest. This is true whether the seizure involves the dominant or non-dominant hemisphere. Isolated focal tonic contraction of a limb is rare but when seen at the beginning of a seizure most often represents a more localized spread into supplementary motor areas with lesions closer to the interhemispheric fissure.[8]

Because of the lower threshold for epileptic discharges, seizures involving the central region can frequently result in focal status epilepticus or epilepsia partialis continua (EPC). These episodes of focal status epilepticus are often associated with very small, discrete and restricted lesions in either the somatomotor or somatosensory cortex and can be very difficult to control pharmacologically. Gliosis and post-inflammatory changes have been implicated in genesis of EPC especially in Rasmussen's encephalitis.[9] The characteristic clinical feature of EPC is focal myoclonus of the distal part of one extremity that may last for minutes, hours, or days. If the epileptic discharges are confined to a small cortical region, then the clonic movements may be confined to a single group of muscles or a single finger. At other times, more extensive muscle segments are involved, and the entire limb may be involved in the synchronous myoclonic jerks. It is common for patients to suffer a transient postictal paresis of minutes to hours.[10]

Rarely, reflex-triggered motor seizures can occur from the rolandic cortex. These are rare conditions provoked by movement or cutaneous stimulation. In these cases, repetitive stimulation of a trigger zone, for example, tooth brushing, or joint movement triggers a focal motor seizure. Generally, the initial seizure manifestations are somatosensory with

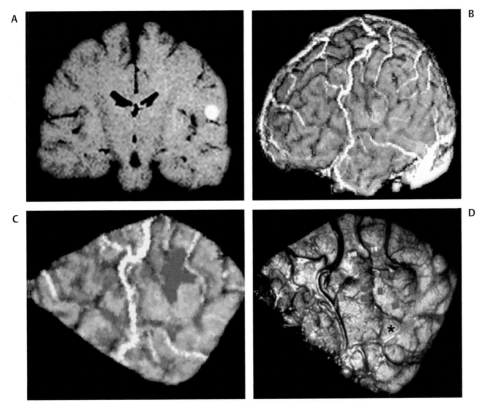

Fig. 6.3 fMRI. **(A)** Coronal view, contrast-enhanced MRI shows an ganglioglioma in the left-frontal lobe. **(B)** Brain lateral surface reconstruction with fMRI activity during a series of language and sensorimotor tasks mapped onto figure. Green indicates areas active during a verb-generation language task. Red indicates primary motor cortex active during tongue movements. Yellow indicates the tumor. **(C)** Detailed view of **(B)**. **(D)** Intraoperative view of the left lateral brain surface, with veins and brain surface exposed. Green tags indicate areas where direct cortical electrical stimulation elicited speech arrest. Red tags indicate cortical areas that created either tongue movement or sensations with stimulation. Asterisk indicates brain tumor.

subsequent tonic activity resulting from spread of the ictal discharge into the motor cortex. The location of the trigger zone or the movement is highly variable but is always in the same location for a given patient.[11]

Etiology of Central Seizures

The etiology of central seizures can be extremely varied and represents a wide variety of pathologies.[12] In the past, tumors and vascular malformations represented approximately half the cause of all forms of central epilepsy. These lesions were generally quite large and extended into the central cortex from adjacent cortical regions. Sometimes small, focal and discrete lesions affecting a specific portion of the rolandic cortex were found at surgery on the basis of electrocorticography (ECoG).[13]

However, with the widespread availability and easy access to MRI scanning, the incidence of infiltrating gliomas and undiagnosed vascular malformations involving the central region is declining, especially in patients with intractable epilepsy. MR imaging, however, has increased the detection of other pathological entities including an increasing number of grade I astrocytomas such as xanthoastrocytoma, ganglioglioma, and dysembryoplastic neuroepithelial tumor. It has also revealed small cortical dysplasias that were previously undetectable. Additionally, one can also define more extensive perisylvian cortical dysplasias and schizencephaly that affect the central cortex and cause seizures. Another major etiology of rolandic seizures has been described as meningocerebral cicatrix due to ischemic or postinfectious etiologies. In these cases there is often neuronal loss, significant gliosis, and atrophy of the central region without a clear etiology. There remain a percentage of cases with no identifiable morphological abnormality, although in the resected specimen there may be evidence of microdysgenesis.[14]

Presurgical Evaluation

The goal of epilepsy surgery in the central region is to identify an abnormal area of cortex from which the seizures originate and remove it without causing any significant functional impairment. The primary components of the presurgical evaluation include a detailed clinical history and physical examination, advanced neuroimaging, video electroencephalogram (EEG) monitoring, neuropsychological testing, and assessment of psychosocial functioning. The major surgical questions one hopes to answer with this evaluation are (1) are the seizures focal and intractable; (2) which part of the central region is involved; (3) is there a lesion associated with the seizures; and (4) if surgery is undertaken, what functional deficits might be anticipated?

Clinical Features

The clinical semiology of seizures originating in the sensorimotor cortex can yield extremely important localizing information to the experienced clinician. Many times, it is the clinical semiology that indicates exactly where in the central region the seizures begin and this can be the most important information of the entire presurgical evaluation.

On examination, the clinician looks for obvious asymmetries of development compatible with an early structural central nervous system lesion and focal neurological abnormalities suggestive of acquired disease (e.g., hemiatrophy of limbs). In the great majority of patients, however, the neurological examination is completely normal.

Neuroimaging

Modern neuroimaging is crucial to surgical decision making. MRI has replaced computed tomography scanning as the imaging study of choice and can detect subtle abnormalities of the brain such as focal atrophy, indolent gliomas, cavernous angiomas, cortical dysplasias, cerebral gliosis, and other small structural lesions of the neocortex. Higher-strength magnets at 3 Tesla have improved signal to noise ratio and may allow for detection of even smaller and less distinct lesions. Three-dimensional surface rendering can also demonstrate abnormalities of cerebral topography and sulcal anatomy. Routine interictal positron emission tomography (PET) and single photon emission tomography (SPECT) studies are rarely useful, but when a patient is experiencing focal status epilepticus, PET or SPECT studies are by definition ictal and can be very helpful in defining the origin and site of the seizures.

Functional MRI (fMRI) can now be used to identify the sensorimotor cortex and create accurate structural and functional models of individual patients' brains. The relationship of the primary motor and sensory areas to local pathology and surrounding areas can be determined preoperatively, which can influence both preoperative and intraoperative decision making.[6] Rapid echoplanar imaging performed while the patient engages in a specific task (e.g., fist clenching, tongue movement, foot wagging) detects small changes in signal intensity related to changes in cerebral blood flow. Intensive computerized image processing can then define the areas of cortex activated by the specific task. Concurrent 3-D rendering of cerebral topography, cortical veins, and related pathology gives an unprecedented display of critical relational anatomy. By combining detailed anatomical information with precise physiological information, fMRI is capable of creating a structural and functional model of an individual's brain.

Electroencephalographic (EEG) Investigation

EEG investigation remains an important part of any presurgical evaluation but is often nonlocalizing in the central epilepsies. Even when a patient is in focal status epilepticus, routine scalp EEG can be completely normal. Even closely spaced electrodes over the area will often not detect electrographic abnormality. This is because of the small volumes of cortex that are involved in the EPC cannot generate sufficient EEG signal to overcome the electrical impedance of the overlying skull and scalp. Continuous video-EEG monitoring should nevertheless be performed, as it allows for detection of the patients habitual or stereotyped events. When EEG abnormality is detected, it is the EEG activity at the very beginning of the seizure before spread to adjacent areas that is most important in terms of localization. If a specific cortical area is involved consistently at the onset, then that area is likely to be the site of seizure origin.

Neuropsychological Testing

Detailed neuropsychological testing is performed to reveal specific focal or multifocal cognitive deficits that might be correlated with the neuroimaging and EEG. In surgery of the central region, this testing has a limited role, although it may still help in localizing an abnormal area of the brain and also serves as a comparison for postsurgical evaluation.

Psychosocial Assessment

Psychosocial evaluation is also important to assess current level of functioning and to ensure realistic goals and attitudes are engendered in both the patient and the family prior to surgery. In many instances, surgery in the central region creates specific sensory or motor deficits that will have varying consequences on patients depending upon their personal and professional circumstances. These issues must be well understood before entering the operating room.

Diagnostic Surgical Options

When the primary epileptogenic region or seizure focus is suspected but remains obscure despite appropriate neuroimaging and scalp (*noninvasive*) video/EEG recordings, some form of implanted (*invasive*) electrodes may be indicated. In general, subdural grids are used for seizures of the central region because the grids can be placed over the dorsolateral convexity covering the primary sensorimotor cortex and the adjacent areas. Rarely, either subdural strips or intracerebral electrodes need to be placed for high vertex lesions or lesions along the interhemispheric fissure. These recordings give more precise EEG information because of their proximity to discharging areas of the brain and the lack of movement or muscle artifact. They can also be used for extraoperative cortical stimulation to map out and confirm specific areas of cortical function. They have the disadvantage, however, of imparting a small but real surgical risk of intracranial hemorrhage and infection. They should only be undertaken after appropriate noninvasive monitoring has been completed.

Therapeutic Surgical Options

Once the epileptic region has been accurately localized, the next objective is to completely excise the seizure focus without causing a neurological deficit. An important determinant of the risk of surgery is the relationship of the lesion to functionally important or "eloquent" brain regions because injury to these eloquent areas can cause irreversible neurological impairment. Because surgery in the central region is by definition in eloquent cortex, resections must be relatively focal and restricted or they will result in irreversible deficits. A variety of strategies have therefore been employed to optimize surgical resection while minimizing risk of injury to functional cortex.

Most surgery in the primary sensorimotor cortex is done under local anesthesia with intravenous sedation. This allows for direct electrical stimulation of the cortex using a handheld bipolar stimulator to map out sensory, motor, and language areas. Rarely, direct cortical stimulation can precipitate a patient's habitual seizures, which can be an important validation of the seizure focus. It also allows for the assessment of function during resection. The patient is carefully evaluated during the resection for loss of either motor or sensory function. In certain areas of the sensorimotor cortex such as the hand, trunk and foot areas, resection will lead to paralysis and therefore only local disconnection procedures can be performed in the form of multiple subpial transections (MST). If the patient has a longstanding preoperative motor or sensory deficit, then more aggressive resections can be considered. Rarely, minute lesions in these primary sensorimotor areas can be resected through a small transgyral corticectomy without permanent deficits. In the inferior portions of the rolandic cortex, resections of the facial region can be performed, especially on the nondominant side. This will result in a 3- to 4-month period of dysarthria but minimal permanent deficits. The superior extent of resection should stop at the motor thumb area. On the dominant hemisphere, similar resections can be performed but special attention has to be paid to prevent encroachment on the deeper white matter pathways, that is, arcuate fasciculus, that connect essential language areas.

After the resection strategy is decided upon, tissue removal is performed using subpial resection techniques. Cortical gray and white matter is carefully removed by bipolar cautery and suction or CUSA Excel (Integra Neurosciences, Plainsboro, NJ) so that the pia remains intact over the adjacent gyri. This tends to form a nonscarring barrier and preserves blood supply to the remaining cortex as well.

Surgical Results of Central Resections

The outcomes of central resections for intractable epilepsy are primarily concerned with two measures: long-term seizure reduction and the absence of significant neurological deficit. Data regarding these outcomes are hard to group together from multiple case series at different surgical centers because of heterogeneous populations and differing surgical techniques and procedures, extent of resections, follow-up periods, and outcome classification scales. Nonetheless, generalizations can be made after review of the larger studies. Seizure frequency reduction (>50% decrease in frequency) occurs in 55 to 75% of patients, and new neurological deficits occur in approximately 15 to 25% when following patients for long-term outcomes postoperatively.[15–17]

Regarding seizure control, the Rasmussen series[15] followed 135 patients who underwent operation at the Montreal Neurologic Institute between 1931 and 1975 for intractable epilepsy from a central or rolandic location. They specified seizure reduction data in the 63 patients who did not have tumor or vascular causes for their lesion. More than 85% of these patients were younger than 30 years old, and more than 40% were younger than 15 years old. After 16 years median follow-up (range 2 to 38 years), 18% were completely seizure free and 40% had rare seizures. The study reports that 43% had "moderate or less reduction" in their seizures. This appears to be a more conservative goal than the typical Engel class I-III cited in other studies. Excluding the glioblastoma patients, the 62 other tumor patients had even better seizure reduction; 70 to 80% of these patients had rare or no seizures in follow-up.

Other series with different outcome scales than in the Rasmussen series show even better seizure reduction. Twenty cases of face sensorimotor cortex localization–related intractable epilepsy showed 90% of patients with >50% reduction in seizure frequency at postoperative follow-up (median follow-up 11 years, ranging from 1 to 34 years).[16] Another cohort of 52 patients with sensorimotor cortex localization–related intractable epilepsy were followed for a mean of 4 years (range 1 to 18 years) postoperatively; 73% had an Engel I-III seizure outcome (ranging from no disabling seizures to worthwhile improvement) at follow-up.[17] Those cases involving localization to the precentral gyrus or inferior central cortex had better postoperative seizure reduction.

Intraoperative and postoperative ECoG has been reported to be helpful in guiding how much cortex to remove. Successful reoperation was guided by ECoG in 4 of 6 patients[16] and the reoperative location (i.e., far from resection site) and high amount of spikes in ECoG were seen to correlate with postoperative long-term seizure reoccurrence.[17] In some of these cases, MST is performed to treat refractory epilepsy where additional cortex cannot be removed due to its elo-

quent nature. MST has shown variable results: 30% of the nine London Health Sciences Center central localization epilepsy patients needing MST had seizure improvement postoperatively[17]; 84% of six patients with sensorimotor cortex seizures had significant seizure reduction[18]; ~65% of 211 patients in a meta-analysis of those needing MST for partial epilepsy had >95% seizure reduction.[19]

Significant moderate or severe permanent neurological deficit after epilepsy surgery in the central region is infrequent in experienced hands but is always a major concern. The deficits are correlated with the location and the extent of resection in the specific central regions. Approximately 20% of patients will have a new and significant neurological deficit that correlates with the removed cortex. Temporary deficits such as dysarthria, weakness, impaired dexterity, sensory loss, and aphasia are common but generally resolve in months. If the postcentral gyrus and/or parietal cortex are removed, often an incidental 2-point discrimination sensory loss is noted on long-term follow-up exam of the contralateral limb. A lower face weakness almost always improves, whereas an upper limb weakness may not completely improve. In the London Health Sciences Center series, 22% of the 52 postoperative patients had new moderate or worse neurological deficit at last follow-up. The deficits in this series included 12 patients with new motor deficits and two patients with speech difficulties. Having the surgery at >25 years of age was seen to increase the odds of a lasting significant postoperative neurological deficit by 4 times.[17]

Conclusion

Intractable epilepsy of the central region or rolandic cortex is a challenging subset of epilepsy due to the highly epileptogenic cortex, refractory nature of the seizures, and the potential for significant deficit after surgery. Careful workup of patients and mapping of function of the involved and neighboring eloquent cortex can help one to select patients who can benefit from surgery with a low risk for significant morbidity.

References

1. Meyer JR, Roychowdhury S, Russell EJ, et al. Localization of the central sulcus via cortical thickness of the pre-central and post-central gyri on MR. AJNR Am J Neuroradiol 1996;17:1699–1706
2. Yousry TA, Schmid UD, Alkadhi H, et al. Localization of the motor hand area to a knob on the precentral gyrus. A new landmark. Brain 1997;120(Pt 1):141–157
3. Brodmann K. *Vergleichende Lokalisationslehre der Grosshirnrinde in ihren Prinzipien dargestellt auf Grund des Zellenbaues (Comparative Localization Studies in the Brain Cortex, Its Fundamentals Represented on the Basis of Its Cellular Architecture).* Leipzig, Germany: Johann Ambrosius Barth Verlag; 1909. English Translation by Garey LJ: *Localisation in the Cerebral Cortex by Korbinian Brodmann.* London: Smith-Gordon; 1994
4. Woolsey CN, Erickson TC, Gilson WE. Localization in somatic sensory

and motor areas of human cerebral cortex as determined by direct recording of evoked potentials and electrical stimulation. J Neurosurg 1979;51(4):476–506
5. Penfield W, Rasmussen T. *The Cerebral Cortex of Man.* New York: Macmillan; 1950
6. Cosgrove GR, Buchbinder BR, Jiang H. Functional magnetic resonance imaging for intracranial navigation. Neurosurg Clin N Am 1996;7: 313–322
7. Jackson JH. On convulsive seizures. Lancet 1890;1:685–688, 735–738, 785–788
8. Chauvel P, Delgado-Escueta AV, Halgren E, et al, eds. *Frontal Lobe Seizures and Epilepsies (Advances in Neurology).* Vol. 57. New York: Raven Press; 1992

9. Rasmussen T, Olszewski J, Lloydsmith D. Focal seizures due to chronic localized encephalitis. Neurology 1958;8(6):435–445

10. Olivier A. Extratemporal cortical resections: principles and methods. In: Lüders HO, ed. *Epilepsy Surgery*. New York: Raven Press; 1992: 559–568

11. Vignal J, Biraben A, Chauvel P, Reutens D. Reflex partial seizures on sensorimotor cortex (including cortical reflex myoclonus and startle epilepsy). In: Zifkin B, Andermann F, Beaumanoir A, Rowan A, eds. *Reflex Epilepsies and Reflex Seizures*. New York: Lippincott-Raven; 1998:207–226

12. Robitaille Y, Rasmussen T, Dubeau F, et al. Histopathology of non-neoplastic lesion sin frontal lobe epilepsy: review of 180 cases with recent MRI and PET correlations. In: Chauvel P, Delgado-Escueta AV, Halgren E, et al, eds. *Frontal Lobe Seizures and Epilepsies (Advances in Neurology)*. Vol. 57. New York: Raven Press; 1992:499–514

13. Rasmussen T. Surgery of frontal lobe epilepsy. In: Purpura DP, Penry JK, Walter RD, eds. *Advances in Neurology*. Vol. 8. New York: Raven Press; 1975:197–205

14. Guerrini R, Anderman F, Canapicchi R, et al, eds. *Dysplasia of Cerebral Cortex and Epilepsy*. Philadelphia: Lippincott-Raven; 1996

15. Rasmussen T. Surgery for epilepsy arising in regions other than the temporal and frontal lobes. In: Purpura DP, Penry JK, Walter RD, eds. *Advances in Neurology*. Vol 8. New York: Raven Press; 1975: 207–226

16. Pondal-Sordo M, Diosy D, Téllez-Zenteno JF, Girvin JP, Wiebe S. Epilepsy surgery involving the sensory-motor cortex. Brain 2006;129: 3307–3314

17. Lehman R, Andermann F, Olivier A, et al. Seizures with onset in the sensorimotor face area: clinical patterns and results of surgical treatment in 20 patients. Epilepsia 1994;35(6):1117–1124

18. Spencer SS, Schramm J, Wyler A. Multiple subpial transaction for intractable partial epilepsy: an international meta-analysis. Epilepsia 2002;43(2):141–145

19. Wyler AR, Wilkus RJ, Rostad SW, Vossler DG. Multiple subpial transaction for partial seizures in sensorimotor cortex. Neurosurgery 1995;37:1122–1128

7 Cortical Resection in Frontal, Parietal, and Occipital Lobe

David W. Roberts and Barbara C. Jobst

Extratemporal epilepsy has been dichotomized from temporal lobe epilepsy historically in large part on account of the considerably more extensive experience and literature associated with the latter. The clinical importance of frontal, parietal, and occipital lobe epilepsy nonetheless is sufficient to warrant full consideration, exploration, and intervention in these epilepsies, and this chapter explores the preoperative evaluation, surgical treatment, and outcomes associated with the spectrum of these seizure disorders.

Frontal Lobe Epilepsy

Diagnosis

Seizure disorders involving the frontal lobes have been thought more likely to be frequent, brief in duration, often nocturnal, and associated with status epilepticus and secondary generalization. In a study of the clinical expression of frontal lobe seizures using video electroencephalogram (EEG) analysis of more than 400 seizures of frontal lobe origin, Jobst et al found that indeed they tended to be frequent (7.1 per week), brief (mean duration 48.3 seconds), preponderantly nocturnal in 58% of patients, associated with status in more than half, and associated with generalized seizures in a quarter of patients.[1] Categorization into various subtypes, reflecting the sometimes distinguishable features associated with the different regions of the frontal lobe, has also been popular, although the same analysis by Jobst et al showed that although such expressions of topography followed trends, such clinical features were often nonspecific.

Seizures arising from the frontal convexity may present with focal clonic activity. Tonic seizures are most often associated with supplementary motor area seizure origin,[1,2] but they can also be observed with frontopolar onset or with propagation to the supplementary motor area from other areas such as the medial parietal cortex.[3] Seizures with oroalimentary automatisms suggestive of temporal lobe epilepsy as well as seizures with hyperactive automatisms can originate in the orbitofrontal region.[1,4] Hyperactive or frenetic motor automatisms, however, are nonspecific with respect to location within the frontal lobe. Interestingly, two-thirds of frontal lobe seizures are associated with aura, most often nonspecific in nature.[1,5]

The traditional evaluation methods of history and neurological exam, imaging studies, scalp EEG, and neuropsychological testing are standard, and with current radiographic tools, including high field-strength magnetic resonance imaging (MRI), ictal and interictal single photon emission computed tomography (SPECT), positron emission tomography (PET), and magnetoencephalography (MEG), sufficient information to enable therapeutic surgical intervention may well be present.

Interictal and ictal scalp EEG can be without definite abnormalities, especially in seizures originating at the medial frontal surface of the cortex.[5] This can lead to misdiagnosis of frontal lobe seizures as nonepileptic psychogenic seizures.[6] Neuropsychological testing may indicate dysfunction of executive function with impulsivity and impersistence.[7] However, neuropsychological testing can rarely lateralize or localize to subregions of the frontal lobes.[7] MRI, ictal and interictal SPECT, PET, and MEG are additional diagnostic tools to localize the seizure onset zone. In those patients in whom imaging does not localize a potentially pathological substrate, further investigation by intracranial recording will likely be required. Should initial evaluation suggest nonlocalizable or multifocal epilepsy, further evaluation by an intracranial study can be avoided.

Intracranial Investigation

EEG recording within the cranium has far greater sensitivity and specificity than its scalp-based counterpart. Its sensitivity will be considerably more spatially limited, of course, and coverage of the brain will always be incomplete. Judgment with respect to how and where an electrode array shall be developed is essential and ideally multidisciplinary. A variety of intracranial electrodes have been developed over many decades, each with respective advantages. Depth electrodes can record well from tissue at essentially any depth, and stereotactic placement can assure accurate placement, at least with respect to preoperative planning. Some groups have used these exclusively with great success, and the Talairach school is a good example.[8] Subdural electrodes, in the form of strips, typically containing four to 12 contacts in a linear array, can be positioned through bur holes and better sample activity on the cortical surface. Subdural grid electrodes, consisting of anywhere from two to eight rows each containing two to eight contacts, obviously require a craniotomy for their insertion, but provide more complete coverage of a specific cortical surface; they also provide a convenient means by which to perform cortical mapping outside the operating room. In practice, most centers utilize all of these types of electrodes, usually in combination. An example of a typical implantation using depth, strip, and grid electrodes is seen in **Fig. 7.1**.

Coverage of the frontal convexity, and particularly of the central region, is well accomplished using large subdural grid arrays; a typical array may consist of one or two 4 × 8 grids or an 8 × 8 grid. Subfrontal coverage is usually achieved using a 4 × 5 grid. Additional coverage, and particularly over the frontal pole, can be obtained with multiple 1 × 8 strips. Medial frontal coverage is less often accomplished using interhemispheric grids, on account of the more difficult exposure required, but in our experience it has been of great utility. Subdural grids in these locations also enable thorough extraoperative functional mapping. Alternatively, multiple depth electrodes may be employed to cover the entire lobe, including access to orbitofrontal, insular, and medial regions, with less extensive exposures.

Additional types of electrodes, including minimally invasive transphenoidal and foramen ovale electrodes as well as PEG electrodes embedded in the cranium itself, have seen effective utilization as well. The efficacy of such intracranial electrode studies in general has been repeatedly demonstrated, and the associated morbidity has been low. A recent review of the experience at the Montreal Neurological Institute over more than two decades revealed the ability to support an indication for surgery in nearly 80% of patients and to exclude a surgical option in 16.5%.[9]

Operative Techniques

Resection of the seizure focus in the frontal lobe, as with other sites, offers the greatest chance of a seizure-free outcome. Published series of frontal resection report a wide range of good outcome,[1,5,10–15] but the diagnostic tools available today enable success in the great majority of patients. Diagnostic imaging of the underlying pathological and pathophysiological substrate, often coupled with intracranial electrode investigation, enables tailored resection. The most common underlying pathological substrates for intractable frontal

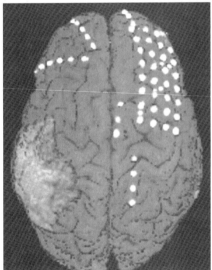

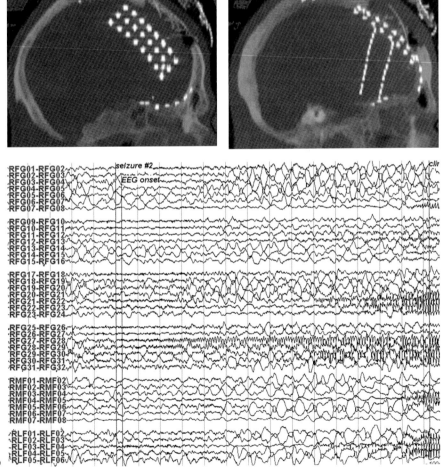

Fig. 7.1 Intracranial electrode implantation in a 22-year-old male with suspected frontal lobe epilepsy. **(A)** Computed tomography (CT) scan reformatted in midsagittal plane, demonstrating a double-sided 3 × 8 subdural grid electrode within the interhemispheric fissure. **(B)** CT scan sagittally reformatted in plane of left frontal depth electrodes. **(C)** CT thresholded to show intracranial electrode contacts co-registered with surface-rendering of MRI. **(D)** EEG recording showing seizure onset in region of contacts RFG28-RFG29 of the right frontal convexity subdural grid electrode.

lobe epilepsy are focal cortical dysplasias, low grade tumors, and posttraumatic encephalomalacia.[16] Subtle dysplasias are not always readily identifiable on routine MRI scanning and may require high field MRI scanning or special reformatting.[17,18] In MRI-normal or nonlesional epilepsy, ictal SPECT, PET, and/or intracranial electrode investigation may also enable good surgical outcomes.[19,20] Co-registration of preoperative studies with the operative field allows preoperative planning of these resective strategies and most importantly their accurate execution. In those instances with lesional substrates, completeness of resection of structural pathology has been associated with better seizure outcome.[21]

Actual resection follows standard microsurgical technique. Adequate exposure of the extent of intended cortical resection is essential, and in those patients in whom eloquent cortex—subserving language and motor function in particular with respect to the frontal lobe—is either involved or adjacent to the resection, recognition of that functional localization is critical. The gold standard of functional mapping has been intraoperative mapping by electrical stimulation technique. For language, this requires an awake craniotomy; for motor function, the ability to map in the anesthetized patient is commonplace. Patients in whom an intracranial electrode investigation has been performed using subdural grid electrodes may be mapped extraoperatively using those same grids, a practice advantaged by the greater ease and less constrained nature of the setting. Traditionally 5-second long 50 Hz stimulation is used for functional mapping intra- and extraoperatively. Due to the propensity for seizures and after-discharges functional motor mapping with high frequency pulse trains and electromyography (EMG) control can be of advantage for motor mapping. Co-registration of imaging studies, including both structural and functional investigations, enables additional localization to be incorporated into the surgical field.

Integration of a surgical plan including identification of both the tissue to be resected as well as that to be preserved delineates the cortical margins of the resection. Corticotomy incisions along the boundary take into account the sulcal topography, and attendance is given to the preservation of vascular structures that may be en passage. The most compelling instance of the latter in frontal lobe resection is that of medial resections, such as that involving the supplementary motor area, where anterior cerebral artery supply to regions posterior to the resection cannot be sacrificed. Resection is generally performed with the aid of the operating microscope, and a combination of en bloc resection (valuable in pathological diagnosis for both therapeutic and prognostic purposes) and subpial dissection is often employed for the removal of tissue. Resections into the ventricular system are avoided, if possible, for minimalization of morbidity including hydrocephalus and subdural hygromas. Hemostasis and closure follow standard surgical techniques.

A considerable surgical experience has now accumulated in the literature, and from these series good outcomes (Engel class I or II) range from as low as 26% to as high as 80%.[1,5,12,14,21–25] Patient selection represents the variable most responsible for such variation, but recent surgical cases have tended to be at the higher end of that range.[1,15,25] Other predictors for a good surgical outcome have been identified. Focal ictal β discharges on scalp EEG,[16,21] focal confined lesions,[14,24] and slow intracranial spread patterns[26] have been identified as favorable prognostic factors.

Unilateral frontal resection is generally well tolerated, with low surgical and neurological morbidity.[27] Supplemental motor area (SMA) resections are often accompanied by well-described post-resection syndrome characterized by decreased spontaneous motor function of the contralateral limbs and, with language-dominant side resection, expressive speech.[28,29] These may last from several days to several weeks but rarely present long-term difficulties.

Nonresective Strategies

Various nonresective surgical strategies have also evolved. There are several reasons why these might be employed, but the most common indications have been in instances where a seizure focus could not be identified or where a focus involved eloquent, nonresectable tissue. Principles of less invasiveness or potentially lower risk may also play a role in selection of a particular procedure.

Corpus callosotomy evolved from the observation that generalization of seizure activity used the callosal commissure as the route of propagation. Seizure-free outcome is not a realistic expectation of the operation, but as a palliative procedure when others are either not options or have failed, it remains a valuable option.[30,31] Of those seizure types most likely to respond, drop attacks have consistently been singled out. As the majority of these have been presumably of frontal lobe origin, anterior section alone may be effective in this application.[12] Surgery has been facilitated by standard microsurgical technique and more recently image guidance. The interhemispheric approach, with the patient positioned either supine or lateral (with gravity assisting retraction of the hemisphere on the side of approach), is now widely used for many other procedures, notably for resection of third ventricular tumors, and will be familiar to most neurosurgeons. Actual callosal division is best performed in the midline, enabling avoidance of ventricular entry, protection of the fornix, and assurance of commissural division. Blunt or aspiration technique is readily performed, and most centers advocate division of the anterior two-thirds to three-quarters of the callosum as an initial procedure as this tends to optimize the efficacy/morbidity ratio. Other commissural structures, targeted in the procedure's earliest descriptions, are no longer divided. The morbidity of anterior section is low, and the neuropsychological consequences rarely exceed the benefits in this patient population.[32] As a palliative procedure, Engel classification of outcome is less useful, but recent surgical series have shown 48 to 78% a significant reduction in seizures with callostomy.[30,33]

In cases in which seizure onset has been localized but lies within unresectable, functional cortex, multiple subpial transection (MST) has been advocated. Technically, the procedure has not changed greatly from its earliest descriptions, with division of the cortical thickness across the width of the gyrus involved with repeat transections at 5-mm intervals.[34–36] Most reports of MST have combined the technique with resection, rendering interpretation of its efficacy difficult.[37,38] A meta-analysis of several centers reported an excellent outcome in 68 to 87% if subpial transections were combined with resection and in 62 to 71% if MST alone was performed.[38] Motor and speech function are generally preserved, but deficits were reported in 19% of patients in the above mentioned meta-analysis.[35,38]

Vagal nerve stimulation (VNS) not surprisingly given its relative noninvasiveness has been widely utilized in difficult cases in which the seizure-free allure of resective procedures is not applicable. Technically, the procedure requires placement of bipolar electrode coils around the vagal nerve in the neck (usually performed on the left side, in an attempt to minimize the risk of cardiac arrhythmia) and then tunneling the electrode to a subcutaneous pocket below the left clavicle where the pulse generator is implanted. Battery life between 3 and 6 years can be expected, and battery replacement requires only a minor, outpatient procedure. In general, 50% of patients have 50% fewer seizures with VNS implantation.[39] There is no particular epilepsy syndrome that responds more favorably than others, but VNS is effective in frontal lobe epilepsy.

Deep brain stimulation has been performed in much smaller numbers generally as part of investigational trials. The equipment and methodology have been directly adopted from surgery for movement disorders and utilize standard stereotactic procedures. Numerous targets have been implanted, the most widely used now being the subthalamic nucleus and the anterior nucleus of the thalamus. Chabardes et al has reported a good outcome in 3 of 5 patient with stimulation of the subthalamic nucleus.[40] Other groups report good results with stimulation of the anterior nucleus of the thalamus and the centromedian nucleus of the thalamus.[41,42] An implantation effect with improvement of seizures regardless of whether the stimulator is on or off has also been observed.[41,43] A large-scale randomized study is currently underway to evaluate the utility of stimulation of the anterior thalamic nucleus in localization-related epilepsy.[44]

Theoretically, stimulation techniques might take advantage of the relatively infrequent occurrence of seizure activity and the frequent ability to detect early the EEG activity associated with the event. Such a conceptual approach underlies NeuroPace, Inc.'s Responsive Neruostimulator (RNS™) system (NeuroPace, Inc., Mountain View, CA), which is currently being evaluated in a multicenter pivotal clinical trial.[45] This system presently consists of two depth or subdural strip electrodes and a cranially implanted, programmable pulse generator with the ability to run a seizure-detection algorithm, and when triggered through such a detection the system sends an electrical stimulus to abort the electrographic seizure. Electrical stimulation has been shown to suppress or alter seizures in patients with subdural electrodes during a preoperative intracranial evaluation,[46] and results of a Phase I and II trial have been promising.

Parietal Lobe Epilepsy

Diagnosis

Without the benefit of immediate motor behavior, seizure onset in the parietal lobe can be less obvious. Further, rapid spread of the epileptic discharge to the temporal or frontal lobes and subsequent first recognized seizure expression reflective of those secondary sites may be misleading. Nevertheless, early sensory symptoms may be highly suggestive of localization.

Somatosensory seizures may have their origin in any portion of the parietal cortex. Most commonly but not exclusively contralateral, any or multiple sensory modality may be involved. Elementary paresthesias are most common[47,48] with initial involvement of a limb or face and often with spread to contiguous regions of the body, analogous to the well-recognized Jacksonian march of motor seizures. Actual motor activity has been reported to occur in approximately half of such sensory seizures.[48–50] Seizures expressed as the sensation of pain, although long recognized, were often thought to be uncommon until Mauguiere and Courjon in 1978 reported them to be the second most common type of somatosensory seizures.[48,51] Thermal sensations, usually described as burning but occasionally as cold, have also been reported.[49,52]

Other seizure manifestations of parietal epilepsy include ideomotor apraxia (ascribed to involvement of the second sensory area) and sexual phenomena (also associated with the temporal and frontal lobes, but when arising from the parietal lobe believed to represent involvement of the paracentral lobule adjacent to the primary somatosensory cortical representation for the genitalia). Disturbances of body image have been described in association with the inferior parietal lobule and the superior aspect of the postcentral gyrus. Ictal anosognosia, apraxia, acalculia, alexia, aphemia, and confusional states may be associated with parietal epilepsy.[53] Gustatory seizures may be either temporal or parietal in origin, with the parietal operculum involved in the latter. All of these seizures may progress to clonic or tonic motor activity depending on the intracranial spread pattern.[54,55]

Operative Techniques

Just as in the frontal lobe epilepsies, evaluation of the medically intractable seizure patient with possible parietal seizure onset may require an intracranial implant for more complete characterization of the seizure onset and possible functional mapping (see **Fig. 7.2**). The methodology for such implantation in the parietal region is the same as that previously

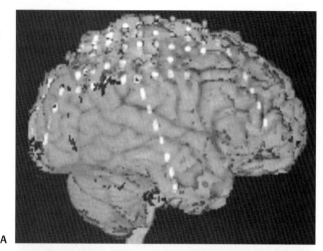

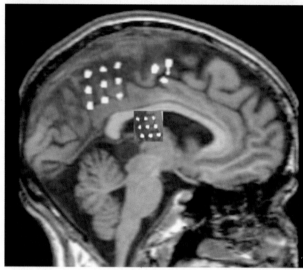

Fig. 7.2 Intracranial electrode implantation in a 44-year-old female with suspected parietal lobe epilepsy. **(A)** Co-registered CT (thresholded to show intracranial electrode contacts) and surface-rendered MRI. **(B)** Co-registered CT and MRI data (the anterior portion of the interhemispheric electrode is depicted in an adjacent sagittal plane, here represented as a composite.

described. However, without a clear lesion it can be difficult to determine a seizure's onset zone in parietal lobe epilepsy as seizures manifestations can be subtle and often a result of propagation.

Resection of the seizure focus similarly follows the methodology outlined in the discussion of frontal lobe epilepsy. Sparing of the postcentral gyrus and its primary somatosensory function and of perisylvian language areas is critically important. Preoperative functional MRI or MEG may assist in identification of the former; alternatively, intraoperative somatosensory evoked potentials (SSEP) mapping has become a standard and reliable technique. Language mapping may be performed extraoperatively in those instances with implanted subdural grid electrodes; alternatively, awake craniotomy with intraoperative language mapping and mon-

itoring is widely used. Care during resection to avoid unnecessarily deep intrusion upon subcortical white matter tracts is equally important, and generation of significant visual field deficits can often be avoided.

One interesting recent report on posterior quadrant epilepsy surgery, including parietal but posterior temporal and occipital lobes as well, describes evolution of a surgical technique from classic resection toward a disconnection procedure, analogous to how functional hemispherectomy has largely replaced actual hemisphere removal.[56]

Results

Epilepsy surgery in the parietal lobes is less successful than in the frontal and temporal lobes, especially in nonlesional cases. The Montreal Neurologic Institute reports successful surgery in 65% of cases over 59 years.[57] In the multiinstitutional report describing a disconnection technique, an Engel's class I seizure outcome was achieved in 12 of 13 patients, with no mortality or major morbidity.[56]

Occipital Lobe Epilepsy

Diagnosis

Less common than either frontal or parietal lobe epilepsy, occipital epilepsy by virtue of this lobe's dominant role in visual perception lends itself well to accurate diagnosis and, when possible, surgical treatment. Elementary visual phenomena, ictal amaurosis, complex visual hallucinations, simple and complex visual illusions, as well as ocular symptoms including epileptic nystagmus, eyelid flutter, and rapid blinking have all been reported with occipital epilepsy.[58,59]

Scalp EEG enabled lateralization of occipital epilepsy in 20 of 41 patients described by Blume and colleagues,[60] but localization within the occipital lobe region generally requires intracranial electrode investigation[60] (see **Fig. 7.3**). Only a preexisting visual field deficit was significantly associated with medial occipital seizure onset. No other clinical sign or seizure manifestation could reliably distinguish between mesial and lateral occipital seizure onset. Occipital lobe seizures propagate anteriorly by several different pathways. A visual aura could be followed by a typical temporal lobe seizure if there is propagation to the temporal lobes, or by typical frontal lobe seizures if there is propagation above the sylvian fissure.[61] Early involvement of the temporal lobe may necessitate an intracranial study.[62] Interestingly, in a study of 20 patients with parietooccipital epilepsy, 35% were found to have ipsilateral hippocampal atrophy. Of the 20 patients, 12 were found to have spread to the temporal lobe, but there was no correlation between temporal spread and hippocampal atrophy.[63]

Surgical Techniques

Surgical decision making in occipital epilepsy is critically influenced by preoperative visual function. Deliberate sacrifice

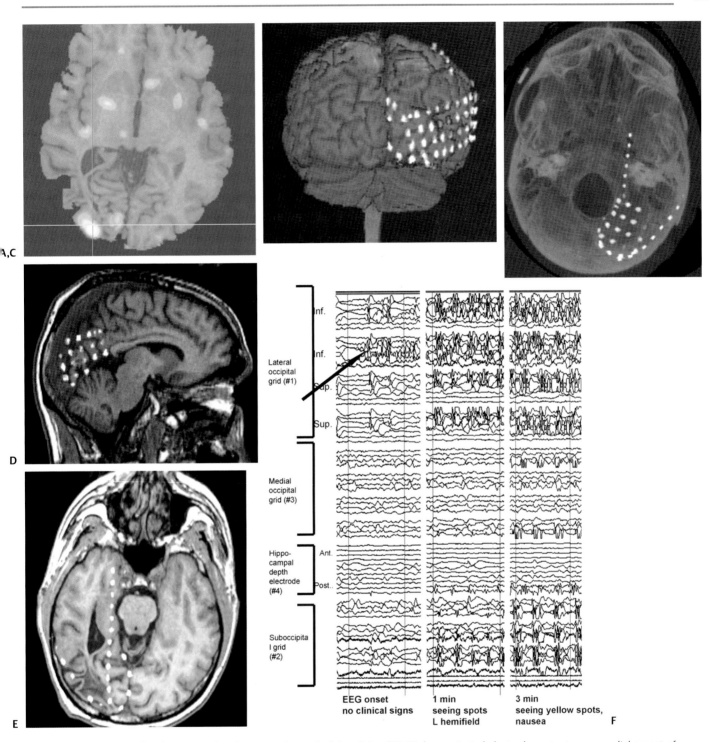

Fig. 7.3   This 42-year-old male presented with seizures 3 months following mycoplasma meningoencephalitis. **(A)** Ictal SPECT during visual hallucination. **(B)** CT-demonstrated electrode contacts over the right occipital lobe, co-registered with surface-rendered MRI. **(C)** CT-demonstrated electrode array covering the inferior aspect of the occipital lobe. **(D)** CT-demonstrated electrode contacts over medial aspect of the occipital lobe. **(E)** CT-depicted contacts of the occipitotemporal depth electrode, also showing a subset of the electrodes over the lateral and medial surfaces of the occipital lobe. **(F)** EEG showing seizure onset beneath the lateral subdural grid electrode.

of primary visual cortex is rarely undertaken. Intracranial investigation of occipital epilepsy can be well approached utilizing subdural grid coverage over the lateral, inferior, and medial surfaces of the lobe. Compared with frontal lobe investigation, the much smaller volume of the occipital lobe as well as the absence of interhemispheric adhesions as account of the posterior falx render electrode placement easier. Such coverage may be essential in understanding the respectability of the affected tissue and in the preservation of visual function. Following delineation of a respectable occipital seizure focus, resection follows standard microsurgical technique.

Results

Guided by localization achieved through intracranial recording, resection of occipital cortex can be effective. Blume et al reported on 32 patients with surgical treated occipital epilepsy and minimum 2-year follow-up: 22% were seizure free, 44% were improved, and 34% were not improved.[60] Kun Lee et al reported 16 (61.5%) of 26 patients who underwent occipital resection as now seizure free.[64] Looking at the relationship of type of underlying pathology to surgical outcome, Aykut-Bingol et al found that patients with developmental abnormalities did significantly worse, with only 45% achieving an excellent or good outcome, compared with 85% of patients with tumor.[13]

Conclusion

Surgery for epilepsy originating in the frontal, parietal, and occipital neocortex is a viable option if seizures cannot be controlled otherwise. In most cases this will require an intracranial study and an extensive presurgical evaluation. In intractable epilepsy this procedure still has the greatest chance to render the patient seizure free, although novel technology such as electrical stimulation may emerge as an effective alternative.

References

1. Jobst BC, Siegel AM, Thadani VM, Roberts DW, Williamson PD. Intractable seizures of frontal lobe origin. Epilepsia 2000;41:1139–1152

2. Morris HHI, Luders H, Dinner DS, Wyllie E, Kramer R. Seizures from the supplementary motor area: clinical and electrographic features. Epilepsia 1987;28:623

3. Aghakhani Y, Rosati A, Olivier A, Gotman J, Andermann F, Dubeau F. The predictive localizing value of tonic limb posturing in supplementary sensorimotor seizures. Neurology 2004;62(12):2256–2261

4. Ludwig B, Ajmone-Marsan C, Van Buren J. Cerebral seizures of probable orbitofrontal origin. Epilepsia 1972;16:141–158

5. Williamson PD, Spencer DD, Spencer SS, Novelly RA, Mattson RH. Complex partial seizures of frontal lobe origin. Ann Neurol 1985;18:497–504

6. Williamson PD, Jobst BC. Frontal lobe epilepsy. In: Williamson PD, Siegel AM, Roberts DW, Thadani VM, Gazzaniga MS,eds. *Advances in Neurology*. Vol. 84. Philadelphia: Lippincott Williams & Wilkins; 2000:215–242

7. Helmstaedter C. Behavioral Aspects of Frontal Lobe Epilepsy. Epilepsy Behav 2001;2(5):384–395

8. Guenot M, Isnard J, Ryvlin P, et al. Neurophysiological monitoring for epilepsy surgery: the Talairach SEEG method, StereoElectroEncephaloGraphy, indications, results, complications and therapeutic applications in a series of 100 consecutive cases. Stereotact Funct Neurosurg 2001;77:29–32

9. De Almeida AN, Olivier A, Quesney F, Dubeau F, Savard G, Andermann F. Efficacy and morbidity associated with stereoencephalography using computerized tomography- or magnetic resonance imaging-guided electrode implantation. J Neurosurg 2006;104:483–487

10. Rasmussen T. Surgery of frontal lobe epilepsy. In: Purpura DP, Penry JK, Walter RD, eds. *Neurosurgical Management of the Epilepsies. Advances in Neurology*. Vol. 8. New York: Raven Press; 1975:197–205

11. Waterman K, Purves SJ, Kosaka B, Strauss E, Wada JA. An epileptic syndrome caused by mesial frontal lobe foci. Neurology 1987;37:577–582

12. Talairach J, Bancaud J, Bonis A, et al. Surgical therapy for frontal epilepsies. Adv Neurol 1992;57:707–732

13. Aykut-Bingol C, Bronen RA, Kim JH, Spencer DD, Spencer SS. Surgical outcome in occipital lobe epilepsy: implications for pathophysiology. Ann Neurol 1998;44(1):60–69

14. Zaatreh MM, Spencer DD, Thompson JL, et al. Frontal lobe tumoral epilepsy: clinical, neurophysiologic features and predictors of surgical outcome. Epilepsia 2002;43(7):727–733

15. Jeha LE, Najm I, Bingaman W, Dinner D, Widdess-Walsh P, Lüders H. Surgical outcome and prognostic factors of frontal lobe epilepsy. Brain 2007;130(Pt 2):574–584

16. Janszky J, Jokeit H, Schulz R, Hoppe M, Ebner A. EEG predicts surgical outcome in lesional frontal lobe epilepsy. Neurology 2000;54(7):1470–1476

17. Bernasconi A. Advanced MRI analysis methods for detection of focal cortical dysplasia. Epileptic Disord 2003;5(Suppl 2):S81–S84

18. Knake S, Triantafyllou C, Wald LL, et al. 3T phased array MRI improves the presurgical evaluation in focal epilepsies: a prospective study. Neurology 2005;65(7):1026–1031

19. Siegel AM, Jobst BC, Thadani VM, et al. Medically intractable, localization-related epilepsy with normal MRI: presurgical evaluation and surgical outcome in 43 patients. Epilepsia 2001;42(7):883–888

20. Chapman K, Wyllie E, Najm I, et al. Seizure outcome after epilepsy surgery in patients with normal preoperative MRI. J Neurol Neurosurg Psychiatry 2005;76(5):710–713

21. Worrell GA, So EL, Kazemi J, et al. Focal ictal beta discharge on scalp EEG predicts excellent outcome of frontal lobe epilepsy surgery. Epilepsia 2002;43(3):277–282

22. Rasmussen T. Surgical therapy of frontal lobe epilepsy. Epilepsia 1963;4:181–198

23. Rasmussen T. Characteristics of a pure culture of frontal lobe epilepsy. Epilepsia 1983;24:482–493

24. Swartz BE, Delgado-Escueta AV, Walsh GO, et al. Surgical outcomes in pure frontal lobe epilepsy and foci that mimic them. Epilepsy Res 1998;29(2):97–108

25. Schramm J, Kral T, Kurthen M, Blumcke I. Surgery to treat focal frontal lobe epilepsy in adults. Neurosurgery 2002;51(3):644–655

26. Kutsy RL, Farrell DF, Ojemann GA. Ictal patterns of neocortical seizures monitored with intracranial electrodes: correlation with surgical outcome. Epilepsia 1999;40(3):257–266

27. Helmstaedter C, Gleissner U, Zentner J, Elger CE. Neuropsychological consequences of epilepsy surgery in frontal lobe epilepsy. Neuropsychologia 1998;36(7):681–689

28. Zentner J, Hufnagel A, Pechstein U, Wolf HK, Schramm J. Functional results after resective procedures involving the supplementary motor area. J Neurosurg 1996;85(4):542–549

29. Jobst BC, Roberts DW, Thadani VM, Williamson PD. Transient postoperative neurologic deficit after supplementary motor area resection. Epilepsia 2002;43(Suppl 7):44

30. Reutens DC, Bye AM, Hopkins IJ, et al. Corpus callosotomy for intractable epilepsy: seizure outcome and prognostic factors. Epilepsia 1993;34(5):904–909

31. Roberts DW, Rayport M, Maxwell RE. Olivier A. Corpus callosotomy. In: Engel JJ, ed. *Surgical treatment of the epilepsies.* 2nd ed. New York: Raven Press, Ltd.; 1993: 519–526

32. Sass KJ, Spencer SS, Westerveld M, Spencer DD. The neuropsychology of corpus callosotomy for epilepsy. In: Bennett TL, ed. *The Neuropsychology of Epilepsy.* New York: Plenum Press; 1992:291–308

33. Fuiks KS, Wyler AR, Hermann BP, Somes G. Seizure outcome from anterior and complete corpus callosotomy. J Neurosurg 1991;74(4):573–578

34. Morrell F, Whisler WW, Bleck TP. Multiple subpial transection, a new approach to the surgical treatment of focal epilepsy. J Neurosurg 1989;70:231–239

35. Wyler AR, Wilkus RJ, Rostad SW, Vossler DG. Multiple subpial transections for partial seizures in sensorimotor cortex. Neurosurgery 1995;37(6):1122–1128

36. Schramm J, Allashkevich AF, Grunwald T. Multiple subpial transections: outcome and complications in 20 patients who did not undergo resection. J Neurosurg 2002;97:39–47

37. Hufnagel A, Zentner J, Fernandez G, Wolf HK, Schramm J, Elger CE. Multiple subpial transection for control of epileptic seizures: effectiveness and safety. Epilepsia 1997;38(6):678–688

38. Spencer SS, Schramm J, Wyler A, et al. Multiple subpial transection for intractable partial epilepsy: an international meta-analysis. Epilepsia 2002;43(2):141–145

39. Vonck K, Thadani V, Gilbert K, et al. Vagus nerve stimulation for refractory epilepsy: a transatlantic experience. J Clin Neurophysiol 2004;21(4):283–289

40. Chabardes S, Kahane P, Minotti L, Koudsie A, Hirsch E, Benabid AL. Deep brain stimulation in epilepsy with particular reference to the subthalamic nucleus. Epileptic Disord 2002;4(Suppl 3):S83–S93

41. Andrade DM, Zumsteg D, Hamani C, et al. Long-term follow-up of patients with thalamic deep brain stimulation for epilepsy. Neurology 2006;66(10):1571–1573

42. Velasco F, Velasco A, Velasco M, Jimenez F, Carrillo-Ruiz JD, Castro G. Deep brain stimulation for treatment of the epilepsies: the centromedian thalamic target. Acta Neurochir Suppl (Wien) 2007;97(Pt 2):337–342

43. Kerrigan JF, Litt B, Fisher RS, et al. Electrical stimulation of the anterior nucleus of the thalamus for the treatment of intractable epilepsy. Epilepsia 2004;45(4):346–354

44. SANTE. Stimulation of the anterior nucleus of the thalamus for epilepsy. Available at: *http://clinicaltrials.gov/ct/show/NCT00101933*

45. RNS™ System Pivotal Clinical Investigation, NeuroPace. Available at: *http://clinicaltrials.gov/ct/show/NCT00264810?order=1*

46. Kossoff EH, Ritzl EK, Politsky JM, et al. Effect of an external responsive neurostimulator on seizures and electrographic discharges during subdural electrode monitoring. Epilepsia 2004;45(12):1560–1567

47. Ajmone-Marsan C, Goldhammer L. Clinical ictal patterns and electrographic data in cases of partial seizures of frontal-central-parietal origin. In: Brazier MAB, ed. *Epilepsy: Its Phenomena in Man.* New York: Academic Press; 1973:236–260

48. Mauguiere F, Courjon J. Somatosensory epilepsy: a review of 127 cases. Brain 1978;101(2):307–332

49. Russell WR, Whitty CW. Studies in traumatic epilepsy, II: focal motor and somatic sensory fits: a study of 85 cases. J Neurol Neurosurg Psychiatry 1953;16:73–97

50. Lende RA, Popp AJ. Sensory Jacksonian seizures. J Neurosurg 1976;44:706–711

51. Siegel AM, Williamson PD, Roberts DW, Thadani VM, Darcey TM. Localized pain associated with seizures originating in the parietal lobe. Epilepsia 1999;40(7):845–855

52. Young GB, Blume WT. Painful epileptic seizures. Brain 1983;106:537–554

53. Sveinbjornsdottir S, Duncan JS. Parietal and occipital lobe epilepsy: a review. Epilepsia 1993;34(3):493–521

54. Williamson PD, Boon PA, Thadani VM, et al. Parietal lobe epilepsy: diagnostic considerations and results of surgery. Ann Neurol 1992;31:193–201

55. Salanova V, Morris H, Van Ness P, Wyllie E, Lüders H. Frontal lobe seizures: electroclinical syndromes. Epilepsia 1995;36:16–24

56. Daniel RT, Meagher-Villemure K, Farmer J-P, Andermann F, Villemure J-G. Posterior quadrantic epilepsy surgery: technical variants, surgical anatomy, and case series. Epilepsia 2007;48:1429–1437

57. Salanova V, Andermann F, Rasmussen T, Olivier A, Quesney LF. Parietal lobe epilepsy: clinical manifestations and outcome in 82 patients treated surgically between 1929 and 1988. Brain 1995;118 (Pt 3):607–627

58. Blume WT. Occipital lobe epilepsies. In: Lüders H, ed. *Epilepsy Surgery.* New York: Raven Press, Ltd.; 1991:167–171

59. Williamson PD, Thadani VM, Darcey TM, Spencer DD, Spencer SS, Mattson RH. Occipital lobe epilepsy: clinical characteristics, seizure spread patterns and results of surgery. Ann Neurol 1992;31:3–13

60. Blume WT, Wiebe S, Tapsell LM. Occipital epilepsy: lateral versus mesial. Brain 2005;128:1209–1225

61. Ajmone-Marsan C, Ralston BL. *The epileptic seizure. Its functional morphology and diagnostic significance.* Springfield, IL: Charles C. Thomas; 1957.

62. Palmini A, Andermann F, Dubeau F, et al. Occipitotemporal epilepsies: evaluation of selected patients requiring depth electrodes studies and rationale for surgical approaches. Epilepsia 1993;34:84–96

63. Lawn N, Londono A, Sawrie S, et al. Occipitoparietal epilepsy, hippocampal atrophy, and congenital developmenta; abnormalities. Epilepsia 2000;41:1546–1553

64. Kun Lee S, Young Lee S, Kim DW, Soo Lee D, Chung CK. Occipital lobe epilepsy: clinical characteristics, surgical outcome, and the role of diagnostic modalities. Epilepsia 2005;46:688–695

8 Insular Resection

Christopher R. Mascott

There has been a rebirth of interest in the insula of Reil from a surgical perspective over the past years. Insular cortex remains somewhat inaccessible because it is buried in the sylvian fissure (**Fig. 8.1**), but this area is clearly of importance in epileptogenesis and is usually considered a "paralimbic" structure.[1-5] Deep to the insular cortex lies the extreme capsule, the claustrum, the external capsule, the putamen, and the pallidum (**Fig. 8.2**). In reports regarding "insular lesions," it is common that these lesions involve these basal ganglia areas as well as the more superficial insular cortex.[6-9] Epilepsy is a common presentation of "insular" lesions. Part of the reason for this can be presumed to be related to the paralimbic nature of insular cortex. In addition, the proximity of piriform cortex and the deep endopiriform area may also play a role in epileptogenesis. The deep endopiriform nucleus was first discovered to be a highly epileptogenic area in rats and termed *area tempestas* (AT).[10-12] The existence of AT was subsequently supported in monkeys,[13] and there are some suggestions of its existence in man.[14] The presumed location in man adjacent to, or within the insular "lobe" may be a further reason for insular involvement in epileptogenesis.

In "nonlesional" limbic-type seizures, there is indirect[15,16] and more recently direct evidence of insular involvement as a component of the epileptogenic network.[17-19] Classic awake intraoperative stimulation studies of the insula resulted in sensory and autonomic phenomenology typical of complex partial seizure semiology.[20] In particular, abdominal rising sensation is thought to be associated with involvement of the amygdala and anterior insula. The stimulation of the an-

teroventral insular cortex has been shown to increase gastrointestinal motility along with other autonomic changes, including changes in heart rate. There has been a wealth of recent data, predominantly from France, on insular involvement in spontaneous seizures in patients.[18,19] This has been derived from invasive electroencephalogram (EEG) recordings during investigation for epilepsy surgery. Most of these studies of stereo-electro-encephalography (SEEG) have been performed according to the technique described by Talairach in the 1950s, in which a stereotactic angiogram is used for frame-based placement of depth electrodes via an orthogonal approach.[21] The angiogram is particularly valuable in the context of insular studies because electrodes need to safely navigate between cortical veins and the branches of the middle cerebral artery (MCA) to safely reach insular cortex. The resulting studies and publications have given us additional insight into insular function by way of stimulation studies of the insular contacts of the electrodes.[17,22,23] Recording spontaneous seizures using the same technology has highlighted insular participation not only in seizure propagation, but occasionally as a locus of primary seizure onset or of early network participation.

Insular Seizure Semiology

With the relatively recent SEEG studies documenting the semiology of seizures with insular onset or participation, **Table 8.1** establishes some criteria for clinically suspecting participation or origin of seizures in insular cortex. Unfortunately, there is considerable overlap in insular seizure

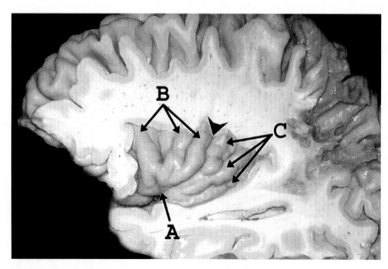

Fig. 8.1 Left cerebral hemisphere with partial frontal, parietal, and temporal lobe removals to expose the insular lobe. The insula has a fan-shaped arrangement centered on the anteroventrally located limen insula **(A)**. The insula is morphologically divided into anterior **(B)** and posterior **(C)** parts by the central insular sulcus (*arrowhead*). Histologically, the limen features three-layer allocortex. Cortex takes on six-layer features as radial distance from the limen increases and the granule cell layers become more defined.

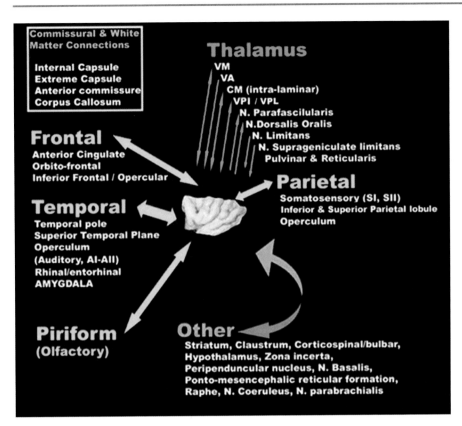

Fig. 8.2 Literature-based summary of insular connections. As with all epilepsy surgery, there is a disconnective component as well as a resective component. This should be kept in mind with regard to seizure origin in or propagation from or to the insula.

semiology with not only typical temporal lobe clinical features,[18] but also with some features thought to be classically implicating the frontal lobe.[24–27] This may in part be due to the fact that there is a histological similarity between the anteroventral insula, the posterior orbitofrontal cortex, the piriform-cortical amygdalar complex and temporopolar cortex. It may also be due to rapid seizure propagation between these areas. Traditionally, nausea, vomiting (ictus emeticus), and autonomic features have been thought to be indicative of insular but also amygdalar involvement.[28] Typical "temporal lobe" semiology such as rising abdominal and thoracic sensation is in fact quite "amygdalo-insular."[29] Throat constriction or abdominal discomfort at seizure onset may be

somewhat more suggestive of insular origin.[19,30] More recently, nocturnal hypermotor seizures, previously thought to be typically of frontal lobe origin, can have an insular origin on SEEG.[26] The search for clinically suggestive features of insular seizures is important in evaluating the necessity for invasive EEG studies with insular coverage.

Insular Anatomy and Physiology

Insular cortex in man is completely hidden within the sylvian fissure, covered by frontoorbital, parietal, and temporal opercular cortices. First described by Johann Christian Reil in 1809, this cortical "island" is triangular in shape and is

Table 8.1 Clinical Correlates for Seizure Origin in Insular Cortex

Semiology	Classic Frontal Lobe Localization	Classic Temporal Lobe Localization	Possible Insular Correlate
Abdominal rising sensation	No	Amygdala	Anteroventral
Abdominal pain	No	Amygdala	Anterodorsal
Throat sensation	No	(Amygdala)	Anterodorsal
Orofacial somatosensory	No	Parietal operculum	Anterior and posterior
Painful somatosenory	No	No	Anterior and posterior
Dysarthria	Motor/premotor/ supplementary motor	No	Anterior and posterior
Hypermotor seizures (+/– nocturnal)	Orbito- and mesiofrontal	No	Anterior and posterior

surrounded by a "circular sulcus" that can also be divided into anterior, superior, and inferior components bordering orbitofrontal, frontoparietal, and temporal opercula, respectively (**Fig. 8.1**). An oblique central insular sulcus (which parallels and is most often an extension of the central sulcus proper) separates the insula into an anterior component consisting of three (to four) short anterior gyrii and the posterior insula consisting of two long gyrii. There are also usually two short transverse gyrii at the orbitofrontal junction. Based on its connections and cytoarchitectonic characteristics, insular cortex has been classified as a paralimbic structure by Mufson and Mesulam, along the same lines as orbitofrontal, temporopolar, and cingulate cortex.[1-4,31] There is immediate proximity between the piriform olfactory cortex (POC) and the limen of the insula (which constitutes the anteroinferior corner of the insula), both areas featuring three-layer allocortex. The cytoarchitectonic features of the cortex progress to six-layer neocortex with increasing distance from the POC with a transitional cortex where the granule cell layer is not yet defined (dysgranular cortex). Within the insula, this change in histology occurs in a radial fashion as distance from the limen increases. As a consequence, the anteroventral aspect of the insula, in closest proximity to the limen insula (LI) is histologically (and functionally) the most "limbic." **Figure 8.2** summarizes the neuroanatomical literature on insular connections. This is indeed the area of the insula with demonstrated autonomic connections and where awake stimulation mapping by Penfield and Faulk has elicited abdominal sensations, increases in gastrointestinal motility, and other autonomic responses.[20] Changes in heart rate have also been elicited from this area, with suggestions that there may be a right insula- left insula difference in cardiac response.[32,33] It is noteworthy that the insula has been implicated as having a possible role in cardiac arrhythmia and death in stroke and as a possible mechanism for sudden unexpected death in epilepsy (SUDEP).[34-39] Regarding the latter, it has been postulated that epileptic activity involving the anteroventral insula may lead to cardiac arrest and SUDEP. It is of surgical importance to be aware of these autonomic effects because cardiac and blood pressure changes can occur during surgery in these areas. Within the context of hemispherectomy variants, these autonomic effects have been implicated as a possible source of instability during surgery of which anesthesiologists should be aware.[40]

Human awake mapping with SEEG has demonstrated gustatory responses in the more dorsal anterior insula.[30] In the posterior insular cortex, sensory responses were evoked including pain responses. This is concordant with many functional imaging (positron emission tomography [PET] and functional magnetic resonance imaging [fMRI]) studies that show insular cortex activation in response to noxious stimuli.[41-45] Conversely, dysarthria but no true dysphasia was elicited by SEEG stimulation.[30] There is considerable literature in functional imaging and stimulation mapping that suggests some speech localization in the insular cortex in the dominant hemisphere.[46,47] That any primary speech

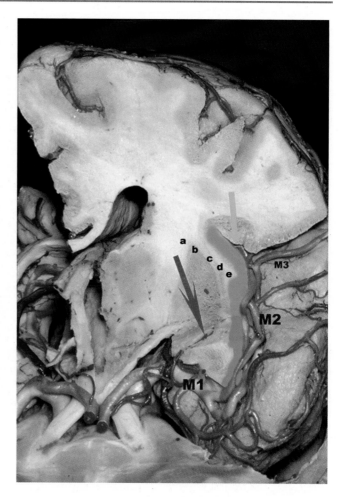

Fig. 8.3 Coronal view of left insular anatomy. **(A)** Internal capsule/corona radiate. **(B)** Putamen. **(C)** External capsule. **(D)** Claustrum. **(E)** Extreme capsule. Insular cortex is highlighted in bright green. Segments of the middle cerebral artery are labeled as M1, M2, and M3. A lateral lenticulostriate branch arising from the M1 segment is dissected out (*red arrow*). A distal perforating artery from the M2 branch is also illustrated (*blue arrow*).

function may be localized in insular cortex is more difficult to establish because surgical resection in the dominant hemisphere affects opercular cortex, where there is definite speech localization and open stimulation studies probably activate white matter deep to insular cortex that may lead to disconnective types of speech disturbance or motor speech interference.[48-51]

Vascular Anatomy and the Insular Lobe

As previously mentioned, access to the insula is restricted by its deep location and by its close relationship to the MCA (**Fig. 8.3**). The insular cortex is vascularized exclusively by the MCA ,and the underlying basal ganglia and internal capsule are supplied to a major degree by the M1 segment of the MCA via the lateral lenticulostriate arteries (LSAs).[52-56] These usually do not extend as far laterally as the actual insular cortex, which is supplied by perforating arteries arising from the overlying M2 segments of the MCA with occasional branches off the distal M1 to the area of the limen before dividing into M2 segments in this location. There are also occasional branches from the opercular M3 segments coursing back to the insular cortex. It is particularly noteworthy that an M2 branch is consistently found in the central sulcus, which subsequently supplies the central sulcus proper, thus the pre- and postcentral gyri. It is therefore particularly important to avoid compromising this artery.

Several detailed anatomical studies have reviewed the vascular anatomy and supply of the insula. From a surgical perspective, it should be noted that a motor deficit from insular surgery that does not directly lesion the internal capsule is most likely to be the result of a vascular injury at one of three levels:

1. The lateral LSAs arise from the M1 segment and enter the basal ganglia via the anterior perforated substance. Because these arteries also supply the internal capsule, vascular compromise can lead to hemiparesis from a vascular capsular insult.
2. Perforating branches from the M2 supply the insular cortex. Anatomical studies estimate that 85 to 90% of these perforating arteries are short, supplying insular cortex and underlying extreme capsule only. Up to 10% of perforators extend further reaching the claustrum and extreme capsule. The functionally worrisome long perforators compose only 3 to 5% of perforators but can go on to supply part of the internal capsule and corona radiata, especially posteriorly.[52]
3. The artery of the central sulcus courses through the central sulcus of the insula. Injury can lead to vascular compromise of primary motor-sensory cortex.

Risk Assessment of Surgical Approaches to the Insula

Based on the previously described anatomical and physiological features, a risk assessment of surgery of the insula can be attempted. In the context of surgery for epilepsy, this must be weighed against the chances of controlling seizures with the planned surgery to establish a likely risk-benefit ratio. Because there are still many unknown aspects regarding insular function, an absolute risk assessment is not possible. The current knowledge with regard to results of insular surgery to control seizures is even less clear.

In the risk assessment of surgical approaches to the insula, it is useful to differentiate between lesional surgery and nonlesional surgery. Lesions that are considered "insular" in the literature most often refer to those not only involving insular cortex but also deeper underlying structures including the basal ganglia. The risks of surgical approaches to these areas is different from an approach to the more superficial insular cortex alone, in that there is additional risk of a motor deficit by direct injury to the internal capsule or

by vascular injury to the same by compromise of the lateral LSAs. This compounds the motor risks of superficial insular approaches where the long perforating arteries from the M2 branches or artery of the central sulcus are at risk.

Assessment of risk to speech function is not as straightforward as that for motor function. Clearly, in the dominant hemisphere, there is a speech risk in the approach itself because frontal, parietal, and temporal opercular cortices are the classic locus for primary speech function. Therefore, any resection, retraction, manipulation, or vascular compromise to opercular cortex in the dominant hemisphere carries a risk to speech function. Stimulation mapping for speech function can help lower risk to speech by helping to define opercular areas lacking obvious language function. Avoidance of resection or retraction of more eloquent opercular cortex should decrease risk to speech.[7,8] As previously mentioned, evidence of primary speech localization to insular cortex itself is less convincing, although several authors who have experience with insular surgery recommend stimulation mapping of the insula itself.[51,57,58] Others do not.[7,59] Some interference with speech function may be more related to a disconnective effect at the level of the external capsule than an actual cortical insular lesion. This author prefers to consider awake speech mapping on a selective, case-by-case basis.

Risk to higher cognitive function is the most difficult of all to discuss regarding insular surgery because the insula is the seat of multimodal integration. Anteroventrally there is evidence of autonomic processing in close conjunction with the amygdalar complex (behavior, motivation, and learning). Dorsally and posteriorly, sensory (including pain), motor, and vestibule-auditory connections exist. Functional imaging also shows insular in the context of more complex auditory processing, pitch perception, and singing.[60–63] In the context of dominant hemisphere insular infarct, loss of verbal memory has been described, but these lesions are unlikely to have involved insular cortex in isolation.[46,64–66] Overall, higher cognitive effects of insular surgery cannot be predicted at present.

Lesional Epilepsy Surgery and the Insula

Because this chapter addresses surgery of the insula to control epilepsy (i.e., chronic intractable seizures), surgery for other indications will not be addressed. Vascular, tumor, and malformative pathologies will be addressed briefly from a practical perspective based on this author's experience and biases.

Vascular

Although arteriovenous malformations (AVMs) that involve the sylvian fissure and the insula can present with chronic seizures, the treatment of these is beyond the scope of this chapter because surgery for AVMs alone is not strictly epilepsy surgery, and other modalities including interventional neuroradiology and radiosurgery play an increasingly important role in AVM management.

Cavernous angiomas, on the other hand, frequently present as "lesional epilepsy" cases and can be localized to the insular cortex or insular lobe.[67-72] There are no large series of insular cavernoma resections for epilepsy, but surgical feasibility of resection has been documented in case reports and series where epilepsy was not the predominant presentation. **Figures 8.4 and 8.5** illustrate some of the surgical considerations involved. This patient has a cavernoma centered deep to the limen insula and has had daily seizures for 12 years. Although the cavernoma does not directly involve insular cortex, there are signal abnormalities in the overlying limen probably due to remote microhemorrhages (**Fig. 8.5**). This patient has not yet had surgery and has had five neurosurgical opinions. She has a high level of function. It was felt that lesion resection would probably improve her daily seizures, but she does have nine other very small cavernous angiomas in other less epileptogenic locations. Video EEG captured 16 events, eight of which showed no EEG changes, the other eight featured left frontotemporal rhythmic theta discharge. Clinical features included initial hyperventilation and frequent gelastic outbursts. A sodium amytal test suggested that major speech localization was in the left hemisphere (but the test was suboptimal). The angiogram performed for the amytal test did not disclose any abnormal displacement of the lateral LSAs or other arteries. Based on this and the three-dimensional (3-D) reconstructions in **Fig. 8.4**, the LSAs are presumed to be draped on the back side of the lesion and particular care would be necessary in this area. Injury to the LSAs represents the major risk to motor function in this case because the lesion is remote from the internal capsule and corona radiata. The artery of the central sulcus and distal M2 perforators should not be subject to much manipulation. Whereas it is unclear whether speech representation in the insula is of significance, circumnavigating the opercular cortex to reach the lesion and LA carry an unequivocal risk to speech. In this context, awake speech mapping would be of value to determine speech localization with a view to selecting the functionally safest approach.

In **Figs. 8.4 and 8.5**, three different angles of approach are illustrated as A, B and C. Approach A is subfrontal and would

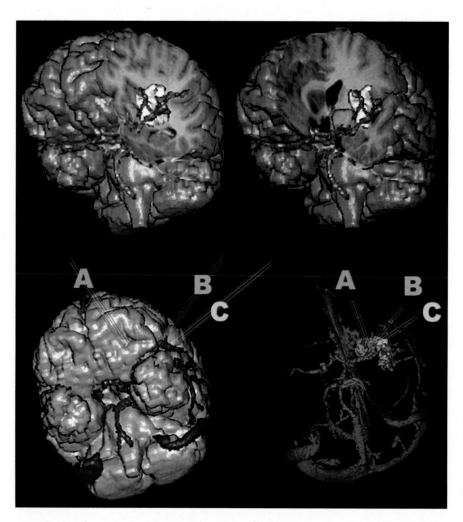

Fig. 8.4 MRI 3-D reconstructions of a patient with a 12-year seizure history and a cavernous angiomas (*in green*) deep to the limen insula. Venous anatomy is in blue; arterial anatomy is in red. **(A–C)** Different surgical angles of approach as detailed in the text.

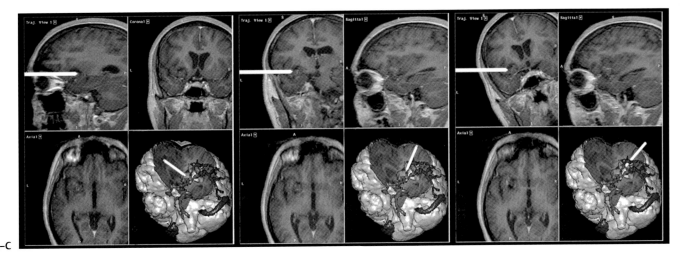

Fig. 8.5 **(A–C)** Same patient as in **Fig. 8.4,** now illustrating MRI trajectory view reformats for approaches.

have the advantage of avoiding manipulation of Broca's area of the frontal operculum. It is the longest approach, however, and in isolation would not permit adequate visualization of the MCA and the LSAs from the M1 segment in particular. The lesion does abut posterior orbitofrontal cortex, which may contribute to the epileptogenic network. Approach B, an anterior transsylvian approach would allow good microsurgical exposure, but manipulation of Broca's area is most likely. This author has avoided self-retaining retractors whenever possible for the past 10 years. Direct retraction on any cortex, but especially highly eloquent cortex, can be detrimental both in the short and long term. Lang et al report a case in their insular tumor series where dominant frontoopercular retraction led to speech dysfunction during awake mapping, which was alleviated by removing the retractor. Approach C represents a more direct transinsular approach to the lesion more removed from presumed Broca's area, but it would be more likely to lead to manipulation of M2 branches, with lesser visualization of the LSAs. A fourth approach (not illustrated) could be a low temporal transamygdalar approach. This approach would avoid opercular cortex, but it would involve removing presumably normal amygdala.

Having pondered the above possibilities, this author would recommend a full frontotemporal craniotomy to allow the flexibility of a change of approach during surgery (the goal is to be minimally invasive to brain, not to skull). Speech mapping would be an advantage, if the patient would tolerate this. Forty-five-degree head position, microsurgical splitting of the sylvian fissure, optimized image guidance, avoidance of self-retaining retractors, identification and protection of the LSAs, resection of the LA along with the cavernous angioma would be the other recommendations. Electrocorticography (ECoG) to specifically address whether resection should be extended to include a limited portion of posterior orbitofrontal cortex is also a consideration. Overall,

the level of risk is nonnegligible but potentially acceptable. Conversely, seizure control benefits seem likely, but difficult to quantify.

Tumor

Over the past 15 years, several reports have detailed strategies to approaching "insular" tumors. It must be noted that the vast majority of these cases involved lesions that extended far beyond the insular cortex to involve deeper structures including the basal ganglia. It is remarkable that the majority of reports stem from "tumor" rather than "epilepsy" surgeons, although acute or chronic seizures seem to be the most common presentation of these lesions. Some series include several "high-grade" gliomas that usually present more acutely with new onset seizures or neurological deficit. It is debatable whether the overall outcome of these more malignant tumors warrants a radical surgical approach, and this topic is beyond the scope of this chapter. Surgery of insular tumors for seizure control is usually restricted to nonenhancing or minimally enhancing tumors of low-grade behavior (although some may show histological evidence of anaplasia), and these shall be addressed here.

In the first large series of limbic and paralimbic tumors (including insular tumors), Yasargil and Reeves reported a seizure-free rate of 84%.[7] Subsequently, several series have been reported, but it is difficult to ascertain how intractable seizures were preoperatively because most reports discuss risk-benefit ratios related to completeness of resection.[8,9,73–75] Overall, there is an impression that better lesionectomy leads to better seizure control.[75] It is important to note, as first pointed out and classified by Yasargil and Reeves,[7] that insular tumors may be "purely" insular (this includes deeper involvement), may be insuloopercular, and may involve other lobes, limbic or paralimbic structures. Similar additional classifications have also been introduced.[73] The surgical implications of tumor infiltration of opercular cortex are obvious, especially in the dominant hemisphere, providing additional incentive for stimulation mapping if these opercular areas are to be resected.

Operative Technique

All of the previously discussed concerns regarding microsurgically defining and respecting the vascular supply (LSAs, central artery, M2 perforators) apply to tumors. Avoidance of retraction when possible and stimulation mapping in the dominant hemisphere are also advisable. In addition, white matter stimulation mapping (under local or general anesthesia) can be considered if the tumor extends to the corona radiata or external capsule. Lang et al reviewed their own experience and provide useful suggestions with regard to using the periinsular sulci and the LSA branches as landmarks to define tumor margins.[8]

In addition to the recommendations above, this author has found the following to be of practical use:

1. Image guidance for conceptual planning preoperatively and optimized accuracy for surgery using skull-implanted fiducials. Fluid-attenuated inversion recovery (FLAIR) MRI sequences are often useful in nonenhancing tumors and can be fused to other sequences.
2. Wide microsurgical splitting of the sylvian fissure. Using large Merocel® pattie strips (Medtronic Xomed, Inc., North Jacksonville, FL) "accordion folded" in lieu of retractors. These swell up gently with irrigation and tend not to adhere to cortex or white matter.
3. Attempting to define superior and inferior tumor planes with image guidance before tumor resection and shift. Again Merocel® pattie strips are left circumferentially in place along these planes.
4. Yasargil has recommended sparing M2 perforating arteries that may be long perforators.[7] This author has found it difficult to determine which perforators these may be. As a precaution, I usually avoid bipolar cautery on any arterial branch altogether unless it is bleeding from a free end. During tumor aspiration (by suction or sometimes ultrasonic aspiration), when bleeding obscures visibility, the area is gently packed with large thrombin-soaked Merocel® patties and resection is performed elsewhere. After a period of time, when the patties are removed, hemorrhage is usually controlled and/or bleeding end-arteries can be better identified and cauterized. The same principle applies to the LSAs, which may also be difficult to identify within the tumor. It is quite common to find the MCA itself imbedded in tumor (**Figs. 8.6 and 8.7**). By adhering to the vascular principles above, the author has not usually found this to be a limiting factor.
5. With regard to vascular manipulation, the author has employed papaverine soaked Gelfoam (Pfizer Inc., New York, NY) on MCA branches to avoid spasm. Dilute hydrogen

peroxide is often used for hemostasis in neurosurgery. The mechanism of action is presumably through vasoconstriction of smaller vessels. This author has observed severe spasm in LSAs due to H_2O_2 in a different (noninsular surgery) context (unpublished observations), and advises strongly against using H_2O_2 in insular surgery.

Figures 8.6 and 8.7 show results in three selected patients with insular tumors.

Dysplasia

When discussing "lesional" versus "nonlesional" epilepsy cases, it is difficult to know where to place cortical malformations. In cortical dysplasia, the MRI-visible lesion may only represent a part of a more widespread histological anomaly, and related surgical planning should probably best be pursued in a similar manner to that on "nonlesional" cases.

Nonlesional Epilepsy Surgery and the Insula

The removal of insular cortex for seizure control has had a recent surge of interest do to the SEEG-documented insular involvement in what were thought to be typical temporal or frontal seizures. On the other hand, only sporadic resections of insular cortex have been reported in recent years.[19,30,76] The last series of insular resections was performed in the context of temporal lobe resections when residual epileptiform activity was found in insular cortex. This was reported by Silfvenius et al in 1964 with previous reports by Guillaume et al.[15,77] Overall, it is unclear at present what the contemporary risk-benefit ratio would be when performing insular corticectomies.

Electrocorticography (ECoG)

Silfvenius et al looked at a series of patients from the Montreal Neurological Institute in whom epileptiform activity was seen in insular cortex when performing intraoperative ECoG after temporal lobe resection.[15] Of these patients, 58 had removal of part or all of accessible insular cortex, whereas 48 did not have insular resection despite the presence of epileptiform activity there. Overall, there was no significant difference between the seizure outcome whether insular cortex was removed or not, although the overall seizure outcome was less favorable in both groups compared with that in patients with no insular epileptiform activity. Paradoxically, better outcomes were obtained in patients who had partial insular removal with subsequent persistent spikes than when no spikes were found. Overall, predicating insular resection on intraoperative spikes alone seems not to improve outcome in this and previous studies. This author has recorded ECoG from the insula in lesional and nonlesional cases, more as an academic exercise, and this has not influenced surgery. Because the majority of this

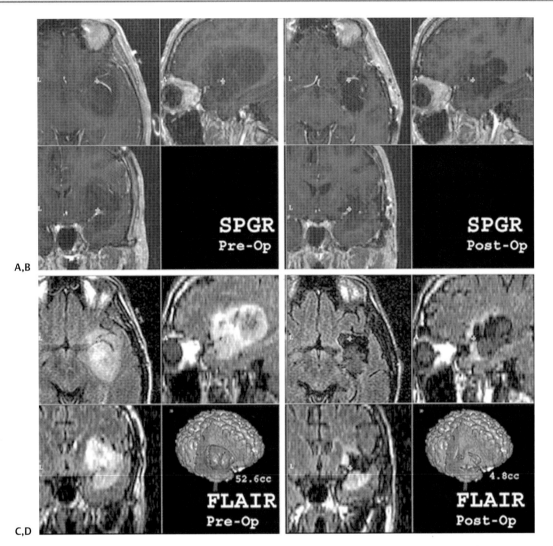

Fig. 8.6 **(A–D)** Left-handed patient with right-sided insular tumor presenting with a 9-month history of very intractable seizures. Amytal testing did not suggest significant right-sided speech localization (surgery was subsequently done under general anesthesia). The (nonenhancing) tumor is particularly well defined on MRI FLAIR sequences both before surgery **(C)** and at 6-month follow-up **(D)**. The FLAIR sequences have been fused to the volumetric SPGR sequences illustrated in the **(A)** and **(B)**. Note that the MCA is encased by tumor (small crosshairs). Following the recommendations in the text, this did not impede surgical resection. A wide split of the sylvian fissure was performed for access. No self-retaining retraction was used, as can be inferred by the absence of postretraction opercular gliosis in the postoperative FLAIR sequences. The patient had no adverse events and insisted on returning to work (against medical advice) on postoperative day 5. He had no seizures in the first year of follow-up (he was subsequently lost to follow-up) despite early cessation of anticonvulsants (also against medical advice). Histology was grade II oligodendroglioma.

author's temporal lobe surgeries involve nontranssylvian selective mesiotemporal resections, ECoG from insular cortex has been rare.

Invasive Studies

Most invasive (SEEG) studies of the insula have come from France (and Italy). From a technical/surgical perspective, there is definitely an advantage to the classic Talairach methodology for stereotactic placement of depth electrodes in insular cortex because direct angiographic visualization of the MCA and cortical veins should make electrode placement safer. Alternately, electrodes can be placed obliquely (**Fig. 8.8**). With the current technological improvements of CT angiography, incorporation of this with optimized (skull-implanted fiducial or stereotactic frame) image guidance may provide a reasonable alternative. Originally, reports of insular involvement, either primarily or early in temporal lobe–type seizures was reported as a poor prognosticator for temporal lobe surgery and a source for possible failure. Overall, seizure onset in the insular contacts of the electrodes was predictive of an unfavorable outcome from temporal lobe surgery alone, whereas early propagation to the insula from the temporal lobe did not imply a lesser prognosis.[18,30]

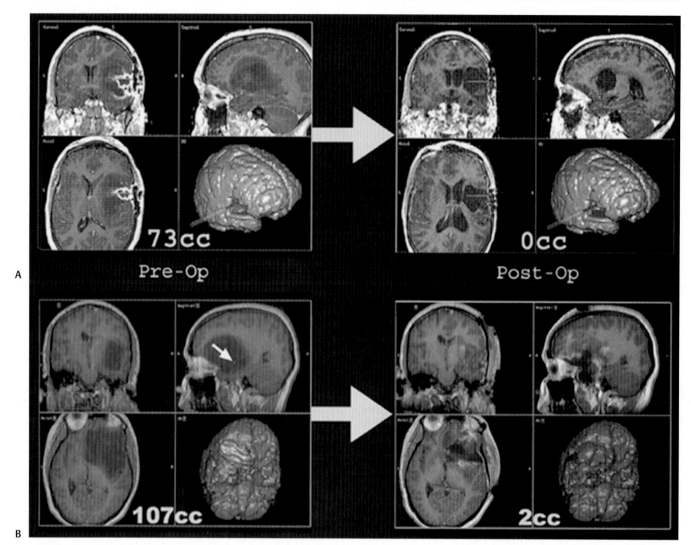

Fig. 8.7 Two additional cases of insular tumors are illustrated. **(A)** The patient presented with several months of simple partial seizures (sensory) and had undergone a frame-guided resection attempt by another surgeon. This was a nonenhancing tumor, and histology from the first surgery came back as a low-grade astrocytoma. The patient was referred shortly after surgery for consideration of further resection. The second surgery was 10 days after the first to avoid scarring. The left upper MRI images show the residual hypointense tumor. The area of bright contrast enhancement delineates the extent of the first surgical resection. Enhancement is due to the known postsurgical blood-brain barrier breakdown, which is maximal at 10 days. Immediate postoperative images had extensive movement artifacts. The postoperative illustration to the left (patient A) was after 1 year.

There is additional atrophy probably due to radiation, which was recommended after areas of anaplasia were found when performing the more radical procedure. There were no postoperative deficits. The patient in **(B)** presented with convulsive seizures. As in **Fig. 8.6,** the MCA can again be visualized encased by tumor. The tumor extends beyond the insula and basal ganglia to involve opercular cortex and orbitofrontal cortex. In the dominant hemisphere, awake speech mapping of the tumor-infiltrated operculum would have been a consideration. This patient was operated on under general anesthesia. There was no postoperative neurological deficit, but hospital stay was protracted by a fever of unknown origin (all cultures negative) probably due to hypothalamic dysregulation (see tumor location). Histology grade II astrocytoma.

Radiofrequency Lesions

To have a therapeutic option in seizures that appeared to have a primary onset in insular cortex in SEEG studies, Guénot et al have used the SEEG electrode implanted for epilepsy to make radiofrequency lesions in the areas of insular cortex where seizure onset was seen (**Fig. 8.9**).[78] This is an interesting option for a selective approach to the insular cortex, although it remains too early to tell whether this will have true impact on surgical outcome.

Resective Surgery

Many aspects of resection of insular cortex must be extrapolated from older literature, from current views on insular function and epileptogenesis, and from recent selective attempts at insular resection. To this author's knowledge there are few reports or cases of resection of insular cortex in isolation.[79] Resection is usually in conjunction with temporal lobe resections or other resective or disconnective surgery including hemispherectomy.

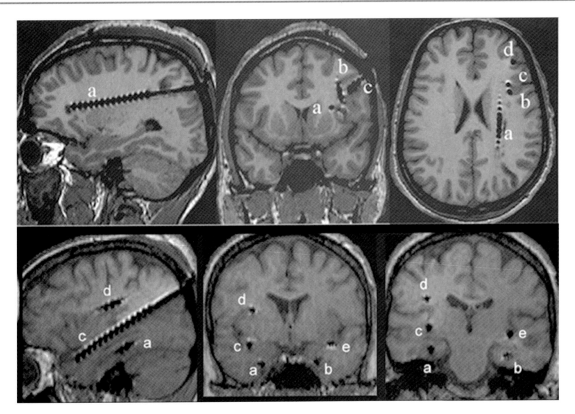

Fig. 8.8 Many electrodes that have targeted the insula during SEEG investigations have been placed using a standard orthogonal "Talairach" approach. MRIs with electrodes in position are usually not obtained in this situation (Marc Guénot, personal communication). An alternative oblique strategy of depth electrode placement is illustrated in this figure. (Courtesy of Santiago Gil Robles and Philippe Coubes.) Upper three images: (a) occipito-insular electrode, (b–d) frontal electrodes; lower three images: (a, b) hippocampal electrodes, (c) right inferior insular electrode; (d) right superior insular electrode, (e) left inferior insular electrode.

Insula and Hemispherectomy

In candidates for hemispherectomy, residual or recurrent postoperative seizures with clinical autonomic features (drooling, abdominal discomfort) suggestive of origin in the residual insular cortex have been reported, prompting a retrospective review of seizure outcome in hemispherectomy without versus with insular corticectomy.[80–82] Among the 56 patients studied, 30 had insular cortex removed, the rest did not. Only a minority had intraoperative ECoG recordings. Essentially, there was no significant difference in seizure outcome whether insular removal was performed or not. Subsequent cases systematically included insular removal

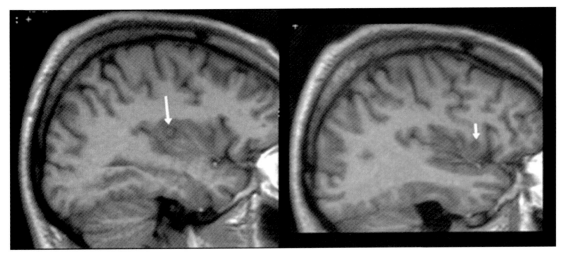

Fig. 8.9 In 2004, Guénot et al published results of radiofrequency (RF) lesions delivered by SEEG electrodes. Three of the 20 cases included lesions in insular cortex. This MRI shows two RF lesions in insular cortex. (Courtesy of Marc Guénot and Jean Isnard.)

on an empirical basis because in the context of functional or anatomical hemispherectomy (including periinsular hemispherotomy), there is no additional functional risk in doing so. It should be noted that some functional hemispherectomy variants, most notably the Delalande hemispherotomy variant, include insular disconnection as part of the original procedure.[83,84]

Operative Technique

This author has technical experience in complete insular cortex removal in the context of periinsular hemispherotomy (**Fig. 8.10**). From this experience, the following technical points can be highlighted:

1. If insular corticectomy is intended, it is easier to split the sylvian fissure primarily. Even if removal of overlying opercular cortex is planned, the usually safe subpial aspiration of this cortex protects the MCA branches, but these are then sandwiched between two layers of relatively hemorrhagic pia mater. The opercular pia needs to be subsequently lifted to expose the MCA and insula, leading to more arterial manipulation than if the sylvian fissure had been split primarily.

2. With a microscope and microsurgical technique, the perforating arteries can be quite well visualized, and usually preserved. Only a minority of perforators supply deeper structures.

3. A very superficial cortical removal is all that is intended in this context. This is not tumor surgery, and small residual areas of gray matter along a perforating artery are probably functionally disconnected.

Obviously, risk to function of insular corticectomy cannot be assessed in the context of hemispherectomy. Most authors cite a 20.6% hemiparesis rate when referring to the 1964 Silfvenius et al article.[15] In the actual article, these motor deficits had cleared in 75% of patients by the time of hospital discharge (usually ~10 days at the time). This would be more indicative of a 5% motor complication rate. Keeping in mind that surgery at the time was performed without a microscope and involved five different surgeons, contemporary microsurgical technique should be able to improve on these figures. With regard to speech dysfunction at the time of hospital discharge, this was documented in 5% of the insulectomy patients and in 17% of the noninsulectomy (control) patients (18% insulectomy, 36% noninsulectomy when assuming the surgery was in the dominant hemisphere). This would im-

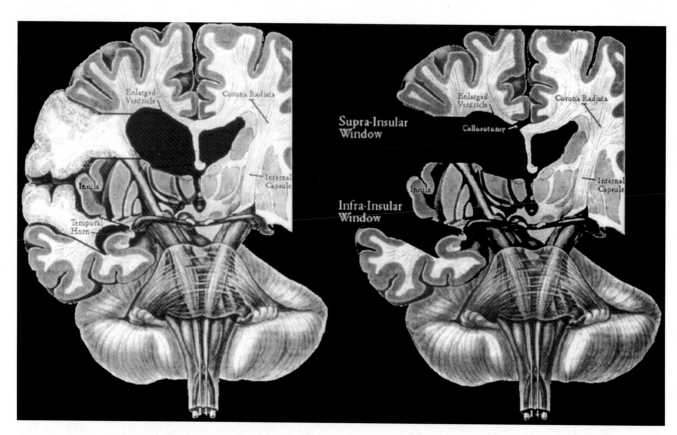

Fig. 8.10 Schematic illustration of periinsular hemispherotomy. As discussed in the text, the exposure of the insula is maximal, but insular cortex resection is facilitated by prior sylvian exposure as opposed to subpial opercular resection. (From Villemure JG, Mascott CR. Periinsular hemispherotomy: surgical principles and anatomy. Neurosurgery 1995;37:975—981. Reprinted with permission.)

ply speech dysfunction associated with dominant temporal lobe resection and not suggest additional speech dysfunction from dominant insular resection. More sophisticated speech processing deficits cannot be extrapolated from this study.

Temporal Plus Epilepsy (TPE)

Successful surgery is not only related to surgical technique, but is predicated on appropriate indications. In this respect, insular corticectomy is a moving target, for clear indications remain to be determined. When discussing insular epilepsy, the concept of temporal plus epilepsy (TPE) introduced by the French groups in Lyon and Grenoble is very important.[84] They basically attribute failure in temporal lobe epilepsy surgery to the subgroup of patients who have seizure onset in extratemporal paralimbic structures including the insular cortex (as documented in SEEG studies in up to 10% of apparently typical TLE).[18] More recently, the same may be said about the frontal lobe, in that frontal lobe "type" hypermotor seizures have also been shown to originate in the insula on some occasions.[26]

Limbic, Paralimbic, and Neocortical Epileptic Networks

The field being complex, this is the author's personal view. The concept of an epilepsy "focus" seems somewhat dated and unrealistic. Seizure origin can occasionally be quite "focal" around a small lesion or in a select area of cortical dysplasia. In the limbic system, and probably elsewhere, things are probably a little more complex. Defining an "epileptogenic zone" is a more contemporary way of looking at surgically treatable epilepsy, but the concept means different things to different authors and does not always correspond to the "what to be resected" zone.[86,87] Also, a zone implies

contiguity of structure, which may be the case, but not always. This author has found it useful to reason in conceptual terms of epileptogenic networks and view surgery in terms of network disruption (by resection, disconnection, and eventually stimulation and other means).[88]

From a functional and histological standpoint, the antero-ventral insula closest to the limen is a paralimbic structure, as is the posterior orbitofrontal cortex and the temporopolar cortex (**Fig. 8.11**). All of these areas can be involved to varying degrees in any individual patient's epileptogenic network, and this should be kept in mind. From a personal standpoint, I would consider SEEG investigations to include the insula in the presence of very suggestive semiology (laryngeal constriction, unpleasant sensory phenomena, or abdominal pain). Seizures can be quite typically temporal on scalp EEG and in semiology and be apparently associated with MRI evidence of mesiotemporal sclerosis, and yet still originate entirely or in part from insular cortex. Nevertheless, this author does not see the justification for systematic invasive monitoring at this time. Insular abnormalities seen on MR spectroscopy (MRS) in TLE do not seem to adversely affect the outcome of temporal lobe surgery.

This author is quite partial to ictal SPECT studies during video EEG workups. It is not uncommon on an early injection to see hyperfixation in the amygdaloinsular area. It remains a subject of controversy whether the amygdala needs to be removed at the time of temporal lobe surgery (whether as part of selective mesial or of more extensive anterior temporal resections).[89,90] This author usually attempts a more radical amygdalar resection when patients have pronounced autonomic semiology and/or amygdaloinsular hyperfixation during ictal SPECT studies. As part of a radical amygdalar approach, it is possible to remove a small area of ventral insula centered around the limen (**Fig. 8.12**). This has not led to any detectable neurological or neuropsychological deficit in the

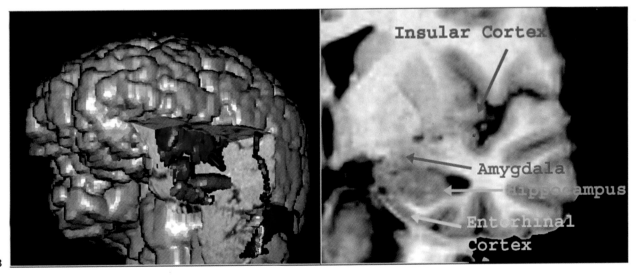

A, B

Fig. 8.11 This figure illustrates the proximity and anatomical relationships of some of the limbic and paralimbic structures discussed.

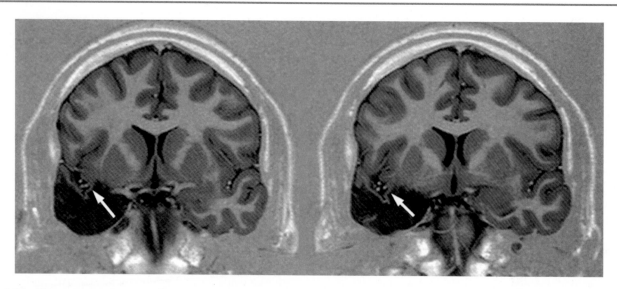

Fig. 8.12 This postoperative coronal inversion recovery sequence MRI illustrates the feasibility of a limited anteroventral insular corti-cectomy (*arrows*) when performing a radical amygdalar removal.

dominant or nondominant hemispheres. Whether this improves outcomes cannot be determined at this point. Without prior SEEG documentation of insular onset, which the author could not justify in the face of quite typical unilateral TLE, this maneuver must be considered empirical.

It is the author's conviction that seizures arising in the posterior and dorsal insula are more akin to neocortical epilepsy than to limbic epilepsy, and represent a distinct entity.

Future Perspectives for the Assessment of Insular Seizures

Should we be assessing all temporal and frontal lobe cases with invasive monitoring including insular electrodes? At present we have limited experience on how to address insular seizures, when documented. The trend has certainly been to perform less invasive studies with the advent of many sophisticated imaging studies, including MRI, MRS, fMRI, EEG-fMRI, magnetic source imaging/ magnetoencephalography (MEG), and nuclear medicine studies. I find the prospect of high-resolution ictal SPECT particularly interesting. In summary, it will be interesting to specifically keep the insula in mind when employing emerging technology and to consider the risk versus benefit ration of SEEG studies in-cluding the insula in selected cases. With regard to lesional insular surgery, there may be an advantage to intraoperative imaging (ultrasound, MRI, CT), but residual nonenhancing tumor may be difficult to distinguish on intraoperative images.

Conclusion

The Insula is an important and, until recently, relatively neglected contributor to intractable seizure disorders. As we recognize situations that call for intervention in this hidden cortical area, surgical options will become more prevalent.

Acknowledgments

The author is indebted to Professor Marc Guénot in Lyon for input and discussions, to Dr. Robert Zatorre of the neuropsychology department at the Montreal Neurological Institute, to Professor Patrick Cheynes in Neurosurgery/Anatomy in Toulouse for brain dissections, and to Dr. Santiago Gil Robles and Professor Philippe Coubes in Montpellier for discussions and illustrations of insular depth electrodes. Finally, a thank you to Professor Jean-Guy Villemure for many things, including getting me interested in the insula in Montreal over 15 years ago.

References

1. Mesulam MM, Mufson EJ. Insula of the old world monkey, III: efferent cortical output and comments on function. J Comp Neurol 1982;212(1):38–52
2. Mesulam MM, Mufson EJ. Insula of the old world monkey. I. Architectonics in the insulo-orbito-temporal component of the paralimbic brain. J Comp Neurol 1982;212(1):1–22
3. Mufson EJ, Mesulam MM. Insula of the old world monkey. II: Afferent cortical input and comments on the claustrum. J Comp Neurol 1982;212(1):23–37
4. Mufson EJ, Mesulam MM, Pandya DN. Insular interconnections with the amygdala in the rhesus monkey. Neuroscience 1981;6(7):1231–1248

5. Augustine JR. Circuitry and functional aspects of the insular lobe in primates including humans. Brain Res Brain Res Rev 1996;22(3):229–244

6. Duffau H, Capelle L, Lopes M, et al. The insular lobe: physiopathological and surgical considerations. Neurosurgery 2000;47(4):801–810

7. Yasargil MG, Reeves JD. Tumours of the limbic and paralimbic systems. Acta Neurochir (Wien) 1992;118(1–2):40–52

8. Lang FF, Olansen NE, DeMonte F, et al. Surgical resection of intrinsic insular tumors: complication avoidance. J Neurosurg 2001;95(4):638–650

9. Zentner J, Meyer B, Stangl A, et al. Intrinsic tumors of the insula: a prospective surgical study of 30 patients. J Neurosurg 1996;85(2):263–271

10. Halonen T, Tortorella A, Zrebeet H, et al. Posterior piriform and perirhinal cortex relay seizures evoked from the area tempestas: role of excitatory and inhibitory amino acid receptors. Brain Res 1994;652(1):145–148

11. Doherty J, Gale K, Eagles DA. Evoked epileptiform discharges in the rat anterior piriform cortex: generation and local propagation. Brain Res 2000;861(1):77–87

12. Piredda S, Gale K. A crucial epileptogenic site in the deep prepiriform cortex. Nature 1985;317(6038):623–625

13. Gunderson VM, Dubach M, Szot P, et al. Development of a model of status epilepticus in pigtailed macaque infant monkeys. Dev Neurosci 1999;21(3–5):352–364

14. Mizobuchi M, Ito N, Tanaka C, et al. Unidirectional olfactory hallucination associated with ipsilateral unruptured intracranial aneurysm. Epilepsia 1999;40(4):516–519

15. Silfvenius H, Gloor P, Rasmussen T. Evaluation of insular ablation in surgical treatment of temporal lobe epilepsy. Epilepsia 1964;157:307–320

16. Guillaume J, Mazars G, Mazars Y. [Surgical indications in the so-called temporal epilepsy.] Bull Med 1953;67(17):387–388

17. Ostrowsky K, Isnard J, Ryvlin P, et al. Functional mapping of the insular cortex: clinical implication in temporal lobe epilepsy. Epilepsia 2000;41(6):681–686

18. Isnard J, Guénot M, Ostrowsky K, et al. The role of the insular cortex in temporal lobe epilepsy. Ann Neurol 2000;48(4):614–623

19. Isnard J, Guénot M, Sindou M, et al. Clinical manifestations of insular lobe seizures: a stereo-electroencephalographic study. Epilepsia 2004;45(9):1079–1090

20. Penfield W, Faulk ME Jr. The insula; further observations on its function. Brain 1955;78(4):445–470

21. Guénot M, Isnard J, Ryvlin P, et al. Neurophysiological monitoring for epilepsy surgery: the Talairach SEEG method. StereoElectroEncephaloGraphy. Indications, results, complications and therapeutic applications in a series of 100 consecutive cases. Stereotact Funct Neurosurg 2001;77(1–4):29–32

22. Krolak-Salmon P, Hénaff MA, Isnard J, et al. An attention modulated response to disgust in human ventral anterior insula. Ann Neurol 2003;53(4):446–453

23. Mazzola L, Isnard J, Mauguiere F. Somatosensory and pain responses to stimulation of the second somatosensory area (SII) in humans. A comparison with SI and insular responses. Cereb Cortex 2006;16(7):960–968

24. Kaido T, Otsuki T, Nakama H, et al. Complex behavioral automatism arising from insular cortex. Epilepsy Behav 2006;8(1):315–319

25. Kaido T, Otsuki T, Nakama H, et al. Hypermotor seizure arising from insular cortex. Epilepsia 2006;47(9):1587–1588

26. Ryvlin P, Minotti L, Demarquay G, et al. Nocturnal hypermotor seizures, suggesting frontal lobe epilepsy, can originate in the insula. Epilepsia 2006;47(4):755–765

27. Ryvlin P. Avoid falling into the depths of the insular trap. Epileptic Disord 2006;8(Suppl 2):37–56

28. Fiol ME, Leppik IE, Mireles R, et al. Ictus emeticus and the insular cortex. Epilepsy Res 1988;2(2):127–131

29. Feindel W. Electrical stimulation of the brain during surgery for epilepsy–historical highlights. Int Anesthesiol Clin 1986;24(3):74–87

30. Guénot M, Isnard J, Sindou M. Surgical anatomy of the insula. Adv Tech Stand Neurosurg 2004;29:265–288

31. Mufson EJ, Mesulam MM. Thalamic connections of the insula in the rhesus monkey and comments on the paralimbic connectivity of the medial pulvinar nucleus. J Comp Neurol 1984;227(1):109–120

32. Oppenheimer SM, Kedem G, Martin WM. Left-insular cortex lesions perturb cardiac autonomic tone in humans. Clin Auton Res 1996;6(3):131–140

33. Oppenheimer SM, Gelb A, Girvin JP, et al. Cardiovascular effects of human insular cortex stimulation. Neurology 1992;42(9):1727–1732

34. Oppenheimer SM, Wilson JX, Guiraudon C, et al. Insular cortex stimulation produces lethal cardiac arrhythmias: a mechanism of sudden death? Brain Res 1991;550(1):115–121

35. Oppenheimer SM, Cechetto DF, Hachinski VC. Cerebrogenic cardiac arrhythmias. Cerebral electrocardiographic influences and their role in sudden death. Arch Neurol 1990;47(5):513–519

36. Oppenheimer SM, Cechetto DF. Cardiac chronotropic organization of the rat insular cortex. Brain Res 1990;533(1):66–72

37. Oppenheimer SM. Neurogenic cardiac effects of cerebrovascular disease. Curr Opin Neurol 1994;7(1):20–24

38. Oppenheimer S. Cerebrogenic cardiac arrhythmias: cortical lateralization and clinical significance. Clin Auton Res 2006;16(1):6–11

39. Oppenheimer S. The anatomy and physiology of cortical mechanisms of cardiac control. Stroke 1993; 24(12, Suppl)I3–I5

40. Brian JE Jr, Deshpande JK, McPherson RW. Management of cerebral hemispherectomy in children. J Clin Anesth 1990;2(2):91–95

41. Peyron R, Frot M, Schneider F, et al. Role of operculoinsular cortices in human pain processing: converging evidence from PET, fMRI, dipole modeling, and intracerebral recordings of evoked potentials. Neuroimage 2002;17(3):1336–1346

42. Oshiro Y, Fujita N, Tanaka H, et al. Functional mapping of pain-related activation with echo-planar MRI: significance of the SII-insular region. Neuroreport 1998;9(10):2285–2289

43. Ploghaus A, Tracey I, Gati JS, et al. Dissociating pain from its anticipation in the human brain. Science 1999;284(5422):1979–1981

44. Peyron R, Schneider F, Faillenot I, et al. An fMRI study of cortical representation of mechanical allodynia in patients with neuropathic pain. Neurology 2004;63(10):1838–1846

45. Peyron R, Laurent B, Garcia-Larrea L. Functional imaging of brain responses to pain. A review and meta-analysis (2000). Neurophysiol Clin 2000;30(5):263–288

46. Shuren J. Insula and aphasia. J Neurol 1993;240(4):216–218

47. Ferro JM, Martins IP, Pinto F, et al. Aphasia following right striato-insular infarction in a left-handed child: a clinico-radiological study. Dev Med Child Neurol 1982;24(2):173–182

48. Duffau H, Bauchet L, Lehéricy S, et al. Functional compensation of the left dominant insula for language. Neuroreport 2001;12(10):2159–2163

49. Duffau H, Capelle L, Sichez N, et al. Intraoperative mapping of the subcortical language pathways using direct stimulations. An anatomo-functional study. Brain 2002;125(Pt 1):199–214

50. Spena G, Gatignol P, Capelle L, et al. Superior longitudinal fasciculus subserves vestibular network in humans. Neuroreport 2006;17(13): 1403–1406

51. Mandonnet E, Nouet A, Gatignol P, et al. Does the left inferior longitudinal fasciculus play a role in language? A brain stimulation study. Brain 2007 130(3):623–629

52. Ture U, Yasargil MG, Al-Mefty O, et al. Arteries of the insula. J Neurosurg 2000;92(4):676–687

53. Ture U, Yasargil MG, Al-Mefty O, et al. Topographic anatomy of the insular region. J Neurosurg 1999;90(4):720–733

54. Varnavas GG, Grand W. The insular cortex: morphological and vascular anatomic characteristics. Neurosurgery 1999;44(1):127–136, discussion 136–8

55. Tanriover N, Rhoton AL Jr, Kawashima M, et al. Microsurgical anatomy of the insula and the sylvian fissure. J Neurosurg 2004;100(5):891–922

56. Tanriover N, Kawashima M, Rhoton AL Jr, et al. Microsurgical anatomy of the early branches of the middle cerebral artery: morphometric analysis and classification with angiographic correlation. J Neurosurg 2003;98(6):1277–1290

57. Gil Robles S, Gatignol P, Capelle L, et al. The role of dominant striatum in language: a study using intraoperative electrical stimulations. J Neurol Neurosurg Psychiatry 2005;76(7):940–946

58. Duffau H, Gatignol P, Mandonnet E, et al. New insights into the anatomo-functional connectivity of the semantic system: a study using cortico-subcortical electrostimulations. Brain 2005;128(Pt 4): 797–810

59. Yasargil MG, Ture U, Yasargil DC. Impact of temporal lobe surgery. J Neurosurg 2004;101(5):725–738

60. Wong PC, Parsons LM, Martinez M, et al. The role of the insular cortex in pitch pattern perception: the effect of linguistic contexts. J Neurosci 2004;24(41):9153–9160

61. Kelly JB. The effects of insular and temporal lesions in cats on two types of auditory pattern discrimination. Brain Res 1973;62(1):71–87

62. Fifer RC. Insular stroke causing unilateral auditory processing disorder: case report. J Am Acad Audiol 1993;4(6):364–369

63. Fallon JH, Benevento LA, Loe PR. Frequency-dependent inhibition to tones in neurons of cat insular cortex (AIV). Brain Res 1978; 145(1):161–167

64. Marien P, Pickut BA, Engelborghs S, et al. Phonological agraphia following a focal anterior insulo-opercular infarction. Neuropsychologia 2001;39(8):845–855

65. Manes F, Springer J, Jorge R, et al. Verbal memory impairment after left insular cortex infarction. J Neurol Neurosurg Psychiatry 1999; 67(4):532–534

66. Kumral E, Ozdemirkiran T, Alper Y. Strokes in the subinsular territory: clinical, topographical, and etiological patterns. Neurology 2004; 63(12):2429–2432

67. Casazza M, Broggi G, Franzini A, et al. Supratentorial cavernous angiomas and epileptic seizures: preoperative course and postoperative outcome. Neurosurgery 1996;39(1):26–32

68. Esposito V, Paolini S, Morace R. Resection of a left insular cavernoma aided by a simple navigational tool. Technical note. Neurosurg Focus 2006;21(1):e16

69. Heffez DS. Stereotactic transsylvian, transinsular approach for deep-seated lesions. Surg Neurol 1997;48(2):113–124

70. Duffau H, Fontaine D. Successful resection of a left insular cavernous angioma using neuronavigation and intraoperative language mapping. Acta Neurochir (Wien) 2005;147(2):205–208, discussion 208

71. Cukiert A, Forster C, Andrioli MS, et al. Insular epilepsy. Similarities to temporal lobe epilepsy. Case report. Arq Neuropsiquiatr 1998; 56(1):126–128

72. Tirakotai W, Sure U, Benes L, et al. Image-guided transsylvian, transinsular approach for insular cavernous angiomas. Neurosurgery 2003; 53(6):1299–1304

73. Hentschel SJ, Lang FF. Surgical resection of intrinsic insular tumors. Neurosurgery 2005; 57(1, Suppl)176–183, discussion 176–83

74. Duffau H, Taillandier L, Gatignol P, et al. The insular lobe and brain plasticity: Lessons from tumor surgery. Clin Neurol Neurosurg 2006;108(6):543–548

75. Duffau H, Capelle L, Lopes M, et al. Medically intractable epilepsy from insular low-grade gliomas: improvement after an extended lesionectomy. Acta Neurochir (Wien) 2002;144(6):563–572

76. Isnard J, Mauguiere F. [The insula in partial epilepsy.] Rev Neurol (Paris) 2005;161(1):17–26

77. Guillaume J, Mazars G, Mazars Y. Surgical indications in so-called temporal epilepsy. Ann Med Psychol (Paris) 1953;111:552–553

78. Guénot M, Isnard J, Ryvlin P, et al. SEEG-guided RF thermocoagulation of epileptic foci: feasibility, safety, and preliminary results. Epilepsia 2004;45(11):1368–1374

79. Dobesberger J, Ortler M, Unterberger I, et al. Successful surgical treatment of insular epilepsy with nocturnal hypermotor seizures. Epilepsia 2008;49(1):159–62

80. Villemure JG, Mascott CR, Andermann F, et al. Is removal of the insular cortex in hemispherectomy necessary? Epilepsia 1989;30:728

81. Villemure JG, Mascott CR. Peri-insular hemispherotomy: surgical principles and anatomy. Neurosurgery 1995;37(5):975–981

82. Mascott C, Villemure JG, Andermann F, et al. Hemispherectomy and the insula. Can J Neurol Sci 1990;17:236

83. Delalande O, Bulteau C, Dellatolas G, et al. Vertical parasagittal hemispherotomy: surgical procedures and clinical long-term outcomes in a population of 83 children. Neurosurgery 2007;60(2, Suppl 1) 19–32

84. De Almeida AN, Marino R, Aguiar PH, et al. Hemispherectomy: a schematic review of the current techniques. Neurosurg Rev 2006;29(2): 97–102

85. Ryvlin P, Kahane P. The hidden causes of surgery-resistant temporal lobe epilepsy: extratemporal or temporal plus? Curr Opin Neurol 2005; 18(2):125–127

86. Kahane P, Landre E, Minotti L, et al. The Bancaud and Talairach view on the epileptogenic zone: a working hypothesis. Epileptic Disord 2006;8(Suppl 2):16–26

87. Chassagnon S, Valenti MP, Sabourdy C, et al. Towards a definition of the "practical" epileptogenic zone: a case of epilepsy with dual pathology. Epileptic Disord 2006;8(Suppl 2):67–76

88. Mascott CR. Epilepsy surgery as disruption of epileptogenic networks rather than focus resection: surgical outcomes following application of a network hypothesis. Acta Neurochir (Wien) 2002;144(10):1083

89. Rasmussen T, Feindel W. Temporal lobectomy: review of 100 cases with major hippocampectomy. Can J Neurol Sci 1991;18(4, Suppl) 601–602

90. Feindel W, Rasmussen T. Temporal lobectomy with amygdalectomy and minimal hippocampal resection: review of 100 cases. Can J Neurol Sci 1991;18(4, Suppl)603–605

9 Hypothalamic Hamartomas

Sandeep Mittal, José Luis Montes, Jean-Pierre Farmer, and Abdulrahman J. Sabbagh

The term *hamartoma* is derived from the Greek word *hamartion* meaning bodily defect. A hamartoma is a focal benign growth in an organ composed of tissue elements normally found at that site but that are growing in a disorganized mass. Hamartomas result from an abnormal formation of normal tissue, although the underlying reasons for the abnormality are not fully understood. Although hamartomas resemble neoplasms, they do not show any particular tendency for neoplastic evolution. Instead, they grow along with, and at the same rate as, the organ from whose tissue they are made, and, unlike cancerous tumors, only rarely invade or compress surrounding structures significantly.

Hypothalamic hamartomas (HHs) are rare, heterotopic masses consisting of an abnormal mixture of neuronal and glial cells. They arise from the floor of the third ventricle, tuber cinerium, or mammillary bodies. These developmental malformations can be diagnosed incidentally during routine autopsy. They are often associated with a range of neurological and endocrine disturbances. In its most disabling form, a progressive epileptic encephalopathy appears in early childhood. In addition to gelastic seizures, which represent the hallmark of HH-related epilepsy, the syndrome is also commonly characterized by other types of medically refractory seizures. As well, patients with HH typically display severe cognitive impairment, pervasive developmental disorders, behavioral disturbances, and psychiatric disorders. A distinct subtype of patients present with central precocious puberty.

Topographic and Functional Anatomy of the Hypothalamus

The hypothalamus is the single most integrative structure in the cerebrum. It lies at the base of the brain, around the third ventricle, extending from a plane immediately anterior to the optic chiasm to one immediately posterior to the mammillary bodies. Its weight in the adult human is less than 2.5 g.[1] In midsagittal section, the human hypothalamus is bound anteriorly by the lamina terminalis, posteriorly by a plane drawn between the posterior commissure and the caudal limit of the mammillary body, and superiorly by the hypothalamic sulcus. Ventrally, the hypothalamus encompasses the floor of the third ventricle, the inferior surface of which is termed the *tuber cinerium* (gray swelling). Laterally, the border is somewhat ill-defined, and the hypothalamus is roughly bounded by the internal capsule, cerebral peduncle, optic tract, and subthalamus.

The hypothalamus can be divided into two longitudinal zones: a densely cellular medial zone and a relatively paucicellular lateral zone roughly separated by a sagittal plane passing through the anterior columns of the fornix. In humans, the majority of named hypothalamic nuclei are in the medial zone. In addition, the hypothalamus is commonly subdivided into regions along its anteroposterior axis (**Fig. 9.1**). The preoptic region extends rostral to the optic chiasm and dorsally to the anterior commissure. The supraoptic region resides above the optic chiasm. The tuberal region lies above and includes the tuber cinerium. Finally, the mammillary region includes the mammillary bodies and the posterior hypothalamic nuclei.

Through its numerous reciprocal afferent and efferent connections, the hypothalamus coordinates autonomic, somatic, endocrine, and behavioral activities of the body. It receives input and in turn projects to a wide distribution of neurons arising in the forebrain, brainstem, and spinal cord. **Figure 9.2** summarizes the major hypothalamic nuclei, their location, and function. Interestingly, the hypothalamus is also implicated in laughter, the behavioral manifestation of mirth.[2,3]

Etiology and Molecular Biology of Hypothalamic Hamartomas

The embryological origin of HHs remains unknown. The true incidence of HH is indefinite, but the estimated prevalence is 0.5 per 100,000.[4] These lesions are usually sporadic, and their exact etiology has not been determined. However, rather than presenting as isolated masses, HHs can be part of a multiple malformation syndrome. In fact, there are several congenital anomaly syndromes in which HHs have been described. Syndromic HHs generally have milder symptoms than do nonsyndromic sporadic HHs, but likely arise from similar pathogenetic mechanisms. The heritable nature of these disorders means that the genes that are mutated in affected patients can be detected. The identification of genes that, in the mutant state, cause HHs, suggests that the normal function of these genes are important for the usual development and function of the hypothalamus.

Pallister-Hall syndrome (PHS), a developmental disorder first described in 1980 in a cohort of six children, is the most extensively studied disorder in terms of the molecular pathology.[5] The syndrome is typically characterized by the presence of an HH in association with multisystem malformations. The spectrum of features also includes central

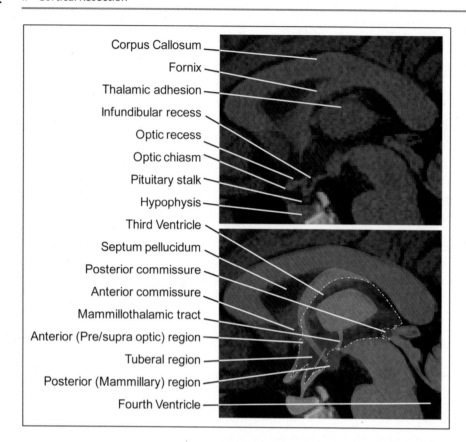

Corpus Callosum
Fornix
Thalamic adhesion
Infundibular recess
Optic recess
Optic chiasm
Pituitary stalk
Hypophysis
Third Ventricle
Septum pellucidum
Posterior commissure
Anterior commissure
Mammillothalamic tract
Anterior (Pre/supra optic) region
Tuberal region
Posterior (Mammillary) region
Fourth Ventricle

Fig. 9.1 Midsagittal diagram of the hypothalamus depicting the surrounding neural structures at the level of the anterior columns of the fornix.

postaxial polydactyly, pituitary hypoplasia or dysfunction, dysplastic nails, bifid epiglottis, and imperforate anus. In some cases, cardiac anomalies, renal defects, and mild mental retardation are seen. Given this characteristic phenotype, PHS is often diagnosed at birth. In familial cases, PHS has been noted to be inherited in an autosomal dominant pattern with variable expressivity. It has been linked with a mutation to a zinc finger transcription factor gene, Gli3, which resides on chromosome 7p13 in some inherited probands.[6] Gli proteins act downstream of the sonic hedgehog (SHH) signaling pathway to regulate target gene expression. SHH plays a critical role in regulating dorsoventral patterning of the developing central nervous system.[7] In the presence of SHH, the Gli3 transcription factor is released intact and migrates to the nucleus to activate downstream genes. In the absence of SHH, Gli3 appears to be processed by a protease into a shorter form that represses downstream genes. In patients with PHS, frameshift mutations in the Gli3 gene cause the production of a truncated version of the protein, which is functionally identical to the processed, repressor form of the protein.[8] Thus, the pathogenetic mutations in patients with PHS remove the ability of SHH to switch Gli3 between the repressor and activator state.

Clinical Characteristics

There appears to be a correlation between the clinical features of HHs and their physical appearance in relation to the normal hypothalamic and surrounding structures. In addition to the classic presentation of gelastic seizures, patients with HHs also commonly develop multiple other seizure types that evolve with age. Other associated symptoms can include precocious puberty, behavioral disturbances, and progressive cognitive decline.

Epileptic Syndromes

The phenomenon of "pressure to laugh" or gelastic epilepsy was first described by Trousseau in 1873.[9] Gelastic seizures, the hallmark of epilepsy related to HHs, typically begin in early childhood, often in the neonatal period, and are invariably followed by development of medically refractory catastrophic seizures. Gelastic fits are characterized by recurrent brief seizures with initial emotionless laughter or grimacing. In addition to ictal laughter, other seizure types commonly occur, which are often more disabling than the gelastic spells.[10,11] Nevertheless, the vast majority of electrophysiological studies have focused on gelastic seizures. Arzimanoglou and colleagues[12] reviewed 16 children with HH and intractable seizures. They found a wide clinical spectrum and variable severity of the epilepsy syndrome. This was in keeping with the findings of Frattali et al[13] and Leal et al[14] who also reported the presence of multiple seizure types, such as generalized tonic-clonic seizures, partial complex seizures, drop attacks, and atypical absences, in the majority of patients. Tassinari et al[15] published the most extensive review of patients with gelastic seizures. The first part of their chapter reported on 60 patients with gelastic seizures without the presence of an HH, suggesting that ictal laughter is not pathognomonic of HH. The second part of the review detailed the profile of another 60 patients with gelastic seizures related to HH. In 51 patients of the latter group, gelastic seizures were the first seizure type to be observed. However, 75% of the patients had other types of intractable seizures, including complex partial seizures with or without secondary generalization in 35.5%, "falling" seizures in 33.3%, tonic seizures in 17.7%, and tonic-clonic seizures in 15.1%. Mullatti[16] and Castro et al[10] observed similar findings in adults with HHs. Castro et al observed two major seizure types other than gelastic seizures in six adults with HH: complex partial seizures and tonic seizures with or without secondary generalization.[10] Mullatti studied 14 adult patients with HH and epilepsy.[16] Only three patients developed seizures in

adult life. She concluded that later onset of epilepsy seems to be associated with a milder epilepsy syndrome with less prominence of gelastic seizures. In addition, cognitive and behavioral difficulties were less common in adults compared with children with HH.

Behavioral and Cognitive Disturbances

An almost constant feature in patients with HH and pharmacoresistant gelastic seizures is development of a severe epileptic encephalopathy and catastrophic epilepsy of childhood. Often this epileptic syndrome is accompanied by profound behavioral problems, with reports of hyperactivity, rage and aggression being common.[17–19] In addition to delinquency and aggressive outbursts, a slowly progressive deterioration in cognitive functions has also been frequently observed in patients with gelastic seizures and HH.[11,12,20]

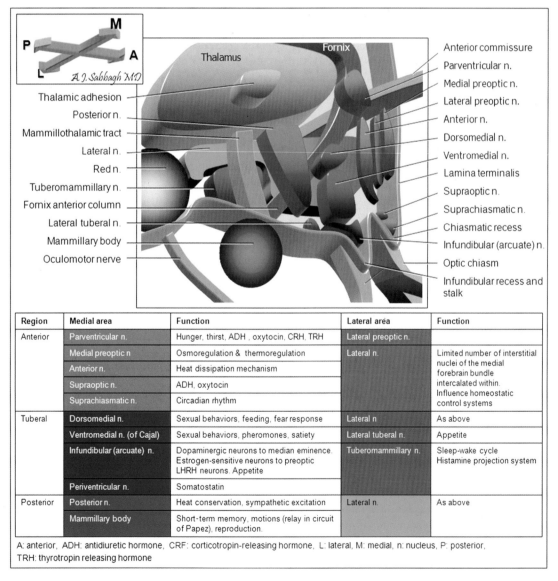

Region	Medial area	Function	Lateral area	Function
Anterior	Parventricular n.	Hunger, thirst, ADH , oxytocin, CRH, TRH	Lateral preoptic n.	
	Medial preoptic n	Osmoregulation & thermoregulation	Lateral n.	Limited number of interstitial nuclei of the medial forebrain bundle intercalated within. Influence homeostatic control systems
	Anterior n.	Heat dissipation mechanism		
	Supraoptic n.	ADH, oxytocin		
	Suprachiasmatic n.	Circadian rhythm		
Tuberal	Dorsomedial n.	Sexual behaviors, feeding, fear response	Lateral n	As above
	Ventromedial n. (of Cajal)	Sexual behaviors, pheromones, satiety	Lateral tuberal n.	Appetite
	Infundibular (arcuate) n.	Dopaminergic neurons to median eminence. Estrogen-sensitive neurons to preoptic LHRH neurons. Appetite	Tuberomammillary n.	Sleep-wake cycle Histamine projection system
	Periventricular n.	Somatostatin		
Posterior	Posterior n.	Heat conservation, sympathetic excitation	Lateral n.	As above
	Mammillary body	Short-term memory, motions (relay in circuit of Papez), reproduction.		

A: anterior, ADH: antidiuretic hormone, CRF: corticotropin-releasing hormone, L: lateral, M: medial, n: nucleus, P: posterior, TRH: thyrotropin releasing hormone

Fig. 9.2 Summary of the major hypothalamic nuclei and their function.

Worsening of the behavioral and cognitive deficits usually parallels the aggravation of epilepsy. In Tassinari's review, mental impairment was reported in 49 of 60 patients (81.6%) with gelastic seizures and HH.[15] In addition, behavioral disturbances were present in 34% of the cases. Arzinmanoglou et al reported progressive development of cognitive and behavioral deterioration in all 16 children.[12] Frattali et al reported mild to severe cognitive deficits in all eight children with HH and refractory epilepsy.[13] Similarly, Mullatti et al reported mild to severe learning difficulties in 14 of 16 patients with childhood-onset seizures.[11] Quiske et al published the first detailed report on cognitive performance in juvenile and adult patients with gelastic seizures and HH.[19] They performed a comprehensive neuropsychological assessment and concluded that more than half of the 13 patients displayed deficits in a broad range of cognitive functions. Most prominent in were impairments in working memory, visual and verbal learning and memory (77% and 62%, respectively), and limitations in global intellectual performance (54%). A considerable number of patients showed below-average functions in cognitive flexibility and speed, concentration, and visuoconstructive abilities. Frattali et al found a significant relation between partial seizure frequency and broad cognitive ability score.[13]

Psychiatric Manifestations

There is also a high prevalence of psychiatric comorbidity in patients with HH.[21] Weissenberger et al evaluated 12 children between 3 and 14 years of age, along with parents and age-matched siblings.[18] They found that children with HH and gelastic seizures had a significantly higher psychiatric morbidity, such as oppositional defiant disorder (83.3%), attention deficit-hyperactivity disorder (75%), conduct disorder (33.3%), and affective disorders (16.7%). Ali et al looked at 10 adult patients with HH and a history of intractable seizures.[22] They also documented a high prevalence of comorbid mood and anxiety disorders with major depressive disorder and social anxiety disorder being the most common.

Precocious Puberty and Other Endocrine Dysfunction

The association between HH and central precocious puberty (CPP) is well established. Pedunculated HH below the third ventricle is rarely associated with seizures but may present with CPP defined as the onset of puberty before age 8 in girls and 9 in boys. CPP tends to occur significantly earlier than idiopathic CPP.[23] The first manifestation of CPP in patients with HH occurs before age 2 in 82% of cases.[23] Several hypotheses have been formulated to explain the potential mechanisms by which HHs cause precocious puberty.[24] One hypothesis suggests that HHs accelerate sexual development by producing bioactive substances that mimic, in an accelerated time-course, the cascade of events underlying the normal initiation of puberty. Alternatively, it has been proposed that because HHs contain key transcriptional and signaling networks required to initiate and sustain a pubertal mode of gonadotropin-releasing hormone (GnRH) release, they are able to trigger the pubertal process at an earlier age. Finally, it is also possible that the developmental abnormalities leading to the formation of HHs result from sporadic defects affecting the same genes and hence the same morphogenic pathways involved in the embryonic development of the ventral hypothalamus and the floor of the third ventricle. The exact mechanisms involved in HH causing CPP remains to be fully elucidated.

Neuroimaging Findings

Plain X-rays

Patients with HHs typically have unremarkable skull x-rays. However, these slowly growing expansile masses can result in local bony erosion at the tip of the dorsum sella. Lin et al (1978) described suprasellar calcification in a patient harboring a histologically proven hamartoma of the tuber cinerium.[25] Diebler and Ponsot (1983) reported a case in which detachment and anterior displacement of the tip of the dorsum sella was seen mimicking a calcified suprasellar craniopharyngioma.[26]

Pneumoencephalography

For historical interest, pneumoencephalography was a sensitive study to define midline lesions and often disclosed a small filling defect in the tip of the infundibular recess (Takeuchi et al, 1979).[27]

Cerebral Angiography

Although an angiographic study has little or no diagnostic value, it may demonstrate slight posterior displacement of the distal basilar artery and anterior pontomesencephalic vein, upward displacement of the A1 segment of the anterior cerebral arteries, and possibly lateral displacement of the posterior communicating arteries. Tumor blush or associated abnormal vessels are typically not encountered.

CT Scan

The computed tomography (CT) findings are dependent on the size of the hamartoma. Plain CT shows a mass in the interpeduncular and suprasellar cistern, which has the same density as normal brain and does not enhance following contrast administration. Obliteration of the suprasellar cistern and anterior third ventricle is commonly observed.[28] Metrizamide CT cisternography showed a filling defect in the suprasellar cistern and greatly improved the diagnostic yield for smaller occult lesions of the hypothalamic-hypophyseal axis by clearly defining the size of the mass as well as its relationship to surrounding neurovascular structures.[29]

MR Imaging

The incidence of HHs has increased since the introduction of high-resolution magnetic resonance (MR) imaging. The detailed imaging of the lesion and its relationship to adjacent structures is of paramount importance in the planning of the surgical approach and during the procedure. High-resolution MRI scanning has therefore largely supplanted all other diagnostic studies and remains the neuroimaging modality of choice for evaluation of patients with lesions of the tuber cinerium. Freeman et al systematically studied the MRI findings of 72 patients with HH and refractory epilepsy.[30] The vast majority of HHs (93%) showed increased T2-weighted signal intensity seen relative to cortical and deep gray matter. Unlike previous studies, which reported signals isointense with gray matter on T1-weighted images,[31-33] the authors found that 53 cases (74%) were hypointense compared with the normal gray matter. The authors explain that this observation may be due to the greater signal intensity contrast among gray matter, white matter, and abnormal tissue obtained with inversion-prepared gradient-echo sequences, compared with conventional spin-echo sequences. The HH did not show contrast enhancement following administration of gadolinium, thereby demonstrating the integrity the blood-brain barrier.

MR Spectroscopy

Magnetic resonance spectroscopy imaging is a highly sensitive method of detective neuronal dysfunction in patients with temporal lobe epilepsy. However, very few studies have reported the spectroscopic properties of HHs. Seven studies with a total of 42 patients underwent magnetic resonance spectroscopy with evaluation of the N-acetylaspartate (NAA), creatine (Cr), choline (Cho), and myoinositol (ml) content within the hamartoma. The group in Montreal was the first to study hypothalamic hamartomas using proton MR spectroscopic imaging.[34] They quantified the amount of neuronal damage in the temporal lobes and hamartomas of five patients with HHs and gelastic seizures. The relative intensity of NAA/Cr was determined for both temporal lobes as well as for the hamartoma. These values were compared with signals from the temporal lobes and hypothalami of normal control subjects. The NAA/Cr ratio was not significantly different from normal control subjects for either temporal lobe, nor was there a significant asymmetry between the two temporal lobes for any of the patients. In contrast, NAA resonance signals were present in the hamartomas, and the ratio of NAA to Cr was significantly decreased in the hamartomas compared with the hypothalami of normal control subjects. This study provided further evidence that gelastic seizures do not originate in the temporal lobes of patients with HHs.

Similarly, Pascual-Castroviejo et al used MR spectroscopy in their patient with an HH to localize and measure in the temporal lobes and in the lesion.[35] The relative intensity of NAA to Cr and NAA to Ch was not significantly different from normal control subjects for either temporal lobes. Within the hamartoma, the ratio NAA/Ch was decreased, however, contrary to the earlier report of Tasch et al,[34] the ratio NAA/Cr was highly increased in the hamartoma in their patient with intractable gelastic seizures.[35]

The altered chemical shift imaging with MR spectrometry in three other patients suggested a biochemical abnormality in the tissue of the HH. Wakai et al[36] found a significant reduction of the NAA/serum creatinine ratio. Wakai et al further demonstrated decreased NAA and increased choline and creatine in the hypothalamic hamartoma. Martin et al found on short-TE proton MR spectra, the NAA concentration in the hamartoma to be lower than in the thalamus but similar to that in the amygdala.[37] In addition, the myoinositol concentration was elevated in the hamartoma compared with that in the amygdala and thalamus.

Recently, two groups reported a larger series of patients with HHs evaluated with MR spectroscopy. In 2004, Freeman and coworkers performed proton MR spectroscopy of the HH in 19 patients and compared it with the metabolite profile of the thalamus in 10 normal children and the frontal lobe in 10 normal adults.[30] They also found reduced NAA and increased myoinositol content. Finally, Amstutz and colleagues studied data from single voxel spectroscopic sequences in 14 patients.[38] They demonstrated a statistically significant decrease in NAA/Cr and an increase in ml/Cr ratios in tumor tissue when compared with values in normal gray matter of the amygdala. In addition, Cho/Cr ratios were also increased when compared with those in normal gray matter controls.

Overall, these results from MR spectroscopy suggest that HHs manifest reduced neuronal density and relative gliosis compared with normal gray matter.

Neurophysiology and Intrinsic Epileptogenesis

The association between the typical severe cases of HHs and epilepsy was obscured by the observation of slow spike and wave electrograph (EEG) patterns with or without multifocal (typically frontal or temporal) epileptiform abnormalities.[31] In addition, some seizures associated with HHs can resemble complex partial seizures of temporal or frontal origin both clinically and with ictal electroencephalography (EEG). Even with ictal recordings with intracranial electrodes (not including the HH itself), the frontal or temporal cortex can appear to be the site of origin of seizures.[39] However, neocortical resection is uniformly ineffective in controlling the seizures.[39]

Depth Electrode Recording

An ictal EEG correlate is frequently lacking during gelastic seizures.[40] This is consistent with ictal onset in a deep-seated structure. Ictal activity may not be captured by scalp electrodes, but it can be seen in the HH when depth electrode recording is used. Munari's group in Grenoble performed the first depth electrode recording directly from the HH in a patient. During the same time period, our group in Montreal implanted electrodes within the HH in 2 patients. These landmark studies provided direct evidence that the ictal events, specifically, the gelastic seizures, are linked to discharge that is confined to the hamartoma itself.[41,42] Over the last decade, ictal EEG recordings derived from a relatively small number of patients who underwent electrode placement within the HH have further confirmed that the ictal events associated with gelastic seizures indeed arise directly from the HH itself.[43–45] Furthermore, electrical stimulation of the depth electrode contacts inserted into the HH lesion provoked the habitual seizures in some of these patients.[41,43,44] Likewise, Choi and colleagues stereotactically implanted depth electrodes within the HH and confirmed the HH-induced epileptic discharges.[45] Interestingly, they observed immediate disappearance of these epileptic discharges on intraoperative or postoperative EEG monitoring following endoscopic disconnection. Clear evidence for the intrinsic epileptogenesis of the hamartoma was further reinforced by metabolic studies.

Positron Emission Tomography (PET) Scan

Palmini et al reported one patient who underwent an interictal [18F]-fluoro-deoxyglucose (FDG) PET scan that showed focal cortical hypometabolism colocalizing with the most prominent scalp EEG abnormalities.[42] Ryvlin et al investigated brain glucose metabolism in patients with epileptogenic HHs, in an attempt to identify signs of focal cortical and subcortical dysfunction that might correlate with other clinical data.[46] They studied five patients with epileptogenic HHs using FDG-PET. The anatomical distribution of interictal FDG-PET abnormalities was compared with that of interictal and ictal electroclinical findings. All five patients demonstrated focal hypometabolism grossly concordant with the cortical regions suspected to participate in the ictal discharges. Epileptogenic HHs are usually associated with focal cortical hypometabolism in regions that might participate in the overall hamartoma-driven epileptic network. Whether these cortical abnormalities only reflect the propagation of ictal discharges or a potentially independent seizure onset zone remains unknown.

Further insight into the intrinsic epileptogenicity of HHs was gained by the study of Palmini and colleagues.[47] They reported the first ictal FDG-PET evidence of the hypothalamic origin of gelastic seizures in a patient with an HH. Ictal FDG-PET was acquired during an episode of status gelasticus with preserved consciousness, in a patient previously operated on for complex partial seizures due to a temporal lobe epileptogenic cyst. Ictal hypermetabolism was localized to the region of the hamartoma during the status gelasticus. This elegant ictal FDG-PET study independently confirmed

that gelastic seizures in patients with HHs do indeed originate in the diencephalic mass.

Single Photon Emission Computerized Tomography (SPECT) Imaging

Further evidence identifying the HH as the focus of seizure generation has been provided by measurements of regional cerebral blood flow during gelastic seizures in patients with HHs. Several studies performed ictal SPECT scans after injection of the tracer [99m]technetium hexamethylpropyleneamine oxime (Tc-HMPAO). These reports consistently demonstrated dramatic ictal hyperperfusion within the hamartoma with normalization during the interictal phase lending further support to the notion that certain types of HHs are inherently epileptogenic in nature.[43,48–53]

Whether the intrinsic epileptogenicity of HHs is responsible for the entire clinical spectrum of epileptic, neuropsychological, and behavioral disorders associated with HH, remains an open issue, in as much as morphologically similar HH can be associated with dramatically different seizure types and cognitive outcomes.

Morphological Characteristics and Topological Classification

A distinction must be made between the two different anatomical subtypes of HHs. The first subtype, referred to as the intrahypothalamic or sessile HH, consists of lesions whose base of attachment within the third ventricle is either partial or complete. These lesions vary significantly in size but typically extend into the third ventricle itself and distort local anatomical structures, including the fornix and mammillary body.[30] Sessile HHs are highly associated with neurological symptoms, including gelastic seizures.[54,55,17,40,56] These lesions typically do not present with precocious puberty, although up to 40% of these patients will develop CPP at some point during their course. The second subtype is referred to as the parahypothalamic, or pedunculated HH. These lesions are attached only to the floor of the third ventricle or suspended from it by a peduncle. In contrast to sessile lesions, pedunculated HHs typically do not present with a catastrophic childhood epilepsy syndrome or neurodevelopmental disorder. Rather, they are commonly associated with CPP as the presenting abnormality. As discussed previously, the interference of HHs with inhibitory pathways onto GnRH neurons has been hypothesized as a possible mechanism for CPP. It is therefore conceivable that HHs are more likely to be associated with CPP if they are located close to the GnRH nerve terminals in the median eminence, as in a parahypothalamic position. Resection of pedunculated lesions causing precocious puberty reverses the hormonal abnormalities.[57,58] However, medical therapy using leuprolide acetate (a long-acting GnRH analog) alone is now the first-line treatment for most of these patients. The majority of HHs can be easily classified as either sessile or pedunculated. However, some intermediary forms have been described; for example a large sessile HH that has a broad base of attachment to the underside of the hypothalamus and that extends into the interpeduncular cistern.

According to Valdueza et al,[55] epilepsy in HHs is observed only in medium and large sessile HH broadly attached to the tuber cinerium or mammillary body. The hypothesis that size, shape, and location of HHs affect the likelihood of clinical presentation is compelling. Jung et al[40] reported that hamartomas inducing gelastic seizures tend to be larger (≥10 mm in diameter) than those with isolated CPP. Sturm et al[59] observed that some patients with small HHs showed pressure to laugh, often without actual laughter, and suggested a dose–response relationship between the size of the HH and the severity of the epilepsy. However, because a significant proportion of patients with a HH of ≥10 mm in diameter presented with isolated sexual precocity, Jung and colleagues[40] emphasized that size cannot be the only characteristic responsible for the induction of these clinical symptoms. **Figure 9.3** outlines the different anatomotopographical classifications of HHs based on MRI findings reported by various authors.

Neuropathological, Neurobiological, and Neurophysiological Findings

The major breakthrough in our understanding of the pathophysiology of HH was the discovery that HHs have intrinsic epileptogenicity. It is believed that through their mamillothalamic tract connections, these lesions predispose to generalized seizures and generalized interictal spike and wave discharges. Until recently, the histopathology of HH was poorly understood. Initial analysis showed that the hamartomas were composed of disorganized networks of neurons and glia similar to the structural lesions associated with epilepsy such as cortical dysplasia. Immunohistochemistry showed that these neurons stained intensely for

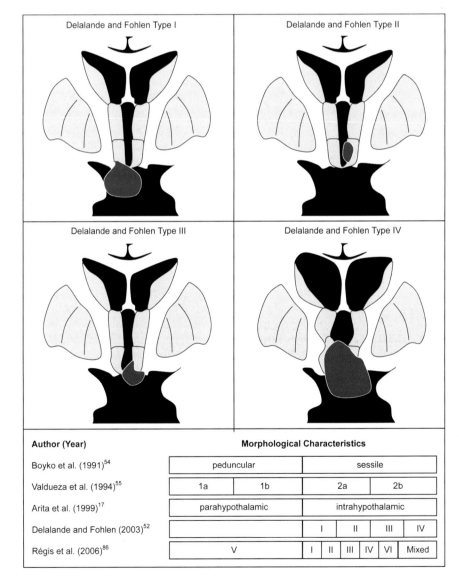

Fig. 9.3 Topological classification of hypothalamic hamartomas based on MRI findings.

NeuN, a marker for mature neurons, and were surrounded by a fine fibrillary matrix positive for synaptophysin immunostaining. Immunocytochemistry with glial fibrillary acidic protein (GFAP) showed scanty astrocytes and oligodendrocytes without neoplastic differentiation.[55] In a recent article, Coons et al[60] provided detailed histopathological analysis of 57 cases of HH. They noted that a consistent feature of all HH specimens examined was the presence of neuronal clusters or nodules that varied in size. The neuronal nodules were composed predominantly of small bipolar neurons interspersed with and surrounded by large pyramidal neurons in an astrocyte-rich neuropil.

Although it is possible that the epileptogenicity of some HHs may be due to intrinsic cellular dysplasia,[61] the striking association between gelastic seizures and the intrahypothalamic position of the HH favors the hypothesis that the epileptogenicity may be due to aberrant connectivity of these heterotopic structures. To determine how the cellular microarchitecture might contribute to seizure generation, Fenoglio et al[62] examined the electrophysiological properties of the small and large neurons and their contribution to network activity in HH brain slices. They noted that the small neurons fired action potentials spontaneously. In addition to a continuous pacemaker-like firing pattern, these small neurons, which express γ-aminobutyric acid (GABA) receptors and likely represent inhibitory interneurons, also exhibit irregular spiking and bursting firing patterns (Wu et al, 2005).[63] In contrast, spontaneous activity was not observed in large HH neurons (Fenoglio et al, 2007). The authors hypothesize that the chronic epileptogenesis of HH tissue requires a network of interconnected neuronal clusters to propagate and synchronize discharges. Based on their data, they propose a model whereby clusters of small GABAergic interneurons exhibit spontaneous firing, which synchronizes the output of large quiescent HH projection neurons. The large neurons, in turn, project to extrahypothalamic structures such as the thalamus and hippocampus, which are well known to play a central role in limbic epilepsies.

Operative Techniques and Results

As described above, patients with HHs suffer from debilitating medically refractory seizures as well as severe progressive cognitive, behavioral, and psychiatric problems. Thus, there has been considerable focus on developing surgical techniques for the treatment of these difficult lesions. Northfield and Russell[64] reported the first successful removal of an HH associated with CPP. Later, Paillas et al[65] provided a detailed account of the clinical, radiographic, and histological data of a patient who underwent excision of an HH. Subsequently, in the 1970s and 1980s, several groups published case reports describing their attempts to control seizures surgically.[66–69] However, interest in the management of HHs expanded considerably in the 1990s with development of high-resolution MRI. The main strategy in the treatment of HHs associated with gelastic seizures has been microsurgical resection using various approaches. Alternatively, good outcomes have also been reported by disconnection of the HH and other minimally invasive techniques including stereotactic radiosurgery. Recent advances have aimed toward minimizing surgical morbidity.

Microsurgical Resection

Pterional and Frontotemporal Approach

The initial clinical series of microsurgical resection of HHs commonly used the frontotemporal or pterional approach.[70,71] Others combined a subfrontal, transsylvian, subtemporal, and other skull-base routes to ameliorate the removal of the diencephalic mass.[72] The major advantage of this familiar approach is that it provides the shortest, most direct route to the suprasellar cistern and hamartoma. However, the surgical corridor may be narrowed by various neurovascular structures (e.g., internal carotid artery, optic nerve and tracts, oculomotor nerve, and pituitary stalk) and thereby limit access into the third ventricle and the intraventricular component of the HH. Furthermore, the boundaries of the lesion may be difficult to identify particularly if there is a broad attachment to the hypothalamus and mammillary bodies. In 2003, Palmini et al[73] observed that 3 of the 13 patients treated using this approach showed complete seizure cessation. The remaining 10 patients had significant (>90%) reduction in seizure frequency. All had improvement in cognition, behavior, and development. However, they reported significant morbidity in seven patients including four thalamocapsular infarcts, transient third nerve palsy in four, and one case each with postsurgical central diabetes insipidus and persistent hyperphagia.

Transcallosal, Interforniceal Approach

The anterior transcallosal, transseptal, interforniceal approach to remove HHs via the third ventricle was pioneered by Rosenfeld and the group in Melbourne.[74] The approach consists of a small anterior callosotomy just behind the genu, between 15 to 20 mm in length, followed by midline transseptal dissection and separation of the fornices. The anterior end of the roof of the third ventricle is entered, and the hamartoma is removed or disconnected. The operative anatomy has been described in detail by Rosenfeld and coworkers.[75] This approach provides a wide exposure to the third ventricle and excellent view of the HH from above. Another advantage of this technique compared with the approaches from below is that the HH can be debulked and/or disconnected while sparing the mammillary bodies when they can be identified and preserving the pituitary stalk and optic chiasm. Also, the avoidance of cranial nerves and blood vessels in the suprasellar cistern and interpeduncular fossa may further reduce the risk of stroke and oculomotor nerve injury. However, there is a risk of short-term memory deficits because of septal, forniceal, or mammillary body injury.

In 2001, the group in Melbourne first reported a series of five patients; two of the patients were seizure free, two others had significant improvement, and one did not benefit from surgery. Two patients developed increased appetite postoperatively. However, no permanent morbidity or mortality was reported. In their follow-up study, Harvey and colleagues[76] presented their experience with 29 patients operated on using the anterior transcallosal, transseptal, interforniceal approach. Patients were followed for a mean of 30 months (range, 12 to 70 months). The resection was complete or near-complete (>95%) in 18 of the 29 patients (62%). Fifteen patients (52%) remained seizure free and seven (24%) had >90% reduction in seizure frequency. Both transient and permanent complications were seen, including, thalamic infarct in two patients, increased appetite in 10 cases (permanent in five), and short-term memory deficits in 14 patients (persistent in four).

The transcallosal interforniceal route has also been utilized by the team at the Barrow Neurological Institute. They first reported their experience in 10 patients with intractable seizures related to HHs.[77] Subsequently, they reported results in 26 patients and showed that completeness of resection of the HH directly correlated with seizure outcome.[78] The mean postoperative follow-up was 20.3 months (range, 13 to 28 months). Fourteen (54%) patients remained seizure free, and nine (35%) had at least a 90% improvement in total seizure frequency. Postoperative improvement in behavior was observed in 23 (88%) patients and in cognition in 17 (65%) patients. Transient postoperative memory disturbance was seen in 15 (58%) patients, but persisted in only two (8%). Two (8%) patients had persisting endocrine disturbance requiring hormone replacement therapy (diabetes insipidus and hypothyroidism in one each). The authors reported that the likelihood of a seizure-free outcome correlated with younger age, shorter lifetime duration of epilepsy, smaller preoperative HH volume, and complete HH resection. The anterior transcallosal, transseptal, interforniceal approach may be a very attractive approach to achieve complete resection of larger HHs in younger patients. However, the authors cautioned that in older patients, because of the increased difficulty in separating the leaves of the septum pellucidum, there is a higher risk of forniceal injury.

Transcallosal, Subchoroidal Approach

The interhemispheric subchoroidal approach has been described as an alternative to the transcallosal interforniceal route.[53] The authors discuss that by eliminating the splitting of the fornices, the subchoroidal access to the third ventricle can lower the risk of permanent postoperative memory deficits.

Endoscopic Transventricular Approach

In 2002, Akai et al[79] presented the case of a 5-year-old-girl with gelastic seizures related to a HH who underwent endoscopic transventricular biopsy of the lesion. Subsequently, she was treated with linear accelerator stereotactic radiosurgery. However, her symptoms remained unchanged for 6 months. She then underwent partial resection and laser coagulation of the tumor by a neuroendoscopic approach. After the procedure, the frequency of her seizures was remarkably decreased, and her violent behavior improved. More recently, Rekate and colleges[80] reported their extensive experience with endoscopic surgery for HHs causing medically refractory gelastic seizures. They treated 44 patients with an endoscopic transventricular approach utilizing frameless stereotaxis. A complete removal of the HH was achieved in 14 (31.8%) patients, 13 of whom remained seizure free after surgery. The remaining patients underwent endoscopic disconnection of the HH (see below).

Open and Endoscopic Disconnection

The possibility that good seizure outcomes could be achieved using an endoscopic approach was first reported by Delalande and Fohlen.[52] They conceptualized that disconnection of the hamartoma would isolate the intrinsically epileptogenic HH and thus lead to favorable seizure outcomes. They reported a series of 17 patients who underwent disconnection of the intraventricular component without resection of the HH.[81] Fourteen patients had an open surgery, three patients became seizure free, and the remaining 11 had significant reduction (>80%) in seizure frequency. Seven of these 11 patients underwent additional endoscopic disconnection of the intraventricular component of which three became seizure free. Three of the 17 children and adolescents underwent endoscopic disconnection only. Two achieved seizure freedom, and the third patient had a second endoscopic disconnection with no marked improvement. Overall, 8 of the 17 patients remained seizure free (47%) and the majority of patient showed improved behavior and social outcome. Postoperative complications included stroke in two patients, meningitis in one patient, and transient diabetes insipidus in two patients. The authors further emphasized that none of the patients who underwent endoscopic disconnection had any postsurgical morbidity and were all discharged from the hospital three days following surgery.

Choi and colleagues[45] reported their experience with four patients who underwent endoscopic disconnection for HH with intractable epilepsy. Depth electrodes were stereotacticly inserted into the HH in three patients at the time of the endoscopic procedure and maintained for 1 week after surgery. As stated above, they confirmed the intrinsic epileptogenesis of the HH and observed immediate disappearance of the epileptic discharges following the disconnection. Interestingly, they did not record any discharges originating from the hamartoma during 1 week after surgery. Two patients became seizure free immediately after endoscopic disconnection and one experienced significant reduction in seizure frequency. The authors caution on the difficulty in completely disconnecting large sessile HH with a broad base connection to the hypothalamus. Also, 3 of the 4 patients suffered transient disconnection-like syndrome including mental dullness, verbal anosmia, unilateral tactile anomia, unilateral constructional apraxia, and lack of somesthetic transfer. All patients had dramatic improvement in behavior during a mean follow-up of 16.8 months (range, 12 to 24 months).

Rekate et al[80] reported their early experience with endoscopic disconnection or complete removal of HHs in 44 patients. Follow-up was too short to allow for adequate analysis of seizure and behavior outcomes. There were no deaths in this large series. Eleven patients (25%) had postsurgical complications. However, only four patients (9.1%) suffered complications that persisted for more than 3 months. In 11 patients (25%), postoperative MRI showed thalamic infarction. In 8 of these 11 patients, the small thalamic infarcts were asymptomatic, whereas three had postoperative hemiparesis. In two patients, the hemiparesis resolved within 1 week of surgery and only one patient had significant weakness after 3 months. Six patients had difficulties with short-term memory that persisted more than 3 months in three patients. No patient suffered a permanent hormonal deficiency.

Overall, both open and endoscopic disconnection surgery appears to be a safe and effective treatment option for small, sessile hamartomas.

Stereotactic Radiosurgery

The concept to radiosurgery, introduced by Lars Leksell at the Karolinska Institute in Stockholm in 1951,[82] involves convergence of narrow ionizing beams focused to a predetermined target using stereotactic guidance and provides minimal radiation to the surrounding structures in a minimally invasive manner. Three approaches to deliver a focused-beam of high-dose radiation have been employed to treat HHs. First, Gamma Knife–based radiosurgery has been used by several groups. Second, linear accelerator (LINAC)-based radiosurgery has been employed others. Finally, stereotactic brachytherapy via intrahypothalamic implantation of radioactive sources has been used by some investigators.

Gamma Knife Radiosurgery

Several groups have reported the use of Gamma Knife radiosurgery (GKRS) for its specific antiepileptic effect in patients with medically refractory epilepsy. The largest and longest experience is from the Marseille group who first employed a stereotactic radiosurgical approach for the management of patients with intractable epilepsy. Régis et al[83] recently reviewed the results of GKRS for mesial temporal lobe epilepsy in a long-term prospective multicenter trial delivering 25 Gy to the 50% isodose line. Analysis of seizure control after a 2-year follow-up showed a reduction of the median number of seizures per month from 6.2 to 0.3, with 13 of 20 patients attaining seizure freedom. Following the promising results obtained in patients with mesial temporal lobe epilepsy, ste-

reotactic radiosurgery was deemed to be very appealing for small, deep-seated lesions such as HH given the significant morbidity and mortality associated with microsurgical techniques as described above.

In 1998, Arita and colleagues[84] first reported a case of successful treatment of gelastic seizures related to HH by GKRS with no side effects. They treated a 25-year-old man with an HH and lifelong history of intractable gelastic and tonic-clonic seizures using 18 Gy to the 50% isodose line. The patient's seizures subsided 3 months following the GKRS, and he remained seizure free at 21 months posttreatment with no neurological or endocrinological complications. MRI performed 12 months after radiosurgery demonstrated complete disappearance of the hamartoma.

In 2000, Régis and colleagues[85] published a multicenter retrospective study evaluating the safety and efficacy of GKRS to treat disabling seizures associated with sessile HHs. They studied 10 patients with a mean age of 14 years (range, 1 to 32 years). The median marginal dose was 15.25 Gy (range, 12 to 20 Gy). Two patients were treated twice (at 19 and 49 months) because of insufficient efficacy. The median follow-up period was 28 months (range, 12 to 71 months). All patients had improved seizure control after GKRS with four patients becoming seizure free, two experiencing rare seizures, and two exhibiting only partial improvement with reductions in the frequency of seizures but persistence of occasional generalized seizures. Two patients, who became seizure free, were considered to exhibit insufficient improvement after the first GKRS procedure and were treated a second time. The authors noted a clear correlation between efficacy and dose. The marginal dose was >17 Gy for all patients in the successful group and <13 Gy for all patients in the improved group. The investigators also reported that complete coverage of the HHs did not seem to be mandatory for good outcome because the dosimetry spared a significant part of the lesion in two patients in the successful group. No major side effects were observed in the 10 patients treated.

In 2002, Dunoyer et al[50] treated two patients with HH and associated epilepsy with GKRS with good results. The first patient was a 4-year-old boy who received 11 Gy at the 85% isodose line and had >90% reduction in seizures at 6 months following radiosurgery. The second patient was a 5-year-old girl who was treated with 14 Gy to the 45% isodose line. She was seizure free at 2.5 months following GKRS. Both patients had improvement in behavior.

In their follow-up prospective study, the authors from Marseille reported the outcome of GKRS in 30 patients with HHs and associated severe epilepsy.[86] The median dose at the 50% isodose line was 17 Gy (range, 14 to 20 Gy). Several of the 19 patients who had follow-up evaluation of more than 6 months had significant improvement of seizure frequency and behavior. Despite these promising results, the study was severely limited because of insufficient duration of follow-up evaluation. Only 6 of the 30 patients were followed for more than 12 months.

In 2006, the Marseille group reported the long-term results of their prospective trial of patients with HH with associated intractable epilepsy treated with GKRS.[87] A total of 60 patients were enrolled in the study. Of the 31 patients evaluated for a minimum of 3 years after radiosurgical treatment, adequate follow-up was available for 27 patients. The median dose at the marginal isodose was 17 Gy (range, 13 to 26 Gy). Beam blocking strategy was used to minimize the dose delivered to critical structures surrounding the HH including mammillary bodies, fornices, tuber cinerium, pituitary stalk, and optic nerve, chiasm, and tract. Ten of the 27 patients (37%) were seizure free and another six (22%) had significant reduction in seizure frequency. Most patients showed dramatic behavioral and cognitive improvement. The vast majority of cases did not have any change on the MRI. Only two patients showed a slight decrease in the size of the lesion. Four patients (15%) experienced temporary worsening of seizures, but none presented with a permanent complication. The authors conclude that GKRS, which can alleviate both the seizures and the behavioral and developmental dysfunction associated with HH, should be considered as first-line treatment for small and medium sized lesions. They advocate a staged approach for large lesions using microsurgical techniques for disconnection (open or endoscopic) of the lower part of the lesion followed by radiosurgery of the small upper part of the HH.

A few other small case series reported their results using GKRS for treating HH. Unger et al[88] reported good outcome (Engel class II) in 3 of the 4 patients treated with margin doses of 12 to 14 Gy to the 50 to 90% isodoses. Barajas et al[89] reported good outcomes at 30 to 50 months following GKRS in three patients with HHs treated with 12.5, 14, and 15 Gy at the 50% isodose line. Mathieu et al[90] also described their experience in treating four patients with HH and seizures with GKRS using a mean of 17.5 Gy at the 50% marginal isodose. After a median follow-up of 22 months, two patients achieved an Engel class II outcome. None had any side effects from radiosurgery.

Overall, these studies clearly show that GKRS can be quite effective in the treatment of epilepsy associated with HHs but can induce neurological sequelae similar to those induced by microsurgical resection. A further disadvantage is that clinical improvements can be very slow, exposing the patient to the risk of persisting seizures for up to 2 years after the procedure. Microsurgery has a definite advantage in this respect because of the immediate postsurgical improvement.

LINAC-Based Radiosurgery

As noted above, in 2002, Akai et al[79] presented the case of a 5-year-old girl with gelastic seizures related to an HH who underwent neuroendoscopic biopsy of the lesion. Subsequently, she was treated with linear accelerator stereotactic radiosurgery. However, her symptoms remained unchanged for 6 months. She then underwent partial resection and laser coagulation of the tumor by a neuroendoscopic approach.

After the procedure, the frequency of her seizures was remarkably decreased, and her violent behavior improved. In 2005, Selch and colleagues[91] reported their experience with linear accelerator stereotactic radiosurgery for the treatment of gelastic seizures due to sessile HH. Three patients received 15 to 18 Gy prescribed at the 90 to 95% isodose line. Two patients remained seizure free at 15 and 17 months, and one patient had significant decline in seizure frequency (Engel class II) 9 months after treatment. None of the four patients developed posttreatment complications.

Stereotactic Brachytherapy

In 2004, Schulze-Bonhage and coworkers[92] published their first report on stereotactic interstitial radiosurgery by intra-hypothalamic implantation of iodine-125 (^{125}I)-seeds. The authors evaluated seven patients with pharmacorefractory gelastic epilepsy due to HHs who underwent stereotactic placement of a single ^{125}I-seed following needle biopsy of the hamartoma via a right frontal approach. The intrahypothalamic hamartoma radioactive seeds were determined to be adequately implanted in 5 of the 7 patients and were removed after a mean period of 24 ± 5.7 days. In one patient, the seed was not placed in the exact center of the hamartoma and in another patient, due to the coarse consistency of the lesion, the seed could not be inserted into the HH. Three patients had to be reimplanted as the first intervention did not lead to complete seizure control. The reference dose was 60 Gy at the outer margin of the hamartoma. Two patients became seizure free within 2 months after seed implantation and two others had only persistent auras. There was no major perioperative morbidity. The authors conclude that stereotactic interstitial radiosurgery is a safe and effective minimally invasive method that compares favorably to GKRS in which a mean latency in seizure cessation of 6 to 9 months has been reported. In addition, the procedure can be done under local anesthesia with combination of stereotactic tissue biopsy and depth electrode recording. In a separate article, they also reported that in 5 of 8 patients who were successfully treated in terms of seizures, there was significant improvement in social and behavioral problems as well as quality of life. In their recent study, the same authors showed that temporary implantation of ^{125}I-seeds within the HH did not produce negative cognitive side effects at 3 months after interstitial radiosurgery (Shulze-Bonhage et al, 2004).[93]

Stereotactic Radiofrequency Ablation

Stereotactic radiofrequency thermocoagulation has been proposed by some groups for lesioning the HH in place of direct microsurgical excision. The technique has been used for the surgical treatment of movement disorders, epilepsy, intractable pain, and metastatic brain tumors.[94,13,95,96]

Kuzniecky and Guthrie[97] reported the results of 12 patients with HHs with progressive epileptic encephalopathy who underwent thermocoagulation with (eight patients) or without endoscopic partial resection (four patients). Of the 12 children, three remained seizure free at a mean follow-up of 27.3 months (range, 18 to 40 months) and another three patients had >90% reduction in seizures at a mean follow-up of 51.6 months (range, 36 to 70 months). Two patients had transient neurological deficits including third nerve palsy and memory loss. One patient had brainstem infarction and died. The authors concluded that a stereotactic thermocoagulation approach should be considered in patients with small lesions.

Similarly, Fujimoto et al[98] reported successful application of radiofrequency ablation to reduce the epileptogenicity and seizure propagation in a 26-year-old man with HH who presented with refractory epilepsy and severe mental retardation from age 6 months. The patient had undergone three prior surgeries yielding partial resection and conventional irradiation treatments. He underwent open radiofrequency ablation of the residual hamartoma via the transcallosal subchoroidal approach using image guidance. This resulted in immediate and remarkable seizure remission without complications. The same group[99] used stereotactic radiofrequency to ablate a large sessile lesion using multiple trajectories with good outcome. Fukuda et al[100] achieved similar results through a single electrode trajectory in treating a 15-year-old girl with a small hamartoma associated with intractable gelastic seizures. They confirmed the intrinsic epiletogenesis in depth electrode studies and the reduction of epileptic discharge after coagulation. Similarly, Parrent[101] presented the case of a patient in whom partial resection of the hamartoma followed by temporal lobectomy and orbitofrontal corticectomy failed to reduce the seizures. Subsequent stereotactic radiofrequency ablation of the hamartoma resulted in progressive improvement in the seizure disorder during a 28-month follow-up period.

Overall, it is proposed that the technique of radiofrequency ablation provides a minimally invasive, low-risk approach for the treatment of HHs. Additionally, the authors add that their approach has an advantage over Gamma Knife radiosurgery in view of the fact that stereotactic radiofrequency ablation can achieve an immediate result. However, the procedure carries several disadvantages, including imprecise volume of tissue ablation and the requirement for multiple trajectories for larger lesions, which inherently carries greater risk of damage to the surrounding structures.

Vagal Nerve Stimulation

Two groups reported their experience with patients with HH and intractable epilepsy who underwent implantation of a vagal nerve stimulator (VNS). The first study by Murphy et al[102] followed six children and noted that none of the patients were seizure free after left vagal nerve stimulation, three had improved seizures, and three were not signifi-

cantly improved. Interestingly, of four patients with severe autistic behavior, all four children had significant improvement in behavior following vagal nerve stimulation. Brandberg and colleagues[4] reported the outcome of five children treated with this technique. None of the patients demonstrated any improvement. We agree with Feiz-Erfan et al[76] that this palliative technique does not effectively control gelastic seizures. As such, we believe that VNS therapy plays a very limited role in the management of gelastic seizures associated with HHs.

Frontal or Temporal Corticectomy

After several years, the seizure semiology in patients with sessile HH usually evolves into focal motor features, autonomic phenomena, and/or secondary generalizations including drop attacks. Scalp EEG typically shows slow spike and wave patterns. Some seizure types suggest the involvement of temporal or frontal lobe. However, resections of temporal or frontal lobe cortex, even in patients carefully investigated with intracranial depth electrode recording demonstrating tonic early involvement of these cortical areas, have invariably failed to control the seizures.[39] Clearly, the intrinsically epileptogenic hamartoma has to be addressed in order to achieve good seizure outcome.

Corpus Callosotomy

Section of the anterior two-thirds of the corpus callosum as a palliative treatment of disabling generalized seizures, including drop attacks, associated with HHs has very limited efficacy. Cascino et al[39] reported on two patients and Pallini et al[103] studied one patient who underwent anterior callosotomy with minimal benefit to the generalized seizure pattern. In our opinion, there is no role for corpus callosotomy in the management of patients with HHs and disabling seizures. However, in circumstances where other first-line strategies, such as microsurgery or radiosurgery have failed and/or are contraindicated, one can consider vagal nerve stimulation instead of callosotomy only as a second- or third-line treatment.

Case Example

A 3-year-old boy was born at 40 weeks gestation by spontaneous vaginal delivery as the older of a set of nonidentical twins. The patient's mother reported an uneventful pregnancy. He had good Apgar scores and had mild neonatal hyperbilirubinemia. He was discharged home within 36 hours of birth. However, in the following days, the patient experienced what later were identified as gelastic seizures. Over the next few months, he continued to have episodes of pathological laughter. It was noted that at 6 months of age, spells typically lasted <5 seconds and occurred up to 20 times per day. These brief but repetitive episodes persisted in the first year of life but remained largely unrecognized until the patient was 18 months old. At that time, he had a usual nonemotional laughing spell lasting a few seconds, but contrary to all previous episodes, this attack was followed by a generalized tonic-clonic seizure. Over the subsequent months, the patient continued to experience ≥20 gelastic seizures and seven to 20 generalized seizures per day. At this time, he was started on vigabatrin. However, not finding any change in the frequency or severity of the seizures, the parents decided to discontinue the anticonvulsant and refused any further antiepileptic medications.

His developmental milestones were also somewhat delayed. He was crawling at 8 months and began walking at 16 months. At that time, his gross and fine motor skills were felt to be marginally below the normal range. From a speech and language developmental perspective, the patient had a vocabulary of six to eight words at 14 months of age. Over the following year, the patient's seizures continued to worsen. In addition to gelastic and secondary tonic-clonic seizures, he started having drop attacks primarily involving the head. During this period, the patient began to regress developmentally. His level of interaction and communication deteriorated. He also failed to develop any new motor or language skills and in fact lost the few words he had spoken previously. Behaviorally, he became very aggressive with frequent temper tantrums. The patient was normocephalic with a slight strabismus with alternating esotropy. The motor and sensory, as well as the rest of the neurological examination, were within normal limits.

EEG video telemetry revealed two electrographic and clinical seizure types. Clinically, the patient appeared afraid and made guttural sounds at seizure onset. This was followed by an emotionless laugh. The patient also had head drops and associated arm extension. Electrographically, an eletrodecremental pattern was observed followed by generalized slow wave and at times intermingled generalized spike and wave complexes. **Figure 9.4** demonstrates rhythmic sharp activity starting in the left frontal region rapidly becoming rhythmic spikes. Head drop attacks were associated with generalized sharp waves. Seizures duration was between 50 and 75 seconds. Interictally, a generalized epileptiform abnormality was observed. Additionally, a bifrontal epileptiform abnormality with right-sided predominance was also noted.

High-resolution MRI scans demonstrated a well-defined, rounded, soft tissue mass in the region of the tuber cinerium (**Fig. 9.5**). The lesion measured 12 mm in diameter and was isointense to gray matter on both T1- and T2-weighted sequences. The lesion did not enhance following administration of gadolinium. The mass showed heterogeneous signal intensities on the fluid-attenuated inversion recovery (FLAIR) images. There was no evidence of restrictive diffusion. There was no hydrocephalus associated with the HH, and no other lesions were identified.

Progressive worsening of cognition and behavior was noted on the formal neuropsychological examination performed at the time of surgery. The evaluation showed moderate mental deficiency, borderline developmental quotients, and delayed speech. In addition, he had behavioral problems that encompassed hyperkinesias, aggressiveness, and autistic features.

Microsurgical excision of the HH was proposed to the patient's parents given the intractability of the seizure disorder, the developmental regression, and behavioral and cognitive disabilities. We have used the traditional surgical approaches such as the transcallosal anterior interforniceal, the pterional, and the subfrontal translaminal terminalis approaches for resection of HHs. Because the main component of the hamartoma was within the third ventricle, it was felt that the interhemispheric, anterior transcallosal route would be best suited for this patient. Craniotomy

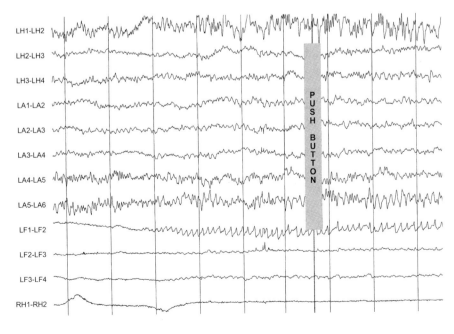

Fig. 9.4 Preoperative scalp EEG showing rhythmic sharp activity at LF1-LF2 rapidly becoming rhythmic spikes with push button denoting clinical seizure.

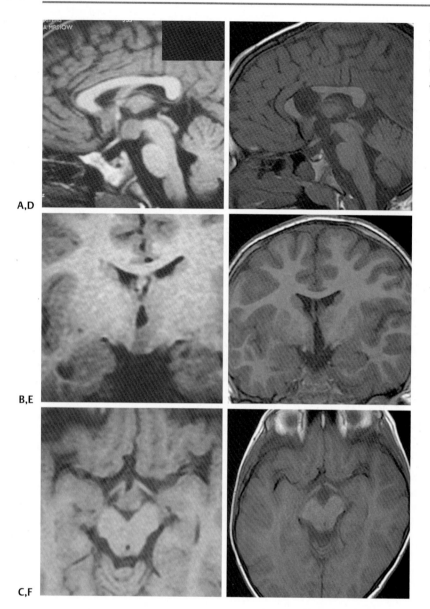

Fig. 9.5 High-resolution MRI scans of demonstrating a well-defined, hypointense, nonenhancing hypothalamic hamartoma measuring 12 mm in diameter. **(A)** Sagittal, **(B)** coronal, and **(C)** axial views obtained preoperatively and following surgery **(D–F)**.

A,D

B,E

C,F

using frameless stereotaxy was performed. Clear and direct visualization of the intraventricular component of the hamartoma was possible. Using a microdissector and an ultrasonic aspirator, complete removal of the lesion was achieved. Differentiation of the hamartoma from the ventricular walls and mamillary bodies can be a challenge. The hamartoma was typically slightly firmer and more gray compared with the surrounding neural structures. The plane of the third ventricle, the mamillary bodies posterolaterally, and the pia above the interpeduncular cistern provided resective surgical margins.

Postoperatively, he became seizure free and is no longer taking any antiepileptic medications. His overall behavioral functioning after surgery was significantly improved. He also showed considerable progress in his cognitive development, both verbal and nonverbal. However, he developed diabetes insipidus requiring desmopressin (DDAVP).

Histological examination of the surgical specimens revealed a disorganized mixture of scattered large neurons similar to those commonly found in the normal tuber cinerium. These mature NeuN-positive hypothalamic neurons were interspersed with clusters of neurocytoid cells with round, monotonous nuclei and clear cytoplasm (**Fig. 9.6**). No mitotic figures were seen with absence of MIB1 positivity. There was no evidence of microvascular proliferation or necrosis.

Conclusion

HHs are rare congenital heterotopic lesions composed of neurons, glia, and myelinated fibers. "Epileptic" HHs are usually sessile and closely associated with the mammillary bodies. Patients classically present with gelastic seizures in early childhood and can progress to a devastating clinical

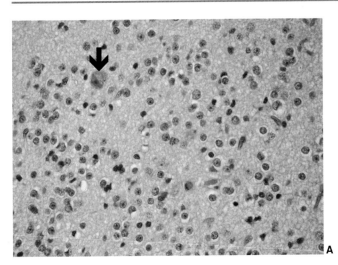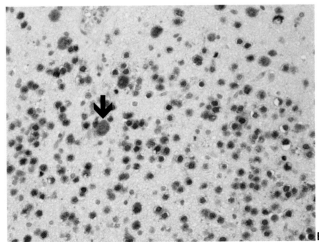

Fig. 9.6 Histology of a hypothalamic hamartoma. **(A)** On a routine hematoxylin and eosin (H&E) stain, there are both large neurons (ganglion cells; *arrow*) and smaller neuronal cells called "neurocytes." They are surrounded by a neurophil-like matrix. **(B)** When stained immunohistochemically with an antibody against NeuN, a neuronal marker, both cell types are intensely positive (*arrow*, ganglion cell). (Original magnification 400x on both images.)

syndrome, which may include various types of refractory seizures with generalization, progressive cognitive decline, and deterioration in behavioral and psychiatric functioning. Contrary to conventional thinking that attributed seizure origin to cortical structures, the hamartoma itself has now been firmly established as the site of intrinsic epileptogenesis for the gelastic seizures characterized by unusual mirth. It also appears that the HH contributes to a phenomenon of secondary epileptogenesis, with eventual cortical seizure onset of multiple types in some patients. Anticonvulsant medications are known to be poorly effective in this disorder. Treatment, including some innovative approaches to surgical resection and/or disconnection, is now targeted directly at the HH itself, with impressive results. Less invasive treatment modalities have also shown to have good outcome in terms of seizure control and improvements in behavior, cognition, and overall development. Younger patients, in particular, may benefit most from an aggressive surgical management in an attempt to minimize or prevent the cognitive and behavioral sequelae commonly associated with this debilitating subcortical epileptic syndrome.

References

1. Daniel PM. Anatomy of the hypothalamus and pituitary gland. J Clin Pathol Suppl (Assoc Clin Pathol) 1976;7:1–7
2. Arroyo S, Lesser RP, Gordon B, et al. Mirth, laughter and gelastic seizures. Brain 1993;116(Pt 4):757–780
3. Freeman JL. The anatomy and embryology of the hypothalamus in relation to hypothalamic hamartomas. Epileptic Disord 2003;5(4):177–186
4. Brandberg G, Raininko R, Eeg-Olofsson O. Hypothalamic hamartoma with gelastic seizures in Swedish children and adolescents. Eur J Paediatr Neurol 2004;8(1):35–44
5. Hall JG, Pallister PD, Clarren SK, et al. Congenital hypothalamic hamartoblastoma, hypopituitarism, imperforate anus and postaxial polydactyly–a new syndrome? Part I: clinical, causal, and pathogenetic considerations. Am J Med Genet 1980;7(1):47–74
6. Kang S, Graham JM Jr, Olney AH, Biesecker LG. GLI3 frameshift mutations cause autosomal dominant Pallister-Hall syndrome. Nat Genet 1997;15(3):266–268
7. Bertrand N, Dahmane N. Sonic hedgehog signaling in forebrain development and its interactions with pathways that modify its effects. Trends Cell Biol 2006;16(11):597–605
8. Lai K, Kaspar BK, Gage FH, Schaffer DV. Sonic hedgehog regulates adult neural progenitor proliferation in vitro and in vivo. Nat Neurosci 2003;6(1):21–27
9. Trousseau A. *Clinique Médicale de l'Hôtel-Dieu de Paris*. 4th ed. Paris: Ballière; 1873

10. Castro LH, Ferreira LK, Teles LR, et al. Epilepsy syndromes associated with hypothalamic hamartomas. Seizure 2007;16(1):50–58
11. Mullatti N, Selway R, Nashef L, et al. The clinical spectrum of epilepsy in children and adults with hypothalamic hamartoma. Epilepsia 2003;44(10):1310–1319
12. Arzimanoglou AA, Hirsch E, Aicardi J. Hypothalamic hamartoma and epilepsy in children: illustrative cases of possible evolutions. Epileptic Disord 2003;5(4):187–199
13. Frattali CM, Liow K, Craig GH, et al. Cognitive deficits in children with gelastic seizures and hypothalamic hamartoma. Neurology 2001;57(1):43–46
14. Leal AJ, Passao V, Calado E, Vieira JP, Silva Cunha JP. Interictal spike EEG source analysis in hypothalamic hamartoma epilepsy. Clin Neurophysiol 2002;113(12):1961–1969
15. Tassinari CA, Riguzzi P, Rizzi R. Gelastic seizures. In: Tuxhorn I, Holthausen H, Boenighk K, eds. *Pediatric Epilepsy Syndromes and Their Surgical Treatment*. London: John Libbey; 1997:429–446
16. Mullatti N. Hypothalamic hamartoma in adults. Epileptic Disord 2003;5(4):201–204
17. Arita K, Ikawa F, Kurisu K, et al. The relationship between magnetic resonance imaging findings and clinical manifestations of hypothalamic hamartoma. J Neurosurg 1999;91(2):212–220
18. Weissenberger AA, Dell ML, Liow K, et al. Aggression and psychiatric comorbidity in children with hypothalamic hamartomas

and their unaffected siblings. J Am Acad Child Adolesc Psychiatry 2001;40(6):696–703

19. Quiske A, Frings L, Wagner K, Unterrainer J, Schulze-Bonhage A. Cognitive functions in juvenile and adult patients with gelastic epilepsy due to hypothalamic hamartoma. Epilepsia 2006;47(1):153–158

20. Berkovic SF, Kuzniecky RI, Andermann F. Human epileptogenesis and hypothalamic hamartomas: new lessons from an experiment of nature. Epilepsia 1997;38(1):1–3

21. Savard G, Bhanji NH, Dubeau F, Andermann F, Sadikot A. Psychiatric aspects of patients with hypothalamic hamartoma and epilepsy. Epileptic Disord 2003;5(4):229–234

22. Ali S, Moriarty J, Mullatti N, David A. Psychiatric comorbidity in adult patients with hypothalamic hamartoma. Epilepsy Behav 2006;9(1):111–118

23. Cassio A, Cacciari E, Zucchini S, Balsamo A, Diegoli M, Orsini F. Central precocious puberty: clinical and imaging aspects. J Pediatr Endocrinol Metab 2000;13(Suppl 1):703–708

24. Jung H, Parent AS, Ojeda SR. Hypothalamic hamartoma: a paradigm/model for studying the onset of puberty. Endocr Dev 2005;8:81–93

25. Lin SR, Bryson MM, Gobien RP, Fitz CR, Lee YY. Radiologic findings of hamartomas of the tuber cinereum and hypothalamus. Radiology 1978;127(3):697–703

26. Diebler C, Ponsot G. Hamartomas of the tuber cinereum. Neuroradiology 1983;25(2):93–101

27. Takeuchi J, Handa H, Miki Y, Munemitsu H, Aso T. Precocious puberty due to a hypothalamic hamartoma. Surg Neurol 1979;11(6):456–460

28. Mori K, Handa H, Takeuchi J, Hanakita J, Nakano Y. Hypothalamic hamartoma. J Comput Assist Tomogr 1981;5(4):519–521

29. Pang D, Rosenbaum AE, Wilberger JE Jr, Gutai JP. Metrizamide computed tomographic cisternography for the diagnosis of occult lesions of the hypothalamic-hypophyseal axis in children. Neurosurgery 1981; 8(5):531–541

30. Freeman JL, Coleman LT, Wellard RM, et al. MR imaging and spectroscopic study of epileptogenic hypothalamic hamartomas: analysis of 72 cases. Am J Neuroradiol 2004;25(3):450–462

31. Berkovic SF, Andermann F, Melanson D, Ethier RE, Feindel W, Gloor P. Hypothalamic hamartomas and ictal laughter: evolution of a characteristic epileptic syndrome and diagnostic value of magnetic resonance imaging. Ann Neurol 1988;23(5):429–439

32. Hahn FJ, Leibrock LG, Huseman CA, Makos MM. The MR appearance of hypothalamic hamartoma. Neuroradiology 1988;30(1):65–68

33. Lona Soto A, Takahashi M, Yamashita Y, Sakamoto Y, Shinzato J, Yoshizumi K. MRI findings of hypothalamic hamartoma: report of five cases and review of the literature. Comput Med Imaging Graph 1991; 15(6):415–421

34. Tasch E, Cendes F, Li LM, et al. Hypothalamic hamartomas and gelastic epilepsy: a spectroscopic study. Neurology 1998;51(4):1046–1050

35. Pascual-Castroviejo I, Moneo JH, Viano J, Garcia-Segura JM, Herguido MJ, Pascual Pascual SI. [Hypothalamic hamartomas: control of seizures after partial removal in one case.] Rev Neurol 2000;31(2):119–122

36. Wakai S, Nikaido K, Nihira H, Kawamoto Y, Hayasaka H. Gelastic seizure with hypothalamic hamartoma: proton magnetic resonance spectrometry and ictal electroencephalographic findings in a 4-year-old girl. J Child Neurol 2002;17(1):44–46

37. Martin DD, Seeger U, Ranke MB, Grodd W. MR imaging and spectroscopy of a tuber cinereum hamartoma in a patient with growth hormone deficiency and hypogonadotropic hypogonadism. Am J Neuroradiol 2003;24(6):1177–1180

38. Amstutz DR, Coons SW, Kerrigan JF, Rekate HL, Heiserman JE. Hypothalamic hamartomas: Correlation of MR imaging and spectroscopic findings with tumor glial content. Am J Neuroradiol 2006;27(4):794–798

39. Cascino GD, Andermann F, Berkovic SF, et al. Gelastic seizures and hypothalamic hamartomas: evaluation of patients undergoing chronic intracranial EEG monitoring and outcome of surgical treatment. Neurology 1993;43(4):747–750

40. Jung H, Neumaier PE, Hauffa BP, Partsch CJ, Dammann O. Association of morphological characteristics with precocious puberty and/or gelastic seizures in hypothalamic hamartoma. J Clin Endocrinol Metab 2003;88(10):4590–4595

41. Munari C, Kahane P, Francione S, et al. Role of the hypothalamic hamartoma in the genesis of gelastic fits (a video-stereo-EEG study). Electroencephalogr Clin Neurophysiol 1995;95(3):154–160

42. Palmini A, Chandler C, Andermann F, et al. Resection of the lesion in patients with hypothalamic hamartomas and catastrophic epilepsy. Neurology 2002;58(9):1338–1347

43. Kuzniecky R, Guthrie B, Mountz J, et al. Intrinsic epileptogenesis of hypothalamic hamartomas in gelastic epilepsy. Ann Neurol 1997;42(1):60–67

44. Kahane P, Ryvlin P, Hoffmann D, Minotti L, Benabid AL. From hypothalamic hamartoma to cortex: what can be learnt from depth recordings and stimulation? Epileptic Disord 2003;5(4):205–217

45. Choi JU, Yang KH, Kim TG, et al. Endoscopic disconnection for hypothalamic hamartoma with intractable seizure. Report of four cases. J Neurosurg 2004;100(5, Suppl)506–511

46. Ryvlin P, Ravier C, Bouvard S, et al. Positron emission tomography in epileptogenic hypothalamic hamartomas. Epileptic Disord 2003;5(4):219–227

47. Palmini A, Van PW, Dupont P, Van LK, Van DG. Status gelasticus after temporal lobectomy: ictal FDG-PET findings and the question of dual pathology involving hypothalamic hamartomas. Epilepsia 2005;46(8):1313–1316

48. Arroyo S, Santamaria J, Sanmarti F, et al. Ictal laughter associated with paroxysmal hypothalamopituitary dysfunction. Epilepsia 1997; 38(1):114–117

49. DiFazio MP, Davis RG. Utility of early single photon emission computed tomography (SPECT) in neonatal gelastic epilepsy associated with hypothalamic hamartoma. J Child Neurol 2000;15(6):414–417

50. Dunoyer C, Ragheb J, Resnick T, et al. The use of stereotactic radiosurgery to treat intractable childhood partial epilepsy. Epilepsia 2002;43(3):292–300

51. Fohlen M, Lellouch A, Delalande O. Hypothalamic hamartoma with refractory epilepsy: surgical procedures and results in 18 patients. Epileptic Disord 2003;5(4):267–273

52. Delalande O, Fohlen M. Disconnecting surgical treatment of hypothalamic hamartoma in children and adults with refractory epilepsy and proposal of a new classification. Neurol Med Chir (Tokyo) 2003; 43(2):61–68

53. Bunyaratavej K, Locharernkul C, Tepmongkol S, Lerdlum S, Shuangshoti S, Khaoroptham S. Successful resection of hypothalamic hamartoma with intractable gelastic seizures–by transcallosal subchoroidal approach. J Med Assoc Thai 2006;89(8):1269–1276

54. Boyko OB, Curnes JT, Oakes WJ, Burger PC. Hamartomas of the tuber cinereum: CT, MR, and pathologic findings. Am J Neuroradiol 1991;12(2):309–314

55. Valdueza JM, Cristante L, Dammann O, et al. Hypothalamic hamartomas: with special reference to gelastic epilepsy and surgery. Neurosurgery 1994;34(6):949–958

56. Kerrigan JF, Ng YT, Chung S, Rekate HL. The hypothalamic hamartoma: a model of subcortical epileptogenesis and encephalopathy. Semin Pediatr Neurol 2005;12(2):119–131

57. Albright AL, Lee PA. Surgery for hypothalamic hamartomas. J Neurosurg 1998;88(2):353

58. Stewart L, Steinbok P, Daaboul J. Role of surgical resection in the treatment of hypothalamic hamartomas causing precocious puberty. Report of six cases. J Neurosurg 1998;88(2):340–345

59. Strum JW, Andermann F, Berkovic SF. "Pressure to laugh": an unsual epileptic symptom associated with small hypothalamic hamartomas, Neurology 2000;54(4):971–973

60. Coons SW, Rekate HL, Prenger EC, et al. The histopathology of hypothalamic hamartomas: study of 57 cases. J Neuropathol Exp Neurol 2007;66(2):131–141

61. Kahane P, Di LM, Hoffmann D, Munari C. Ictal bradycardia in a patient with a hypothalamic hamartoma: a stereo-EEG study. Epilepsia 1999;40(4):522–527

62. Fenoglio KA, Wu J, Kim DY, et al. Hypothalamic hamartoma: basic mechanisms of intrinsic epileptogenesis. Semin Pediatr Neurol 2007;14(2):51–59

63. Wu J, Xu L, Kim DY, et al. Electrophysiological properties of human hypothalamic hamartomas. Ann Neurol 2005;58(3):371–382

64. Northfield DW, Russell DS. Pubertas praecox due to hypothalamic hamartoma: report of two cases surviving surgical removal of the tumour. J Neurol Neurosurg Psychiatry 1967;30(2):166–173

65. Paillas JE, Roger J, Toga M, et al. Hamartome de l'hypothalamus. Étude clinique, radiologique, histologique. Résultats de l'exérèse. Rev Neurol (Paris) 1969;120(3):177–194

66. Pendl G. Gelastic epilepsy in tumors of the hypothalamic region. Adv Neurosurg 1975;3:442–449

67. Ponsot G, Diebler C, Plouin P, et al. [Hypothalamic hamartoma and gelastic crises. Apropos of 7 cases.] Arch Fr Pediatr 1983;40(10):757–761

68. Sato M, Ushio Y, Arita N, Mogami H. Hypothalamic hamartoma: report of two cases. Neurosurgery 1985;16(2):198–206

69. Nishio S, Fujiwara S, Aiko Y, Takeshita I, Fukui M. Hypothalamic hamartoma. Report of two cases. J Neurosurg 1989;70(4):640–645

70. Machado HR, Hoffman HJ, Hwang PA. Gelastic seizures treated by resection of a hypothalamic hamartoma. Childs Nerv Syst 1991;7(8):462–465

71. Nishio S, Shigeto H, Fukui M. Hypothalamic hamartoma: the role of surgery. Neurosurg Rev 1993;16(2):157–160

72. Miranda P, Esparza J, Cabrera A, Hinojosa J. Giant hypothalamic hamartoma operated through subfrontal approach with orbitary rim osteotomy. Pediatr Neurosurg 2006;42(4):254–257

73. Palmini A, Paglioli-Neto E, Montes J, Farmer JP. The treatment of patients with hypothalamic hamartomas, epilepsy and behavioural abnormalities: facts and hypotheses. Epileptic Disord 2003;5(4):249–255

74. Rosenfeld JV, Harvey AS, Wrennall J, Zacharin M, Berkovic SF. Transcallosal resection of hypothalamic hamartomas, with control of seizures, in children with gelastic epilepsy. Neurosurgery 2001;48(1):108–118

75. Rosenfeld JV, Freeman JL, Harvey AS. Operative technique: the anterior transcallosal transseptal interforniceal approach to the third ventricle and resection of hypothalamic hamartomas. J Clin Neurosci 2004;11(7):738–744

76. Harvey AS, Freeman JL, Berkovic SF, Rosenfeld JV. Transcallosal resection of hypothalamic hamartomas in patients with intractable epilepsy. Epileptic Disord 2003;5(4):257–265

77. Feiz-Erfan I, Horn EM, Rekate HL, et al. Surgical strategies for approaching hypothalamic hamartomas causing gelastic seizures in the pediatric population: transventricular compared with skull base approaches. J Neurosurg 2005;103(4, Suppl)325–332

78. Ng YT, Rekate HL, Prenger EC, et al. Transcallosal resection of hypothalamic hamartoma for intractable epilepsy. Epilepsia 2006;47(7):1192–1202

79. Akai T, Okamoto K, Iizuka H, Kakinuma H, Nojima T. Treatments of hamartoma with neuroendoscopic surgery and stereotactic radiosurgery: a case report. Minim Invasive Neurosurg 2002;45(4):235–239

80. Rekate HL, Feiz-Erfan I, Ng YT, Gonzalez LF, Kerrigan JF. Endoscopic surgery for hypothalamic hamartomas causing medically refractory gelastic epilepsy. Childs Nerv Syst 2006;22(8):874–880

81. Fohlen M, Lellouch A, Delalande O. Hypothalamic hamartoma with refractory epilepsy: surgical procedures and results in 18 patients. Epileptic Disord 2003;5(4):267–273

82. Leksell L. The stereotaxic method and radiosurgery of the brain. Acta Chir Scand 1951;102(4):316–319

83. Régis J, Rey M, Bartolomei F, et al. Gamma knife surgery in mesial temporal lobe epilepsy: a prospective multicenter study. Epilepsia 2004;45(5):504–515

84. Arita K, Kurisu K, Iida K, et al. Subsidence of seizure induced by stereotactic radiation in a patient with hypothalamic hamartoma. Case report. J Neurosurg 1998;89(4):645–648

85. Régis J, Bartolomei F, de Toffol B, et al. Gamma knife surgery for epilepsy related to hypothalamic hamartomas. Neurosurgery 2000;47(6):1343–1351

86. Régis J, Hayashi M, Eupierre LP, et al. Gamma knife surgery for epilepsy related to hypothalamic hamartoma. Acta Neurochir Suppl 2004;91:33–50

87. Régis J, Scavarda D, Tamura M, et al. Epilepsy related to hypothalamic hamartomas: surgical management with special reference to gamma knife surgery. Childs Nerv Syst 2006;22(8):881–895

88. Unger F, Schrottner O, Feichtinger M, Bone G, Haselsberger K, Sutter B. Stereotactic radiosurgery for hypothalamic hamartomas. Acta Neurochir Suppl 2002;84:57–63

89. Barajas MA, Ramirez-Guzman MG, Rodriguez-Vazquez C, Toledo-Buenrostro V, Cuevas-Solorzano A, Rodriguez-Hernandez G. Gamma knife surgery for hypothalamic hamartomas accompanied by medically intractable epilepsy and precocious puberty: experience in Mexico. J Neurosurg 2005;102(Suppl):53–55

90. Mathieu D, Kondziolka D, Niranjan A, Flickinger J, Lunsford LD. Gamma knife radiosurgery for refractory epilepsy caused by hypothalamic hamartomas. Stereotact Funct Neurosurg 2006;84(2–3):82–87

91. Selch MT, Gorgulho A, Mattozo C, Solberg TD, Cabatan-Awang C, DeSalles AA. Linear accelerator stereotactic radiosurgery for the treatment of gelastic seizures due to hypothalamic hamartoma. Minim Invasive Neurosurg 2005;48(5):310–314

92. Schulze-Bonhage A, Homberg V, Trippel M, et al. Interstitial radiosurgery in the treatment of gelastic epilepsy due to hypothalamic hamartomas. Neurology 2004;62(4):644–647

93. Schulze-Bonhage A, Quiske A, Homberg V, et al. Effect of interstitial stereotactic radiosurgery on behavior and subjective handicap of epilepsy in patients with gelastic epilepsy. Epilepsy Behav 2004;5(1):94–101

94. Anzai Y, Lufkin R, DeSalles A, Hamilton DR, Farahani K, Black KL. Preliminary experience with MR-guided thermal ablation of brain tumors. Am J Neuroradiol 1995;16(1):39–48

95. Patil AA, Andrews R, Torkelson R. Stereotactic volumetric radiofrequency lesioning of intracranial structures for control of intractable seizures. Stereotact Funct Neurosurg 1995;64(3):123–133

96. Parrent AG, Blume WT. Stereotactic amygdalohippocampotomy for the treatment of medial temporal lobe epilepsy. Epilepsia 1999;40(10):1408–1416

97. Kuzniecky RI, Guthrie BL. Stereotactic surgical approach to hypothalamic hamartomas. Epileptic Disord 2003;5(4):275–280

98. Fujimoto Y, Kato A, Saitoh Y, et al. Open radiofrequency ablation for the management of intractable epilepsy associated with sessile

hypothalamic hamartoma. Minim Invasive Neurosurg 2005;48(3): 132–135

99. Fujimoto Y, Kato A, Saitoh Y, et al. Stereotactic radiofrequency ablation for sessile hypothalamic hamartoma with an image fusion technique. Acta Neurochir 2003;145(8):697–700

100. Fukuda M, Kameyama S, Wachi M, Tanaka R. Stereotaxy for hypothalamic hamartoma with intractable gelastic seizures: technical case report. Neurosurgery 1999;44(6):1347–1350

101. Parrent AG. Stereotactic radiofrequency ablation for the treatment of gelastic seizures associated with hypothalamic hamartoma. Case report. J Neurosurg 1999;91(5):881–884

102. Murphy JV, Wheless JW, Schmoll CM. Left vagal nerve stimulation in six patients with hypothalamic hamartomas. Pediatr Neurol 2000;23(2):167–168

103. Pallini R, Bozzini V, Colicchio G, Lauretti L, Scerrati M, Rossi GF. Callosotomy for generalized seizures associated with hypothalamic hamartoma. Neurol Res 1993;15(2):139–141

10 Multiple Subpial Transections

Albert E. Telfeian

The initiation and propagation of epileptiform discharges in the brain divides the problem of focal epilepsy into two parts: one, the generation of epileptiform activity, and two, the spread of epileptiform activity throughout the brain. Most successful epilepsy surgery is directed at resective techniques, that is, removing the seizure generator. Multiple subpial transection (MST) is a nonresective technique developed for the surgical interruption of the seizure process in areas of the brain where resective techniques would result in undesirable complications.

Scientific Rationale

Understanding the rationale behind MSTs is critical for the practitioner to perform them effectively. Morrell and Hambrey[1] and Morrell et al[2] conceived of the procedure of MSTs after an eruption in the understanding of multicellular neurophysiology. The concept of the cortical column developed in visual, auditory, somatosensory, and motor cortex physiology. Five millimeter–wide columns of neurons appeared to act as functional modules responsible for processing behavioral tasks. Vertically oriented neuronal processes such as apical and basal dendrites, as well as centrifugal and centripetal axonal process, appeared to be the necessary and sufficient building blocks for cortical function. Morrell cited experiments reported by Sperry and Miner[3] and Sperry et al[4] to support the rational behind MSTs. In Sperry's experiments, subpial transections or the insertion of mica plates in cat visual cortex were used to surgically create isolated vertical cortical columns; visual function did not appear to be interrupted. Morrell hypothesized that if these columns were the minimal units for function, then transecting the brain to no less than these 5 mm units might be enough to prevent seizure initiation and propagation. Morrell proposed parceling neocortex into its minimal functional volumes to undermine the initiation of seizure activity by reducing the volumes of cortex to neuron numbers not sufficient to generate the synchronized activity to trigger a seizure. With this cortical disconnection, even if synchronization occurred in an isolated cortical cube, it would not be able to propagate horizontally, synchronizing other neurons.

Technique

Seizure Localization

MSTs are applied, generally, to nonlesional cortical tissue after electrocorticography is used in an awake monitoring unit for seizure localization. During intraoperative electrode implantation, digital photography should be used to correlate surface anatomy with electrode position. Frameless stereotactic magnetic resonance imaging (MRI)-guidance is also important for co-localization, especially in lesional cases. After video monitoring, photographic maps are used to register epileptogenic areas as well as co-register information from awake motor and sensory mapping done in the epilepsy monitoring unit. These cortical maps are then used in the operating room at the time of surgery and refined with further motor and sensory mapping (**Fig. 10.1**). At the second surgery for removal of electrodes and performance of MSTs and resection, additional photographs are taken to demonstrate the actual area where the resection and transections were performed. Postoperative MRI is useful to demonstrate no postoperative complications, the removal of lesional cortex for lesional cases, and to demonstrate the depth and area of the MSTs (**Fig. 10.2**). The neurologist and neurosurgeon can use the intraoperative images in the forum of the preoperative epilepsy planning conference to discuss the possible risks, benefits, and options of the extent of resection and whether to substitute MSTs for surgical resection in areas that might be eloquent.

Operative Technique

Reports from different centers describe multiple variations on the technique of MSTs.[2,5–8] Generally, a small hole is made in the pia for the insertion of the transector. A no. 11 blade can be used or a hypodermic needle of various gauges. We coagulate the surface of the pia, only briefly and at low amplitude, with an irrigating bipolar coagulator before inserting a 25-gauge needle to provide the point of entry for the transector. Different centers also report various points of entry for the transector. Morrell et al described the point of entry for the transector at the sulcal border of the gyrus, where they inserted the transector as deep into the sulcus as possible.[2] Our preference is to make the point of entry in the middle of the gyrus. The transector is then inserted twice into the same point of entry and swept toward opposite sulci. We avoid the sulcal border as a point of entry because of its vascularity. The transector can be a microsurgical ball probe, stainless steel wire bent appropriately and held on a hemostat, or a commercially available product such as those developed for the procedure (e.g., AD-Tech Medical Instrument Corp., Racine WI). Transectors of various levels of sharpness and angle have been described. Our preference is to use a 5-mm blunt microsurgical probe bent at ~100 degrees. The

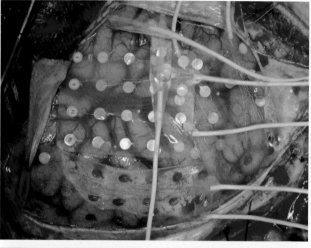
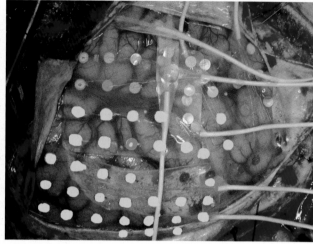

A,B

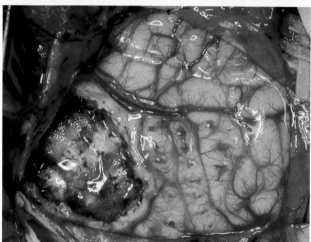

C

Fig. 10.1   Intraoperative digital photography is used to create cortical maps to record electrode positions, correlate sensory and motor mapping with electrode recordings and frameless stereotactic lesion localization, and communicate to the neurology team intraoperative findings. **(A)** Right frontotemporal-parietal craniotomy. Grid and strip electrodes are positioned to obtain maximal recording coverage. Photograph is oriented with temporal lobe superior and frontal lobe anterior. **(B)** Yellow dots indicate the epileptic areas recorded in the epilepsy monitoring unit. The green and yellow dot is the lesional area presumed to be cortical dysplasia from the MRI, localized using MR-guided frameless stereotaxy. **(C)** Postresection and MST. The resection cavity is seen on the left bordered to the right by the motor and sensory areas, treated with MSTs (note the punctuate hemorrhages frequently seen).

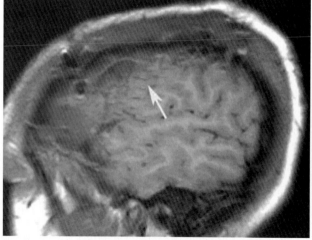
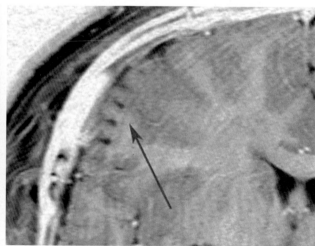

A,B

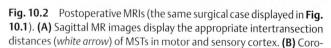

Fig. 10.2   Postoperative MRIs (the same surgical case displayed in **Fig. 10.1**). **(A)** Sagittal MR images display the appropriate intertransection distances (*white arrow*) of MSTs in motor and sensory cortex. **(B)** Coronal MR images display the appropriate depths (*black arrow*) through the gray matter of MSTs.

length of the probe should be kept to 4 to 5 mm to avoid penetrating deeply into the white matter and disrupting cortical blood supply. We do not recommend a sharp probe so as not to pierce the pia on sweeping the transector backward or not to catch on sulcal vessels. We occasionally also use longer-tipped transectors with more obtuse angles to reach deeper along sulci when necessary. Transections should be performed every 5 mm along a sulcus perpendicular to the gyri. As much as possible, coagulation should be avoided in eloquent areas. Using thrombin-soaked Gelfoam (Pfizer Inc., New York, NY) over the entry point of the transection stops most bleeding.

Electrocorticography

After transections, surface electrocorticography (ECoG) must be performed and MSTs repeated until abnormal ECoG activity arrests. If transections are performed every 5 mm and abnormal ECoG activity persists, then the surgeon should look to repeat the transection so as to disconnect what may be a deeper sulcus than first imagined. If MSTs are performed in conjunction with a lesionectomy, the MSTs should be performed after initially performing an adjacent focal lesionectomy to avoid reading an ECoG-active post-MST site as active as a result of transmitted activity from the lesion.

Indications for MST

MSTs are useful for the treatment of seizure activity arising from cortex serving indispensable function, such as motor, sensory, vision, and language areas. Most often, MSTs will be used in conjunction with a resection done for a lesional or nonlesional case when the ECoG-active area extends into nonresectable cortex. Most cases involving MSTs should, if possible, at least include a small cortical biopsy for diagnostic purposes.

MSTs are also useful specifically for epilepsia partialis continua (EPC) that originates from motor cortex. Activity similar to EPC that arises in the early stages of Rasmussen's encephalitis, a progressive inflammatory disorder, can be treated in a palliative way with MSTs when Rasmussen's is in its early stages, before hemiparesis makes hemispherectomy the appropriate treatment.

Landau-Kleffner syndrome (LKS) is a rare, acquired epileptiform aphasia thought to be secondary to epileptiform activity in perisylvian or intrasylvian areas; children with developed speech become mute. Several small studies of LKS patients have indicated that applying MSTs can reverse the aphasia.[8,9,10] In LKS, children achieve a normal developmental speech pattern and then regress in receptive and expressive language. Epileptiform activity is recorded in cortical language areas, especially during sleep. True clinical epileptic activity may not be seen and can usually be controlled with medication. The aphasia, however, is medically refractory. If seizure onset is unilateral rather than bilateral, which can be tested with a methohexital suppression test, MSTs can be applied. The technique is the same, coupling transections with ECoG to test posttransected areas, except that the area treated requires opening the sylvian fissure to obtain access to the affected cortex.

Results

Seizure Control and Complications

MSTs have been shown to be an effective surgical method for controlling seizures. Small patient numbers in individual series reported variabilities in the pathologies treated, and uncoupling the impact of a procedure most often done in conjunction with resection has made it difficult to convincingly report the efficacy of MSTs.[2,5,7,10] An international meta-analysis was published by Spencer et al in 2002 that included more than 200 patients and showed for MSTs performed with resection a >95% reduction of seizure frequency in 87% of patients with generalized seizures, 68% for complex partial seizures, and 68% for simple partial seizures.[11] For the patients who underwent MSTs without resection the same improvement in seizure frequency was almost as good: 71% for generalized, 62% for complex partial, and 63% for simple partial. In the same meta-analysis the complication rate for MSTs alone (19%) was comparable, overall, to MSTs coupled with resection (23%). Complications included memory loss, hemiparesis, and visual field loss. For LKS, Morrell et al have reported their experience with MTS in 16 children; 75% were seizure free, 44% had recovered age-appropriate language, and an additional 38% displayed a significant improvement in language function.[8] For the six patients in that study who required opening the sylvian fissure, two had subcortical infarcts demonstrable on MRI likely secondary to vascular manipulation.

Functional Impact

MST success has generally been accepted as a reduction in the seizure frequency without a paresis, aphasia, or significant visual field cut. Although MSTs usually induce minimal long-term postoperative functional deficits, transient deficits are not unusual. Several studies using functional MRI[12] and positron emission tomography[6] have indicated that during the recovery period and even long term, multiple and bilateral areas become co-activated to subserve the function of the selectively lesioned cortex. Very little has been done to assess the higher-level functional impact of MSTs in short- or long-term studies. Studies of pre- and postoperative neuropsychological testing have not been presented. Certainly MSTs would not be expected to have a worse functional impact than resection and, as is a general tenet of epilepsy surgery, significant seizure reduction leads to an overall improvement in quality of life.

Failures

It is likely that after transecting cortical tissue into 5-mm cubes, individual cubes can still support epileptiform activity. In vitro slices of neocortex only half a millimeter wide can support synchronous epileptiform discharges under certain conditions. If a 5-mm cube of cortex is sufficient to support epileptiform activity, eliminating the horizontal connectivity of these cubes is the likely mechanism of this technique.

The question then should be asked, which horizontal connections are important for seizure propagation? Mammalian neocortex is a six-layer structure. If only the most superficial layers are important to seizure spread, perhaps secondary to a technical error these are incompletely transected and deeper areas less necessary to seizure propagation are senselessly disconnected. Using rat neocortical slices we investigated local circuits for epileptiform propagation.[13] Making vertical cuts in slices of rat neocortex and creating laminar cortical bridges, it appeared that lower layer 5, the location of large pyramidal neurons with extensive basal dendritic trees, was the preferred layer to support the horizontal propagation of epileptiform activity. In just threshold levels of convulsant medium, an intact lower layer 5 bridge was both necessary and sufficient for seizure propagation. A particular excitatory neurotransmitter receptor system did not seem to distinguish layer 5 as important for the horizontal propagation of seizure activity because in both N-methyl-D-aspartic acid (NMDA) and non-NMDA dependent convulsant medium, lower layer 5 was the preferred path for seizure propagation.[14] The length of effective axonal connections in layer 5 also did not appear to be what distinguished layer 5 as particularly important in seizure spread. In comparing layer 2–3 and layer 5 projecting axonal connections, 2 mm appeared to be the greatest effective length for propagating monosynaptic inputs.[15] We had hypothesized that the intrinsic bursting characteristic of some of these lower layer 5 neurons may be what distinguishes them from other layers, but in human brain slice experiments, using cortical tissue removed from patients undergoing epilepsy surgery, we did not find neurons with intrinsic burst characteristics.[16]

If layer 5 neurons are important in the propagation of epileptic activity, what light does this shed on why MSTs sometimes fail to completely eliminate seizure activity? Kaufman et al provide many important details on how MSTs actually work and might not work in their histological analysis of human temporal lobe tissue removed after MSTs.[17] First, MSTs created acute pyknosis and tissue edema in 1- to 3-mm columnar blocks around each transection. Second, additional deep tissue damage, in up to a third of specimens, was seen that severed afferent and efferent connections; in addition to horizontal desynchronization, deafferentation may be one part of reducing epileptic activity. Third, transections often involved oblique cuts, disrupting dendrites and vertical axons. And fourth, secondary to limitations of the technique and variations in cortical thickness, such as those seen secondary to small gyri superimposed on major lobar gyri, transections missing deeper layers were regularly noted. In fact, 41% of MSTs transected down only as far as layers 3 and 4; only 35% of transections disconnected deeper cortex corresponding to layer 5 and 6. Certainly the perceived depth of transections performed only with a surface cortical view is only partially accurate and may make a very significant impact on the technique's effectiveness if lower cortical layers are indeed the important layers for the horizontal propagation of seizure activity.

Future Improvements for MST

If transections too superficial to layer 5 are less effective, and transections deep into the white matter are dangerous because they interrupt the vascular supply, MSTs may depend too strongly on a surgical technique that is limited by not being able to visualize the great variability in cortical laminar contours below the surface. Robotics is a science that has advanced but has found very few applications in neurosurgery. Coupling higher-resolution MRI, frameless-stereotactic MRI guidance, and robotics with this technique has clear possible applications. The surgeon and neurologist could sketch the most desirable subpial transection along the actual irregular cortical gyral laminations on high-resolution MR images on a cortical tablet, insert a microinstrument on a robot arm, and press a button to complete the best transection. MST is a "smart" technique in functional neurosurgery. Understanding its shortcoming is necessary to improve it.

References

1. Morrell R, Hanbrey JW. A new surgical technique for the treatment of focal cortical epilepsy. Electroencephalogr Clin Neurophysiol 1969; 26:120

2. Morrell F, Whisler WW, Bleck TP. Multiple subpial transection: a new approach to the surgical treatment of focal epilepsy. J Neurosurg 1989;70(2):231–239

3. Sperry RW, Miner N. Pattern perception following insertion of mica plates into visual cortex. J Comp Physiol Psychol 1955;48:463–469

4. Sperry RW, Miner N, Myers RE. Visual pattern perception following subpial slicing and tantalum wire implantations in visual cortex. J Comp Physiol Psychol 1955;48:50–58

5. Hufnagel A, Zentner J, Fernandez G, Wolf HK, Schramm J, Elger CE. Multiple subpial transection for control of epileptic seizures: effectiveness and safety. Epilepsia 1997;38(6):678–688

6. Leonhardt G, Spiekermann G, Muller S, Zentner J, Hufnagel A. Cortical reorganization following multiple subpial transection in human brain—a study with positron emission tomography. Neurosci Lett 2000;292(1):63–65

7. Morrell F, Kanner AM, de Toledo-Morrell L, Hoeppner T, Whisler WW. Multiple subpial transection. Adv Neurol 1999;81:259–270

8. Morrell F, Whisler WW, Smith MC, et al. Landau-Kleffner syndrome. Treatment with subpial intracortical transection. Brain 1995;118(Pt 6):1529–1546

9. Grote CL, Van Slyke P, Hoeppner JA. Language outcome following multiple subpial transection for Landau-Kleffner syndrome. Brain 1999;122(Pt 3):561–566

10. Sawhney IM, Robertson IJ, Polkey CE, Binnie CD, Elwes RD. Multiple subpial transection: a review of 21 cases. J Neurol Neurosurg Psychiatry 1995;58(3):344–349

11. Spencer SS, Schramm J, Wyler A, et al. Multiple subpial transection for intractable partial epilepsy: an international meta-analysis. Epilepsia 2002;43(2):141–145

12. Moo LR, Slotnick SD, Krauss G, Hart J. A prospective study of motor recovery following multiple subpial transections. Neuroreport 2002;13(5):665–669

13. Telfeian AE, Connors BW. Layer-specific pathways for the horizontal propagation of epileptiform discharges in neocortex. Epilepsia 1998;39(7):700–708

14. Telfeian AE, Connors BW. Epileptiform propagation patterns mediated by NMDA and non-NMDA receptors in rat neocortex. Epilepsia 1999;40(11):1499–1506

15. Telfeian AE, Connors BW. Widely integrative properties of layer 5 pyramidal cells support a role for processing of extralaminar synaptic inputs in rat neocortex. Neurosci Lett 2003;343(2):121–124

16. Telfeian AE, Spencer DD, Williamson A. Lack of correlation between neuronal hyperexcitability and electrocorticographic responsiveness in epileptogenic human neocortex. J Neurosurg 1999;90(5):939–945

17. Kaufmann WE, Krauss GL, Uematsu S, Lesser RP. Treatment of epilepsy with multiple subpial transections: an acute histologic analysis in human subjects. Epilepsia 1996;37(4):342–352

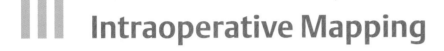

III Intraoperative Mapping

11 Corticography

Douglas Maus and Brian Litt

Detecting the intrinsic electrical activity of the brain remarkably followed, rather than preceded, electrically stimulating the brain. In the late 19th century, individuals such as Richard Caton, Gustav Fritsch, and Edward Hitzig electrically stimulated the cerebral cortex of man and animals, and began to demonstrate that such stimulation could induce motor activity. It was soon apparent that cortex capable of transducing such stimuli into motor actions was surprisingly localized. By the early 1900s, some surgeons were reporting the use of electrical stimulation to map the motor cortex.[1] In the next decades, this technique spread among neurosurgeons, with Wilder Penfield being one of the early pioneers of mapping wider expanses of cortex via stimulation.

In parallel, in 1920s Germany, Hans Berger began to report his recordings of the spontaneous electrical activity of the brain using scalp electrodes, now known as electroencephalography (EEG).[2] Berger even performed the first direct cortical recordings with silver needle electrodes on patients who had undergone craniotomies for tumors. The extension from intraoperative stimulation to direct intraoperative cortical recording (electrocorticography, ECoG) was quickly made.[3] Also in the early 1930s, the aberrant electrical activity detectable on scalp EEG during seizures and even interictally was noted by neurologists such as Gibbs et al.[4] Penfield recruited the neurologist and electroencephalographer Herbert Jasper to the Montreal Neurological Institute, where these two men took their place among the pioneers who synthesized the techniques of EEG, ECoG, and brain stimulation for the examination of cortex in what was to become standard practice worldwide as functional surgery for epilepsy.[5]

ECoG reached what was to be its apogee in utility, until recent years, in the early 1950s. Early resections for temporal lobe epilepsy had focused on the lateral temporal cortex.[6] However, these early series of surgical outcomes were decidedly underwhelming, with success rates of around 50% of patients being rendered seizure free. Stimulation and ECoG played a pivotal role in demonstrating that stimulation of mesial structures (amygdala and hippocampus) could recapitulate the electrographic and clinical manifestations of seizures, and that epileptiform discharges were present in these mesial temporal structures. After this discovery, resections were expanded to include the mesial temporal structures as well, specifically the amygdala and hippocampus, resulting in a much greater proportion of seizure freedom for patients.[7]

Once this crucial role of mesial structures in temporal lobe epilepsy was realized, the role for intraoperative ECoG waned. As early as 1958, prominent neurosurgeons such as Murray Falconer suggested that with "adequate" preoperative studies, intraoperative ECoG was "unnecessary" for the surgical treatment of temporal lobe epilepsy.[8]

Since the 1950s, ECoG and functional brain stimulation continue to be used during evaluation for epilepsy surgery, as well as to map brain function during surgery and other treatments for tumors, movement disorders, or other brain disorders. Cortical recording has also extended beyond the operating room, employed via chronic implantation of subdural electrodes for localization of epileptic networks spanning days to weeks. In addition, recording of field potentials, small collections of neurons (multi-unit), and even single neurons (single-unit) is performed routinely during placement of brain stimulating electrodes to treat an expanding array of brain disorders. This chapter, however, will be restricted to intraoperative ECoG, focusing on use in epilepsy surgery to guide resection.

The use of intraoperative ECoG for epilepsy surgery has certainly waxed and waned over the years, and practices vary greatly from center to center worldwide. It is difficult to be optimistic about its traditional role in epilepsy surgery because the only consensus about its use is that the evidence supporting it is divergent, though at this chapter's end we will discuss new exciting applications of these techniques that may herald their return to mainstream clinical practice. The bulk of this chapter will focus on specific advice for implementation, offering a fair exposition of the evidence regarding the role of ECoG during routine clinical practice, and leaves the decision on its applicability to the individual surgeon, for each particular case.

Equipment and Procedure

Preoperative Planning

Many facets of intraoperative planning must be considered and coordinated prior to surgery. Choice of anesthetic needs to be made with some forethought, depending on such general factors as need for awake-patient testing. More specifically, choice of anesthetic must be coordinated with the goals of ECoG. Anesthetics have drastically different effects on ECoG. Some decrease the interictal epileptiform discharge (IED) frequency, whereas others increase the rate, some even increasing the likelihood of seizure. The effect depends significantly on the dose of the anesthetic (as well as other factors such as CO_2 tension), often with increased discharge rate at moderate dosages, then decreased rate as global cerebral activity is generally depressed. Dramatic depression of discharge rates would obviously hamper their detection and localization by ECoG. On the other hand, agents that increase IEDs have been advocated to shorten the time of required monitoring. However, one must recognize some studies have raised suspicion that the discharges elicited by these "activating" agents may be falsely localizing.

Of note, Modica and colleagues present an overview of much contradictory evidence on the pro- and anticonvulsant effects of anesthetics, which, although dated, remains useful because the evidence remains conflicting.[9]

Inhaled Anesthetics

- **Nitrous oxide.** A systematic crossover study of nitrous oxide effect on ECoG in epilepsy surgery patients reported no significant difference in IED rates between on-nitrous and off-nitrous.[10]
- **Halothane.** There are few systematic reports on the effect of halothane on ECoG in epileptic patients. It is believed not to significantly affect IED rates.
- **Enflurane** (Ethrane®). As reviewed in Modica et al,[9] there are multiple reports of ictogenic effects of enflurane,[11] in patients with preexisting epilepsy, and also those without a history of epilepsy. The lack of selectivity of this effect limits the utility of enflurane with ECoG.
- **Isoflurane** (Forane®). A specific study of the effect of isoflurane on the ECoG of epilepsy surgery patients reported that high-dose (1.5 MAC, near burst-suppression), isoflurane provoked increased IED rate compared with low-dose (0.3 MAC), which seemed to suppress IED rates (none or <1 per 10 seconds).[12]
- **Sevoflurane** (Ultane®). The above study with isoflurane also included sevoflurane, which was found to increase the IED rate, and was argued to be specific: 6 of 10 patients had a single IED focus, whereas in 3 of the remaining 4 with multiple foci, the prime focus was "consistent with the location of the seizure origin."[12]
- **Desflurane** (Suprane®). No reports of the effect of desflurane on ECoG are available. One report indicates that on scalp EEG of nonepileptic patients, although sevoflurane provoked epileptiform discharges, desflurane had no such effect.[13]

Analgesics (Opioids)

- **Fentanyl.** A study in temporal lobe epilepsy patients with chronic subdural electrodes reported that fentanyl provoked electrographic seizures in 8 of 9 patients, but in 4 of these 8, the provoked seizure was contralateral to the seizure origin.[14] Certainly, localization of provoked seizures with fentanyl must be cautiously interpreted.

- **Sufentanil** (Sufenta®). In another study examining both fentanyl and sufentanil in nonepileptic patients, these were both found to induce epileptiform discharges at moderate dosages, then suppression at higher concentrations.[15]
- **Alfentanil** (Alfenta®). In one study of ECoG in temporal lobe epilepsy patients, alfentanil significantly increased the mesial temporal mean "spike frequency" (but did not affect the rate in extratemporal regions.)[16] In another study of ECoG in epilepsy surgery patients, alfentanil was found to activate IED, at a higher rate than remifantanil.[17]
- **Remifentanil** (Ultiva®). The aforementioned study comparing alfentanil and remifentanil reported provoked IEDs at a higher rate with alfentanil.[17] Another study examining only reminfentanil found it to activate IEDs, and emphasized the advantages of its shorter elimination half-life, particularly in neurological patients in whom neurological examination is important postoperatively.

Sedatives

- **Droperidol** (Dropletan®). Droperidol had been used extensively for conscious sedation in the past, but the FDA "black box" warning regarding long QT intervals and increased risk of sudden death has significantly reduced its use, though the basis for this warning is debated.[18]
- **Propofol** (Diprivan®). Propofol has been often presumed to be anticonvulsant and even used at anesthetic doses for termination of status epilepticus. One study specifically of ECoG in epilepsy patients reported no interference between propofol and ECoG monitoring, provided it is suspended 15 minutes before recording.[19]
- **Methohexital** (Brevital®). Methohexital has long been advocated for activating IEDs.[20] However, some have cautioned that it may yield misleading results, in that it was shown to induce "new" spike (IED) foci in a significant number of epilepsy patients.[21] Brevital activation of the EEG during ECoG was, in the past, standard procedure in some institutions. Concern over activating new regions of epileptiform activity has curtailed its use for this purpose in recent years.

Recommendations

The practice of purposefully activating the EEG with anesthetic agents to enhance recordings of interictal epileptiform activity has fallen out of favor in recent years. Procedures in which EEG recording is essential in the operating room are usually done with agents such as fentanyl, nitrous oxide, and on some occasions, with propofol as an ancillary agent, provided it is turned off for >15 minutes prior to cortical mapping/ECoG.

Recording

In its early years, traditional ECoG employed spherical metal electrodes supported by thin, flexible metal cylinders mounted to a frame that was typically clamped to the patient's (exposed) calvaria. This set-up had the advantage of easy adjustment of electrode position and ease of visualization of underlying anatomy. Disadvantages included the fact that the relative location of electrodes were not fixed or standardized, leading to ambiguity of amplitude measurements with bipolar montages. These electrodes could be reused with appropriate sterilization.

Currently, most ECoG is performed with strips or grids of inert metal disk electrodes embedded at fixed intervals in flexible transparent Silastic sheets. Typical grids have platinum or stainless steel electrodes of a diameter of 4.0 mm (exposed diameter 2.3 mm), in a square lattice separated by 10.0 mm center-to-center distance. Dimensions of subdural electrode strips and grids vary, depending upon the coverage required, and usually range from one row of four contacts (i.e., 1 × 4) to sheets of 64 electrodes in a single square array of eight contacts in each row and column (i.e., 8 × 8) (**Fig. 11.1**), to custom grid arrays in asymmetric sizes, depending upon the application. Choosing the right electrode configuration permits adequate movement (with vascular pulsations) and permits underlying anatomy to be fairly visualized. However, precise placement at multiple anatomical landmarks is not generally possible. Subdural strip or grid electrodes are used only once (disposable), and as such can become expensive for frequent use. It is also important to note that depth electrodes can be used to map epileptiform activity and for brain stimulation. As in the calculations described below, electrode surface area, impedance, and placement are key to interpreting information gathered by passive recording and through electrical stimulation.

Because ECoG is generally performed when localization of the epileptic network is nebulous, a large extended craniectomy is often required, unless stereotaxic placement of depth electrodes is used, which can be done through bur holes. After opening the dura and exposing the pial surface, subdural electrode strips or grids are placed with visual guidance over the regions/lobes of interest. A reference electrode is typically placed on the skin of the neck in the midline, though contacts on the grid or additional strips may be used as an electrical reference and isoground.

Traditionally, the electroencephalographer does not significantly alter the electrical characteristics of the recording apparatus from routine scalp EEG recordings, though more recent research suggests that mapping of high-frequency oscillations may be of some utility (see section on nonlesional extratemporal epilepsy below). For most current digital data acquisitions, the pre-digitization analog low-pass (anti-aliasing) filter remains at 70 to 100 Hz. Most centers use digitization rates of 200 to 400 samples per second (per channel). The absolute voltages recorded (relative to the "machine" reference) are not so different from typical scalp

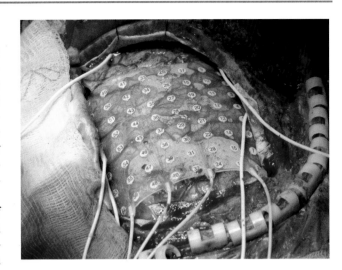

Fig. 11.1 An example of an electrode grid, arranged in a square lattice 8 x 8, with labeled contacts 1 through 64.

recordings to necessitate changes to digitizer voltage input scale. On the other hand, being recorded directly from cortex and cleared of many sources of artifact, the relative voltages (especially in bipolar montages) are much larger, on the order of hundreds of microvolts (μV). Therefore, the voltage scale of the display must be adjusted accordingly, and the display sensitivity is usually decreased to 50 to 100 μV per millimeter (from 7 μV per millimeter on typical scalp EEG). As with scalp EEG, attention must be paid to electrode placement, particularly to having good contact with the brain surface, no air bubbles beneath the electrodes, and electrodes of importance should be kept off blood vessels, to insure good signal quality. Electrode impedance should be less than or equal to 10 kΩ, and preferably in the 5 to 10 kΩ range.

In typical situations, there will be many electrodes simultaneously implanted during evaluation for epilepsy surgery, in cases where localization of epileptic networks is the motivation for electrode placement and ECoG, more than can be usefully displayed at one time. Montages should be created in which spatially close electrodes (or electrode pairs, in bipolar montages) are visually close as well. Montages can be created that, for example, display electrodes (or electrode pairs) over individual lobes. As in scalp EEG, referential montages are useful in spatially restricted events of interest, whereas bipolar montages can be very useful in identifying relative maxima of spatially broad events. As with other types of electroencephalography, montages should be balanced and symmetrical when possible, so that electrode distances are comparable and signal amplitude is comparable from channel to channel.

A flowchart representing the authors' basic protocol for recording intraoperative ECoG is shown in **Fig. 11.2**.

Stimulation

The surgeon must be aware of (and pay special attention to) the stimulation protocol to prevent irreversible injury to the

IntraOperative ECoG Recording

Plan (before OR):
- Suspected location of seizures (to plan for craniotomy)
- Agree on whether single resection after recording, or performing iterative "tailored" resections based on post-resection recording

Prepare (ready for OR):
- ECoG recording machine
- Cables for strip/grid/depth electrodes
- Sterile, writable paper for labeling regions ("brain labels")
- Template brain maps to document locations of electrodes (either paper or with computer drawings)
- (Digital) camera to document locations of electrodes

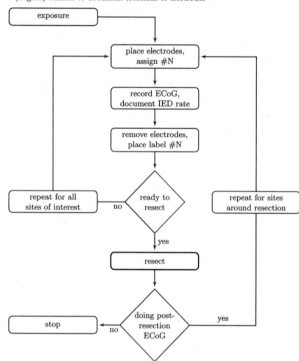

Fig. 11.2 Checklist and flowchart for performing iterative ECoG and resection.

cortex. Several parameters are key. Some basic relations to consider:

When discussing electric currents applied to biologic systems, an important parameter is the energy delivered per unit area of tissue. Energy is measured in joules (J). However, it is difficult to gain a practical feeling for this unit of measurement. A related figure is power, whose units have a somewhat more familiar value, namely watts (W). Power is the rate of energy transfer, or energy per unit time. 1 watt ≡ 1 joule per second. Thus, a source delivering 1 watt and maintained for 1 second, delivers a net total energy of 1 joule (= 1 W · 1 second = 1 J/s · 1 second). Values of energy for electrical currents are fairly straightforward. For DC electrical currents, power = voltage · current, ($P = V \cdot i$), where 1 volt · ampere (V · A) ≡ 1 watt. Thus, a resistor of 10,000 Ω (ohms), with an applied voltage of 100 volts (V), by Ohm's law for resistors ($V = i \cdot R$) will pass 0.01 amperes (A), or 10 mA. The power dissipated in the resistor will then be 100 volts · 0.01 amperes = 1 (V · A) = 1 watt. Such a current flowing through

this resistor over 1 second will then dissipate (convert from electrical to thermal) an energy of 1 joule.

This measurement is somewhat more complicated in electrical circuits that do not have constant (DC) currents. For a typical sine wave, the net voltage across, or current through, an element (a resistor), when averaged over many cycles, will obviously be 0. Clearly, this will not reflect the fact that real power and energy are dissipated in these elements. The key is to recognize that the power reflects the product of the voltage at a given time and the current at the same time.

$$P(t_k) = V(t_k) \cdot i(t_k)$$

When the voltage is reversed for the second half of the cycle, the current is also reversed, and the product of these two negatives still results in a positive value, so the sum or average over a whole cycle will be a positive real value. For a simple resistor, $i(t) = V(t)/R$, so

$$P(t) = V(t) \cdot i(t) = \frac{V(t) \cdot V(t)}{R} = \frac{V^2(t)}{R}$$

For a sinusoidal voltage source: $V(t) = V_0 \sin(\omega t)$, then

$$P(t) = \frac{V_0^2 \cdot \sin^2(\omega t)}{R}$$

By the trigonometric identity $\sin^2 + \cos^2 = 1$, the average over 1 cycle of $\sin^2 = \frac{1}{2}$. By comparison with the above DC example, a sine wave voltage source with a peak (V_0) of 100 V, applied to a 10,000 Ω resistor will deliver 0.5 W

$$P = \frac{[(100V)^2 \cdot 1/2]}{10,000\Omega}$$

exactly half as much as the constant 100 V applied to the same resistor.

Another concern is delivered charge and charge density. Charge is measured in coulombs (C). Current, measured in amperes, is a measure of rate of flow of charge: 1 ampere ≡ 1 coulomb per second (1 coulomb of charge passing a point in 1 second.) In other words, if the current is known to be 10 mA, then this current maintained for 1 second will deliver 10 mC of charge. Charge density is calculated by dividing the charge delivered by the surface area of the electrode. For typical subdural strips and grids, the exposed electrode has a diameter of 2.3 mm, thus (neglecting edge effects, treating just the single side) a surface area of $\pi \cdot (1.15 \text{ mm})^2 = \pi \cdot 1.3 \text{ mm}^2 = 4.1 \text{ mm}^2$ or 0.041 cm². For a current of 8 mA delivered for 0.3 milliseconds, over a surface area of 0.041 cm², the charge delivered is 2.4 μC, and the charge density is 2.4 μC/0.041 cm² = 58 μC/cm².

Energy delivered usually shows the best correlation with biological injury, and so an equivalent amount of energy can be delivered by either higher power for briefer time, or lower power maintained for longer duration. One watt maintained for 1 second is generally comparable to 2 W for 0.5 seconds.

However, stimuli are typically delivered with constant-current stimulator units, with currents on the order of 1 to 10 mA. Though resistances between a pair of ECoG electrodes are typically on the order of 10 kΩ, these resistances and the necessary applied voltages can be quite variable, making the voltages, and consequently the power and energy, difficult to determine or track. Thus, most research into the thermal damage from electrical stimuli has focused on the charge density. Delivered charge will roughly correspond to delivered energy, in the sense that it, too, reflects the product of "intensity" and duration. That is, 1 mA for 1 second will result in the same delivered charge as 10 mA for 0.1 second. Charge density accounts for spatial focusing of the delivered stimulus.

Most stimuli are supplied in biphasic pulses to minimize irreversible cellular damage.[22] Maintaining charge balance probably prevents buildup of potentially damaging electrolysis products, such as acids and oxidized metal.[23]

Stimuli may be delivered via several different methods. Often, the train of biphasic pulses may be delivered to two of the contacts on a grid. The leads from the two chosen contacts are disconnected from the ECoG recording apparatus and connected to the stimulation units. The ECoG from the remaining electrodes should continue to be monitored, to examine for possible induced seizures, or for afterdischarges. One must be careful in re-connecting the electrode leads to maintain acquisition of documented contacts. For more precise delivery of stimulation, some surgeons employ handheld probes. There are electrically two different types: a combined bipolar probe (**Fig. 11.3**), in which the two closely spaced (5 to 10 mm) contacts constitute the origin and return path, respectively, or a "unipolar" probe, in which case the current return path is via a distantly placed dermal patch electrode.

The complete pulse train in typical use consists of biphasic pulses with currents ranging from 1 to 15 mA, each phase lasting 0.3 milliseconds. These biphasic pulses are repeated at 50 Hz. The total duration of the trains is typically 1 to 5 seconds (**Fig. 11.4**).[24,25]

Gordon et al have studied the effect of such electrical stimuli to cortex (in which cortex that was known to be later resected was first stimulated with various settings), and found that such trains with charge densities up to 55 μC/cm²/phase were deemed safe,[26] though other investigators have exceeded this limit safely with shorter train durations. More detailed studies taking total stimulation dose over longer periods of time, for example summing up trains that last up to 5 seconds or more, are needed to better resolve the relationship between tissue damage, aberrant fiber sprouting, and long-term safety.

Finally, it is important, as with all electronic devices connected to patients, that stimulation equipment be adequately isolated to prevent DC shock to the patient.

A flowchart representing the authors' protocol for electrical cortical stimulation is shown in **Fig. 11.5**.

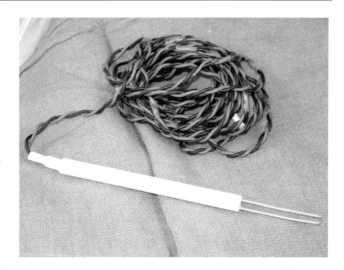

Fig. 11.3 A bipolar stimulator.

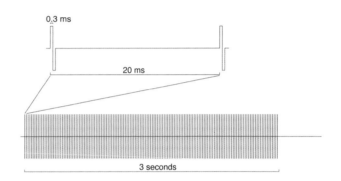

Fig. 11.4 Diagram of a stimulation pulse train. Note the pulses are biphasic, with equal but opposite current and equal durations.

Applications

Using ECoG to Map Interictal Spiking

Interictal spikes have been the focus of many decades of interest in tailoring epilepsy surgery resections. Older studies and applications for mapping interictal epileptiform discharges (see **Fig. 11.6**) fall broadly into preresection and postresection analysis, and the traditional metrics involve spatial localization, spike rate, and spike amplitude (some centers also attempt to determine "primary" versus "secondary" spikes based on intervals between spike maxima). In situations in which there has been no preoperative identification of the most likely ictogenic zone, initial surgical resection may rely entirely on ECoG spike localization, as employed at some centers. More commonly, the likely ictogenic zone is identified preoperatively, either by a lesion visible on radiographic imaging, or via scalp ictal EEG findings, and ECoG is used to refine localization and, in some centers, to tailor surgical resection to individual patients. In the cases of identified lesions, because it has been thought that the

IntraOperative Cortical Stimulation

Plan (before stimulation):
- Identify regions of suspected eloquence
- Identify regions of interictal epileptiform discharges
- Identify regions of seizure onset (if any)

Prepare (ready for stimulation):
- Stimulation train generator
- Hand-held stimulator, if desired
- ECoG recording machine
- Cables for strip/grid/depth electrodes
- Sterile, writable paper for labeling regions ("brain labels")
- Materials for clinical testing (pictures/objects for naming, etc.)
- Cold saline (OR) and lorazepam available to abort seizures

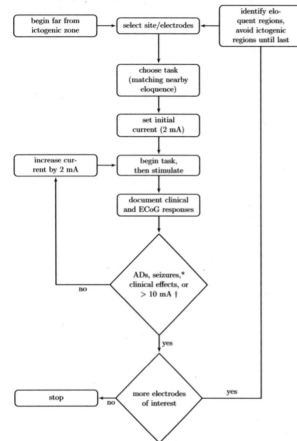

Notes:
ADs = After-Discharges
★ If after-discharges persist longer than 3–5 sec, or clear seizure begins, cold saline squirted onto the cortex may abort these. If a seizure spreads widely or develops clinical signs, lorazepam or midazolam is recommended.
† Some centers routinely increase the current up to 18–20 mAmps, though most limit the maximum current to 10 mAmps. One should also account for different sizes of electrode contact areas and be aware of the current density per phase, as in the report by Gordon et al.

Fig. 11.5 Checklist and flowchart for performing electrical stimulation.

ictogenic (seizure generating) zone is often somewhere on the periphery of the visible lesion, some practitioners may examine the preresection ECoG and remove the lesion and those regions surrounding the lesion that are spiking most actively. More recent literature suggests that this approach may be particularly beneficial in resecting regions of cortical dysplasia, whose total removal has been associated, by some investigators, with better outcome, specifically with better seizure reduction. In the cases where a putative ic-

togenic zone has been identified by scalp EEG, preresection ECoG may be used to confirm this suspicion, to help guide the placement of subdural electrodes for spontaneous ictal recording.

After tissue has been resected, mapping and counting the postresection spike rate to help localize regions important to the epileptic network is employed in some centers, though this approach is much more controversial. In this scheme, resection margins are expanded in an iterative fashion until spike rates fall below some "threshold" value felt to be important to seizure generation. The debate here is that some investigators express concern that the tissue injury from the resection itself may be responsible for acutely generating epileptiform activity in tissue that would not otherwise do so, and that this approach may be less useful. In addition, visible interictal epileptiform activity may be electrically conducted to regions at the resection site from distant sites, which cannot be easily determined or resolved due to limited recording in the region of resection. Finally, the criteria for determining quantitative thresholds for interictal spiking requiring resection are not well specified, and there is often an empirical flavor to how this idea is implemented, from center to center, in practice. It is important to note that this "standard" method of performing interictal ECoG during surgical resection now varies widely from center to center, and its utility is difficult to assess, given the absence of sufficient class I data with regard to these practices (see specific applications, below). For these reasons, ECoG as an important tool for guiding surgical resection in the operating room has largely fallen out of favor in recent years. New data derived from higher frequency recording and specific cases, such as cortical dysplasia and refractory partial status epilepticus, may initiate a revival of such techniques, in a more rigorous, quantitative way.

Specific Clinical Applications

Nonlesional Mesial-Temporal Epilepsy

As Chatrian et al have recently reviewed,[27] although this has been extensively studied, there is little firm support that ECoG examinations of interictal spiking add anything to the percentage of patients rendered seizure free following standard resective surgery for mesial-temporal epilepsy. Chatrian et al also concludes that such studies do not provide reliable prognostic information. Indeed, as Engel et al reported,[28] many centers no longer used ECoG in temporal lobe epilepsy surgery in the early 1970s, and even fewer do today. Still, some practicioners maintain that ECoG may play some role in tailoring such temporal amygdalohippocampectomies.[29] The assumption that the location of maximal interictal spikes co-localizes with the ictogenic zone is probably flawed. Older literature distinguishing between mesial temporal and temporal neocortical epilepsy using depth electrode studies of interictal epileptiform activity are still

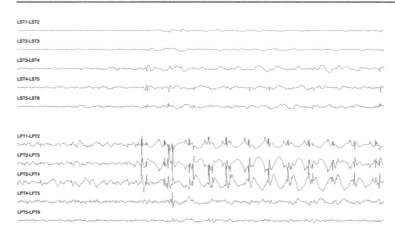

Fig. 11.6 ECoG showing epileptiform discharges progressing to a seizure. Duration of traces is 10 seconds. The LST series is from a six-contact strip placed (L)eft (S)ub-(T)emporal, and the LPT series is from a six-contact strip placed (L)eft (P)osterior-(T)emporal. The traces are displayed in a bipolar montage. LST1–2 reflects the LST contact 1 minus LST contact 2. Note the rhythmic epileptiform discharges on LPT1–2, LPT2–3, and LPT3–4 representing incipient focal seizure. There are independent epileptiform discharges at LST3–4, and LST4–5.

likely valid, but this technique has largely been supplanted by chronic invasive ictal recording, outside of the operating room, with implanted depth and strip electrodes in patients whose seizures are not clearly due to the syndrome of mesial temporal sclerosis.

Nonlesional Extratemporal Epilepsy

ECoG in nonlesional extratemporal (neocortical) epilepsy has few documented studies. In general, this situation is handled in most centers with chronic intracranial (extraoperative) recordings to identify the ictogenic zone. Newer, more exciting studies in recent years have focused on using ECoG in more specialized circumstances in extratemporal epilepsy. These include resection of cortical dysplasia and tumors, in which removing localized margins of significant spiking, and particularly focal seizure-like bursts ("beta buzzes"), has been associated with better outcome.[30,31,32,33] Similar information is available, though mostly in the form of isolated case reports, of dramatic outcome following intraoperative resection of seizing tissue in cases of severe, refractory partial status epilepticus, localized by ECoG[34] (and personal communication, Peter Crino and Brian Litt). Again, in all of these cases, the substrate for seizure generation is presumed to be focal functional lesions that are silent on current radiologic imaging, due to the lack of ability of structural imaging to pick up what are likely network abnormalities. The addition of functional magnetic resonance imaging (fMRI) has promise to demonstrate functional lesions that may better steer ECoG studies in the operating room; however, this research also remains experimental at this time.

More recently, there is increasing interest in mapping epileptic networks through recording specific high-frequency oscillations that may be associated with epileptic networks.[35,36] Although no studies currently exist using this application, our group has begun to investigate mapping these high-frequency oscillations (HFEOs in standard intracranial EEG, and ripples and fast ripples in microwire recordings), to define functional ictogenic networks. This work remains

purely research at this time, but preliminary work is promising, and more investigation is needed.

Lesional Epilepsy

Lesional epilepsy is currently the area of most controversy regarding ECoG. As opposed to mesial-temporal epilepsy, where the epileptic network is probably fairly stereotyped, explaining why standard anatomical resections yield good outcomes, the epileptic network associated with lesions is much less well defined, let alone understood. Each lesion and associated epileptic network is likely unique, and the limits of resection may vary quite a bit in constraint depending on proximity of eloquent cortex. What is clear from much of the ECoG literature, with regard to structural lesions such as easily visualized dysplastic or neoplastic tissue as well as regions of old head trauma and other lesions, is that ictogenic tissue is commonly found outside of lesion margins. The debate then is whether intraoperative ECoG is sufficient to best define the extent of network dysfunction responsible for seizure generation in these patients, or whether chronic intracranial monitoring and ictal recording are required. Most centers, at present, focus on the latter technique, preferring to record multiple seizures, as well as interictal activity, and plan resective surgery to remove ictogenic regions and so-called primary tissue generating interictal epileptiform activity. The definition of "primary" in this case varies from center to center, though its usual meaning is regions generating very frequent interictal spikes, or interictal activity that transitions into seizures at the time of onset. Again, there are no good, statistically sound studies that test the hypotheses implicit in these techniques, which is remarkable, given that the majority of epilepsy centers base their surgical resections upon this approach.

Stimulation: Afterdischarges

As stimulation current is increased, at some (individually variable) threshold, spontaneously occurring epileptiform discharges distinct from the background are often seen, usually localized near the stimulation site. In the past, these "after-discharges" were thought to be more prominent in locations near the spontaneous ictogenic zone, and some investigators felt that the occurrence of this response to stimulation could be used to localize the ictogenic, or seizure-generating, zone. This idea has fallen into disfavor, primarily because of reports that afterdischarges are easily provoked in normal cortex that otherwise has no evidence of ictogenic potential, depending upon stimulation current, waveform, etc.[37] It has been reported that single-pulse stimulation may induce late–afterdischarges, which may be useful in identifying ictogenic cortex, especially in frontal lobe epilepsies.[38,39] It is well recognized that stimulations that provoke afterdischarges can frequently lead to induced seizures. It is standard protocol that cortical stimulation for functional localization/brain mapping is always performed at currents below that which precipitates afterdischarges, also known as the "afterdischarge threshold."

Afterdischarges following cortical stimulation are common, more so in regions near the seizure onset zone. Although, as noted above, using the afterdischarge threshold to map candidate regions for surgical resection has not borne fruit, it is important to test regions near the seizure onset zone last, meaning during cortical stimulation mapping. It is also important to establish a stimulation afterdischarge threshold for each electrode pair being tested, as this may vary greatly from one brain area to another. Although some centers may use stimulation currents of up to 18 mA in some stimulation protocols, our experience is that stimulation currents above 10 mA are not generally necessary. Our experience is that above 10 mA may just spread currents spatially, and not yield added information about the region directly beneath the electrode contact.

Seizure Induction

Historically, seizure induction was useful to the early practioners in guiding their resections. The theory behind this is that if focal brain stimulation could produce a patient's typical seizures at low stimulation currents, it was likely that the regions so localized were involved in seizure generation. Because spontaneous seizures are rather rare intraoperatively, various techniques were devised to promote seizures, and aid in localization of ictogenic regions. For example, antiepileptic medications were tapered prior to surgery. Electrical stimulation was intensified until seizures were provoked. In some cases, frankly proconvulsant agents such as pentylene tetrazole (PTZ) or bemegride were used. These techniques have fallen out of favor (thankfully), due to poor utility and potential morbidity associated with their use. With electrical stimulation of seizures, or PTZ/bemegride seizure induction, the location of the seizure onset was determined by ECoG, and the clinical manifestation of these provoked seizures was compared with the patient's typical events. This information was used in decisions of what regions to resect. In many cases, seizure outcome after surgery with these techniques was suboptimal. This has been thought to be due to false-localization—that is, the seizures provoked by these measures were often generated in other regions, even when the clinical manifestations were similar. This has seemed to suggest that many of the apparent manifestations of seizures reflect activity in cortex that is spatially removed from the actual ictogenic zone. Experienced surgical epileptologists are familiar with this finding, as often seizures are clinically silent, despite clear appearance on the intracranial EEG, until they reach a clinically "eloquent" region, which generates symptoms.

Conclusion

Intraoperative ECoG and brain stimulation have a long, rich history that traces and is largely responsible for the evolution of modern epilepsy surgery. It is a story of wonderful collaborations between elecrophysiologists, neurologists, and neurosurgeons to understand the nature of brain networks that generate normal function over distributed regions. It also provides a window onto the nature of dysfunction associated with focal lesions and processes silent on brain imaging that generate seizures and other clinical manifestations of circuits programmed by nature that have gone awry. Once thought to be essential to resective surgery, these techniques largely fell out of favor over the past 20 years, due to improvements in brain imaging, better definitions of epilepsy syndromes amenable to surgery with good outcome (e.g., mesial temporal sclerosis), and better patient selection for surgery at specialty epilepsy centers. These surgical candidates were suggested to have lesions or discrete "epileptic foci," though more recent research suggests that networks causing seizures are also likely distributed in these patients, but sufficient tissue resection (such as standard temporal lobectomies) is often sufficient to keep seizures at bay, at least for a while with continued administration of antiepileptic drugs. Early ECoG studies were also often based upon empirical findings and interpretation of electrophysiology that were more an art than hypothesis-driven, statistically sound science.

More recent information from state-of-the-art electrophysiology, particularly high-frequency intracranial EEG and recordings of multi-unit and single-unit activity, has changed our impression of what constitutes epileptic networks, and what might be required to make patients seizure free, even those with poorly defined, nonlesional, extratemporal neocortical epilepsy. Although this work remains primarily research at this time, there is some suggestion that these new techniques, coupled with rigorous statistical analysis and functional imaging, may allow us to better map epileptic networks, and perhaps bring on a resurgence of ECoG-based studies, both in and outside of the operating room. It is clear that this field remains very much alive, and will likely be an important component of moving epilepsy surgical techniques forward. The difference is that no longer are electrophysiological techniques an art to be handed down from master to student, at the foot or head of the patient. Rather, the electroencephalographers of now and the future, who do research in this area, will need to be mathematically sophisticated, with expertise in engineering, signal processing, and statistics, and have a deep understanding of clinical epileptology and neurophysiology.

References

1. Horsley V. The function of the so-called motor cortex of the brain. BMJ 1909;2:125–132
2. Berger H. Über das elektrenkephalogramm des menschen. Arch Psychiatr Nervenkr 1929;87:527–570
3. Foerster O, Altenburger H. Elektrobiologische vorgange and der menschlichen hirnrinde. Dtsch Z Nervenheilkd 1935;135:277–288
4. Gibbs FA, Davis H, Lennox WG. The electro-encephalogram in epilepsy and in conditions of impaired consciousness. Arch Neurol Psychiatry 1935;34:1133–1148
5. Jasper HH. History of the early development of electroencephalography and clinical neurophysiology at the Montreal Neurological Institute: the first 25 years 1939–1964. Can J Neurol Sci 1991;18:533–548
6. Bailey P, Gibbs FA. The surgical treatment of psychomotor epilepsy. J Am Med Assoc 1951;145:365–370
7. Feindel W, Penfield W. Localization of discharge in temporal lobe automatism. Arch Neurol Psychiatry 1954;72:605–630
8. Falconer MA. Discussion. In: Baldwin M, Bailey P, eds. *Temporal Lobe Epilepsy*. Springfield, IL: C.C. Thomas; 1958:483–499
9. Modica PA, Tempelhoff R, White PF. Pro- and anticonvulsant effects of anesthetics (parts I and II). Anesth Analg 1990;70:303–315
10. Hosain S, Nagarajan L, Fraser R, Van Poznak A, Labar D. Effects of nitrous oxide on electrocorticography during epilepsy surgery. Electroencephalogr Clin Neurophysiol 1997;102:340–342
11. Niejadlik K, Galindo A. Electrocorticographic seizure activity during enflurane anesthesia. Anesth Analg 1975;54:722–724
12. Watts AD, Herrick IA, McLachlan RS, Craen RA, Gelb AW. The effect of sevoflurane and isoflurane anesthesia on interictal spike activity among patients with refractory epilepsy. Anesth Analg 1999;89:1275–1281
13. Vakkuri AP, Seitsonen E, Jäntti V, et al. A Rapid increase in the inspired concentration of desflurane is not associated with epileptiform encephalogram. Anesth Analg 2005;101:396–400
14. Tempelhoff R, Modica PA, Bernardo KL, Edwards I. Fentanyl-induced electrocorticographic seizures in patients with complex partial epilepsy. J Neurosurg 1992;77(10):201–208
15. Kearse LA Jr, Koski G, Husain MV, Philbin DM, McPeck K. Epileptiform activity during opioid anesthesia. Electroencephalogr Clin Neurophysiol 1993;87:374–379
16. Cascino GD, So EL, Sharbrough FW, et al. Alfentanil-induced epileptiform activity in patients with partial epilepsy. J Clin Neurophysiol 1993;10(4):520–525
17. McGuire G, El-Beheiry H, Manninen P, Lozano A, Wennberg R. Activation of electrocorticographic activity with remifetanil and alfentanil during neurosurgical excision of epileptogenic focus. Br J Anaesth 2003;91:651–655
18. Habib AS, Gan TJ. Food and Drug Administration black box warning on the perioperative use of droperidol: a review of the cases. Anesth Analg 2003;96:1377–1379
19. Herrick IA, Craen RA, Gelb AW, et al. Propofol sedation during awake craniotomy for seizures: electrocorticographic and epileptogenic effects. Anesth Analg 1997;84:1280–1284
20. Musella L, Wilder BJ, Schmidt RP. Electroencephalographic activation with intravenous methohexital in psychomotor epilepsy. Neurology 1971;21(6):594–602
21. Fiol ME, Torres F, Gates JR, Maxwell RE. Methohexital (Brevital) effect on electrocorticogram may be misleading. Epilepsia 1990;31(5):524–528
22. Lilly JC, Hughes JR, Alvord EC Jr, Galkin TW. Brief, noninjurious electric waveform for stimulation of the brain. Science 1955;121:468–469
23. Brummer SB, Turner MJ. Electrochemical considerations for safe electrical stimulation of the nervous system with platinum electrodes. IEEE Trans Biomed Eng 1977;24:59–63
24. Ojemann GA, Sutherling WW, Lesser RP, Dinner DS, Jayakar P, Saint-Hilaire J. Cortical Stimulation. In: Engel J Jr, ed. Surgical Treatment of the Epilepsies. 2nd ed. New York: Raven Press, Ltd.; 1993:chap 32
25. Riviello JJ, Kull L, Troup C, Holmes G. Cortical stimulation in children: techniques and precautions. Tech Neurosurg 2001;7(1):12–18
26. Gordon B, Lesser RP, Rance NE, et al. Parameters for direct cortical electrical stimulation in the human histopathologic confirmatio n. Electroencephalogr Clin Neurophysiol 1990;75:371–377
27. Chatrian GE, Tsai ML, Temkin NR, Holmes MD, Pauri F, Ojemann GA. Role of the ECoG in tailored temporal lobe resection: the University of Washington experience. Electroencephalogr Clin Neurophysiol Suppl 1998;48:24–43
28. Engel J Jr, Driver MV, Falconer MA. Electrophysiological correlates of pathology and surgical results in temporal lobe epilepsy. Brain 1975;98:129–156
29. McKhann GM II, Schoenfeld-McNeill J, Born DE, Haglund MM, Ojemann GA. Intraoperative hippocampal electrocorticography to predict the extent of hippocampal resection in temporal lobe epilepsy surgery. J Neurosurg 2000;93:44–52
30. Ferrier CH, Aronica E, Leijten FS, et al. Electrocorticographic discharge patterns in glioneuronal tumors and focal cortical dysplasia. Epilepsia 2006;47(9):1477–1486
31. Mikuni N, Ikeda A, Takahashi JA, et al. A step-by-step resection guided by electrocorticography for non-malignant brain tumors associated with long-term intractable epilepsy. Epilepsy Behav 2006;8:560–564
32. Hader WJ, Mackay M, Otsubo H, et al. Cortical dysplastic lesions in children with intractable epilepsy: role of complete resection. J Neurosurg 2004;100:110–117
33. Zumsteg D, Wieser HG. Presurgical evaluation: current role of invasive EEG. Epilepsia 2000;41(Supp 3):S55–S60
34. Kamada K, Isu T, Takahashi T, Tanaka T. Remote epileptogenic focus detected by electrocorticogram in a case of cavernous angioma. Acta Neurochir (Wien) 1994;127(3–4):236–239

35. Bragin A, Engel J Jr, Wilson C, Fried I, Mathern GW. Hippocaompal and entorhinal cortex high-frequency oscillations (100–500 Hz) in human epileptic brain and in kainic acid-treated rats with chronic seizures. Epilepsia 1999;40(2):127–137

36. Worrell GA, Parish L, Cranstoun SD, Jonas R, Baltuch G, Litt B. High-frequency oscillations and seizure generation in neocortical epilepsy. Brain 2004;127(Pt 7):1496–1506

37. Gloor P. Contributions of electroencephalography and electrocorti-cography to the neurosurgical treatment of the epilepsies. Adv Neurol 1975;8:59–105

38. Valentin A, Anderson M, Alarcon G, et al. Responses to single pulse electrical stimulation identify epileptogenesis in the human brain. Brain 2002;125:1709–1718

39. Valentin A, Alarcon G, Garcia-Seoane JJ, et al. Single-pulse electrical stimulation identifies epileptogenic frontal cortex in the human brain. Neurology 2005;65:426–435

12 Motor/Sensory/Language Mapping

James Schuster

Electrical cortical stimulation was first reported by Bartholow in 1874.[1] Cushing, Penfield, Rasmussen, and others greatly refined these techniques with regard to intraoperative stimulation and recording.[2-4] Additionally, refinements in these techniques have led to a better understanding of cortical organization and function.[4-6] These techniques are now routinely applied to allow precise localization of structures intraoperatively.[7,8]

Accurate localization of functional brain regions such as rolandic cortex and language areas can potentially maximize resections of tumors, vascular lesions, and epileptic foci while reducing postoperative deficits.[9] Preoperative localization with high resolution magnetic resonance imaging (MRI), functional MRI (fMRI), magnetoencephalography (MEG), and diffusion tensor imaging (DTI) allow detailed preoperative planning.[10-15] These studies can also be utilized with mono- and multimodality frameless stereotactic navigation for intraoperative localization.[10,12] However, it remains to be seen if preoperative imaging can completely replace intraoperative stimulation especially with regard to language function, as intraoperative mapping provides more precise localization when brain shift lessens the accuracy of frameless navigation. This chapter is intended to provide an introduction to preoperative and intraoperative functional mapping. We will discuss the strengths and weaknesses of the various techniques as well as common pitfalls inherent in these techniques.

Preoperative Functional Localization

Anatomical

High-resolution MRI techniques give excellent anatomical visualization and resolution. Berger et al showed that axial MRI images consistently localized the central sulcus based on the marginal ramus of the cingulated sulcus (**Fig. 12.1**). Parasagittal and far lateral sagittal images readily identified rolandic (sensorimotor) cortex as a functional unit.[16] Quinones-Hinojosa et al showed that an anatomical analysis of the sulcal pattern of the dominant hemisphere frontal operculum correlated with intraoperative language mapping, facilitating prediction of the approximate location of Broca's area. This information can then be used to determine the necessity of an awake craniotomy.[17]

Functional Imaging

Functional imaging modalities such as fMRI, MEG, and DTI can be utilized alone or in combination to localize rolandic cortex

and language areas. Motor evoked responses, for example, from a finger tapping paradigm or a vibrotactile stimulator,[18,19] can be utilized to localize motor cortex by fMRI (**Fig. 12.2**). However, fMRI localization depends on the indirect effect of neuronal activity on local blood flow. Neuronal activity changes the magnetic susceptibility of blood, producing the BOLD (blood oxygen level dependent) contrast.[20] This is limited by the varying degrees of hemodynamic response to neuronal activity, especially in pathological conditions. Additionally, the BOLD activity represents blood flow from not just the activated area but also from the whole territory drained by the veins in the sampled area.[20,21] Comparisons of fMRI with MEG, which depends on measurement of direct neuronal current flow, show that MEG more accurately localizes motor cortex when compared with intraoperative mapping.[21-23] Recently, DTI techniques have been utilized to map white matter tracts. DTI measures the diffusion displacement properties of water in three-dimensional (3-D) space. The technique takes advantage of the difference in restricted diffusion between water perpendicular and parallel to white matter tracts. This directional variation is termed

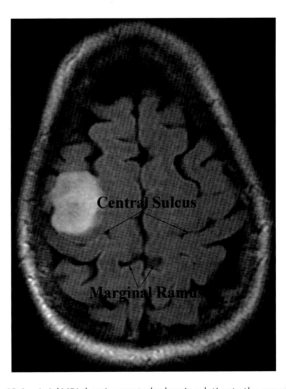

Fig. 12.1 Axial MRI showing central sulcus in relation to the marginal ramus.

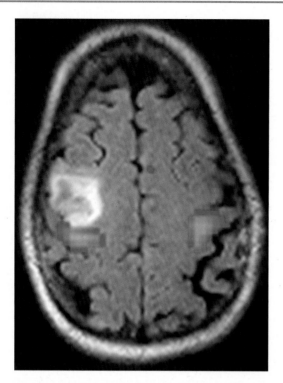

Fig. 12.2   Functional MRI (fMRI) showing bilateral localization of motor cortex.

diffusion anisotrophy.[15] DTI allows visualization of subcortical white matter tracts and is useful for preoperative planning in patients with intrinsic lesions (**Fig. 12.3**). This technique has also been utilized to identify primary motor cortex[24] and has been used with other modalities such as MEG and fMRI to give a more global picture of motor cortex including subcortical tracts.[12]

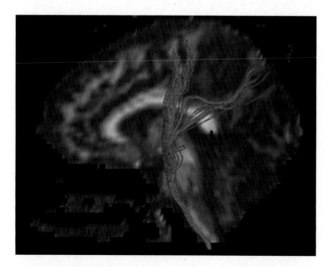

Fig. 12.3   Sagittal MRI showing reconstruction of subcortical white matter tracts by diffusion tensor imaging (DTI).

Language Testing

Amobarbitol (Amytal) Wada testing has long been the gold standard for determining language hemispheric dominance and lateralizing memory function.[25–27] However, it is invasive, carrying the inherent risks of angiography. Additionally, the presence of significant vascular shunting as with a tumor or arteriovenous malformation (AVM), can make the interpretation difficult.[28] Functional magnetic resonance imaging has been used extensively to localize language.[29,30] It compares favorably with Wada in determining language hemispheric dominance[29,30] especially in combination with MEG and DTI.[31,32] However, the localization of specific language sites within the dominant hemisphere is less precise.[33] This is due in part to inconsistencies in the language maps produced by different activation protocols.[34] Additionally, as with all language localization, fMRI may identify language involved areas but not necessarily essential areas, which may effect surgical planning. However, recently Kamanda and colleagues reported more precise localization of specific language sites using MEG, DTI, and fMRI in combination.[31,32]

There have also been reports that mesial temporal memory activation detected by fMRI during complex visual scene encoding correlates with postsurgical memory outcome.[13] However, the authors suggest that the reliability of these determinations needs to be further evaluated.

Intraoperative Mapping

Frameless Navigation

Multimodality, preoperative imaging techniques are being combined and used in frameless stereotaxy to guide resections near eloquent cortex. Kamada et al report utilizing fMRI, MEG, in combination with DTI, and 3-D anatomical MRI to visualize both cortical and subcortical structures for use with neuronavigation-guided tumor resections. Again, the limitation of this technique is that during surgery there can be significant brain shift, negating the accuracy of these techniques. This perhaps can theoretically be addressed with intraoperative "re-registration" using intraoperative MRI.

Stimulation Mapping

Intraoperative stimulation mapping remains the gold standard for localization of functional cortex including motor/sensory and language areas. However, successful mapping requires a thorough understanding of the benefits and shortcomings of the various mapping modalities, as well as accurate interpretation of mapping data. As with many clinical decisions, patient selection is paramount in determining the feasibility and success of mapping. Somatosensory evoked potentials (SSEP) and cortical stimulation mapping of motor cortex can be performed under general or local anesthesia.

Intraoperative language mapping and stimulation mapping of sensory cortex require an awake and cooperative patient. Awake procedures in patients with psychiatric disorders and/or developmental delay should generally be avoided. Additionally, although there is no specific age cutoff, awake mapping has been reported in children as young as 4 years of age.[7,35] Physiological abnormalities such as obesity or pulmonary conditions such as sleep apnea are relative contraindications for awake procedures, as airway management is paramount. If an awake procedure is not feasible, language mapping can still be performed by placement of a subdural or epidural grid electrode for extraoperative functional mapping and seizure monitoring.[36,37] This requires an additional operation, but this does not necessarily detract from the utility of this procedure.

Anesthesia

When performing SSEP monitoring under general anesthesia, halogenated anesthetic agents should not be utilized as they increase the latency of cortical SSEP.[38] Agents that lead to burst suppression such as barbiturates or high-dose propofol are also generally contraindicated. Propofol in combination with a short-acting opiate such as remifentanyl have been shown to work well for these procedures.[39,40] Pharmacological paralysis must be avoided or completely reversed for motor mapping. Finally, higher stimulation currents may be required for patients under general anesthesia.

Awake language or sensory mapping requires an awake, cooperative patient. Generally, the patient is anesthetized for the initial scalp/bone work and then allowed to awaken for the mapping. Benzodiazopines are avoided if intraoperative electrocorticography is to be utilized. Propofol works well for this portion of the procedure as it is quickly reversible. However, it is not an adequate analgesic and so a short-acting narcotic such as remifentanyl can be added.[41] Also, a generous regional field block is utilized, using short- and long-acting local anesthetics (1% lidocaine, 0.25% bupivacaine, 1:200,000 epinephrine).[8] The surgeon should discuss the tolerable dose of local anesthetic for any individual patient (based on weight) with the anesthesia team. A small amount injected with a small-bore needle into the dura at the skull base near the middle meningeal artery also helps with pain control. Pin skull fixation is well tolerated with local anesthetic but is not required. When pin fixation is not used, a skull clamp can be attached to the bone edge to control the head as the patient awakens from general anesthesia, and serve as an attachment for self-retaining retractors and as a support for an electrocorticography harness.

Airway issues are a prime concern with a nonsecured airway. Strategies include temporary use of a laryngeal mask or nasal airways/nasal cannula.[42,43] There is also significant variability with regard to the time to awakening from propofol anesthesia after it is discontinued, as well as the patient's cooperativeness during this awakening period. Therefore, it is often advisable to open the dura only after the patient is awake and cooperative.

Urinary catheters can be placed preoperatively; however, they can be a distraction, especially to male patients. An alternative is to allow male patients to use a urine bottle on request during the procedure.

Finally, with stimulation mapping there is a risk of intraoperative seizures, and possible intraoperative brain swelling. Therefore, anticonvulsant levels need to be optimized preoperatively. Intraoperative seizures can be terminated with cold irrigation solution applied to the cortex, administration of a short-acting benzodiazepine, and/or deeper levels of general anesthetic in patients with endotracheal intubation.[44]

Somatosensory Evoked Potentials

In our opinion, intraoperative SSEP is an extremely useful and underutilized functional mapping technique. SSEP provide a straightforward and accurate way of identifying the primary somatosensory/postcentral gyrus, and then indirectly the motor/precentral gyrus. SSEP localization can be utilized in patients of all ages and under either general anesthesia or in an awake patient. Another primary advantage of SSEP over direct stimulation methods is that seizures cannot be evoked with SSEP.[45]

Intraoperative SSEP techniques involve stimulation of the median and/or tibial nerves as this will give strong cortical surface recordings.[46] Stimulation is generally performed at 2 to 5 Hz, with a 0.1 to 0.3 millisecond pulse duration. The current is adjusted to give a minimal but not painful muscle twitch. The use of mechanical and thermal stimulation have also been reported.[47] The stimulus provides a signal thought to be carried by the spinothalamic fibers to the thalamus by way of the medial lemniscus, subsequently ending in the contralateral somatosensory cortex. Recording from the cortical surface tends to have much higher voltages than scalp recordings. Generally, trials of 100 to 200 stimuli are needed to produce well-defined responses from somatosensory cortex. Cortical responses can be positive (P) or negative (N) when compared with the reference electrode. The number following the polarity designation is the latency of the peak in milliseconds. As an example, stimulation of the median nerve at the wrist generally produces an initial N20 component followed by a P25 peak in the contralateral cortex.[48]

Two types of recording configurations or montages can be utilized. A *referential montage* is one in which all cortical electrodes are referenced to an electrode off the cortical surface. The second type is a *bipolar montage*, in which each electrode is referenced to the adjacent electrodes. When using a referential montage, the somatosensory cortex is located beneath the electrode with the highest recorded amplitude. In a bipolar montage, a recorded phase reversal occurs across the somatosensory cortex (**Fig. 12.4**).[48]

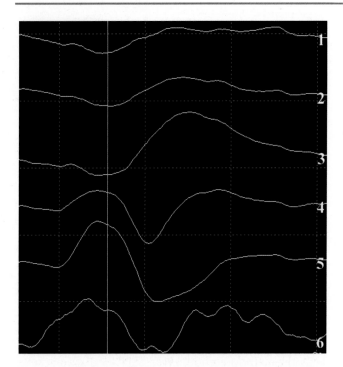

Fig. 12.4 SSEP with bipolar montage demonstrating phase reversal between electrodes 3 and 4.

Intraoperatively, after the craniotomy and durotomy, a strip electrode (four to eight contacts) is placed on the surface of the brain in a transverse orientation to the presumed rolandic cortex (4 cm above the sylvian fissure for the median nerve and at or just past the vertex for the tibial nerve). It is generally easier to use the median nerve signal for localization. The orientation and location of the strip can be changed to optimize the signals as well as to verify the localization.[46] This information can then be utilized to extrapolate the position of motor cortex and correlated with surface anatomy and perhaps with frameless navigational localization.

Electrodes can also be placed over the dura for recording. This is especially helpful in re-operative cases or postinfectious cases where the dura may be densely adherent to the underlying cortical surface.[49] Additionally, if the craniotomy does not directly expose rolandic cortex, a strip electrode can be placed under the bone edge to localize rolandic cortex.

As stated previously, SSEP provides a quick and accurate way of localizing Rolandic cortex. It can be used as a primary localization entity or used to correlate and/or verify localization from anatomical or functional imaging modalities (MRI, fMRI, MEG) utilizing frameless navigation. Even when direct stimulation motor mapping is planned, preliminary localization using SSEP can streamline the process and can be used to verify direct stimulation localization. Utilization of continuous SSEP monitoring during resection of parietal neoplasms near primary somatosensory cortex has been described as a method to avoid postoperative deficits.[46]

Optimal and safe utilization of SSEP requires a thorough familiarity with interpretation of cortical SSEP by both the surgeon and electrophysiology team. This includes an understanding of the anesthetic requirements for successful SSEP. Verification of localization with differing strip electrode positions is advisable. There is also evidence to suggest that the presence of large central or postcentral tumors can reduce the likelihood of obtaining adequate SSEP localization.[50] Additionally, physiological and or anatomical abnormalities along the SSEP course from stimulation site to cortex (peripheral neuropathy, myelopathy) may effect SSEP localization.

Cortical Stimulation Motor and Sensory Mapping

Functional localization by cortical stimulation mapping can be a powerful and reliable surgical adjunct but again requires a thorough familiarity with the technique including potential pitfalls, and constant communication by all members of the surgical team (surgeons, anesthesiologists, electrophysiologists). Reliable responses can be difficult to obtain in children and in adults under general anesthesia. Stimulation mapping of somatosensory cortex requires an awake patient, but motor cortex stimulation can be performed under general anesthesia. The major consideration in direct stimulation mapping of motor/sensory cortex is that unless the exact location of rolandic cortex is identified, lack of response in an area of interest cannot be interpreted as a lack of function in that area. Additionally, it is important to remember that repetitive cortical stimulation at or near the same area, or with high current, can cause seizure activity that may generalize. Therefore, preoperative serum anticonvulsant levels must be optimized and a short-acting anticonvulsant (midazolam, lorazepam) should be on hand. Additionally, as stated previously, irrigation of the brain with cold saline has been shown to terminate seizures and may be preferable as a first choice in conditions where benzodiazopines may not be optimal (intraoperative electroencephalography [EEG]).[44]

For motor mapping, the patient is positioned so that the motor areas of interest are visible to an observer. It is generally advised to avoid obscuring and or distracting lines or devices on the side of interest. Ojemann and others describe utilizing a constant current, biphasic square wave, 60-Hz, bipolar stimulator (Ojemann stimulator, 5-mm interelectrode distance; Integra Lifesciences, Plainsboro, NJ) for direct cortical stimulation.[5,51] Higher-current settings may be required in younger children, patients under general anesthesia, and when stimulating through the dura.[52] Generally, stimulation is initiated at lower-current settings (2 mA in an awake patient, 4mA in a patient under general anesthesia). Current is incrementally increased in 2 mA steps and applied in brief pulse trains until the desired response is obtained (generally up to 10 mA). It has been observed that increased stimulation efficiency is obtained with stimulation nearer the central sulcus.[5,7,8]

Direct stimulation motor mapping is also useful for guiding resections below the cortical surface within the subcortical white matter. This technique is used to identify and spare descending white matter motor tracts. When utilizing this technique is it useful to intermittently recheck cortical motor stimulation, especially if there is any question regarding subcortical stimulation. Generally, the current level required for subcortical mapping is equal to or less than the current required for cortical mapping. Resections near functional cortex require frequent restimulation as the penetration depth of the current is generally 2 to 3 mm.[51]

Language Cortex Mapping

Surgical resections in the dominant cerebral hemisphere put language function at risk. Altered language function can be an especially disabling and demoralizing complication for patients and families. Direct stimulation mapping remains the gold standard for language localization for several reasons: (1) Because of the tremendous individual variability with regard to the number and location of essential language sites, standard anatomical resections don't always spare language. (2) Functional imaging is useful for determining the side of language dominance, but is not as useful for accurately localizing language sites within the dominant hemisphere.

However, as with other mapping techniques, the surgical team must be very familiar with the limitations and pitfalls inherent to language mapping. First, language mapping is unique in comparison with sensory/motor mapping in that it depends on blockade of function instead of elicitation of a response.[5,8] Second, both direct stimulation and functional MRI localization may localize language involved but not necessarily language essential areas. As stimulation of face motor cortex can cause speech arrest, it is usually necessary to localize face motor cortex so that it is not mistaken for an expressive language area such as Broca's area.

Speech mapping often requires higher stimulation currents to obtain a response. Therefore, stimulation is often done at the highest tolerable current as determined by afterdischarge threshold potentials (ADP) utilizing electrocorticography to identify propagation of depolarization into nearby cortical regions. Higher currents are often utilized, as again lack of a response does not imply lack of underlying function, especially if normal speech areas cannot be identified.

After opening the scalp and removing the bone, the patient is allowed to recover fully from anesthesia. The dura is subsequently opened. Motor mapping can then be undertaken to identify face motor cortex. One method of determining afterdischarge potentials is to use a series of electrodes spaced ~10 to 20 mm apart over the cortical surface or with strip electrodes placed at the edges of the exposed cortex. Bipolar stimulation is then utilized starting at a current of 2 mA. The current is gradually increased in 0.5 to 1 mA increments until the spread of afterdischarge potentials are determined. The current used for language mapping is then set 0.5 to 1.0 mA below the afterdischarge threshold. The duration of stimulus for determining the ADP is the

same as for mapping, essentially the duration of each slide presentation.[5,8]

For the mapping procedure, 15 to 20 perisylvian sites are marked with small number tags. Sites for stimulation are randomly selected to cover the areas of presumed language areas as well as the planned resection area. The patient is shown images of simple objects to identify using either a computer or slide projector. A new image is projected every 2 to 4 seconds. Cortical stimulation is applied before the presentation of each image and is continued until there is a correct response or the next image is presented. Each site is stimulated three to four times but never twice in succession. Sites where there is consistent speech arrest or anomia are marked as essential language areas. It has been demonstrated that resections within 10 mm of essential language areas may lead to transient postoperative speech difficulties.[5,8] With resections within 2 cm of identified language areas, one strategy is to have the patient name continuously during the resection. The resection should proceed slowly with cessation if naming errors are detected.[5,8] Intraoperative stimulation mapping using memory specific paradigms have also been correlated with postoperative memory deficits.[53]

Difficulty arises if language areas cannot be identified and no language deficits are elicited over the planned resection site. The decision to carry out the resection may put language function at risk. In these cases secondary determinants such as anatomical and functional imaging data may be considered.

As stated previously, there is significant individual variability with regard to the topography of essential language. Standard anatomical temporal lobe resections do not always spare language function.[5] Ojemann and others have also demonstrated that bilingual patients show language-specific localization in which case mapping may need to be performed in each language.[54,55] We cannot overemphasize that the inability to identify functional cortex in an area of interest does not imply that it is safe to resect in that area. With regard to speech there may be more than one essential speech area.[5,8] Therefore the entire area to be resected should be mapped (mapping should not be stopped because a speech area has been identified). Again, for resections near primary speech cortex, it is often helpful to have the patient continuously name objects during the resection as the resection is performed 1 to 2 mm at a time to avoid injuring essential cortex.

Conclusion

As with any surgical adjunct, the limitations and pitfalls of cortical mapping must be considered. Both functional imaging and direct stimulation may identify involved cortex and not necessarily essential cortex. Conversely, the inability to identify functional cortex does not necessarily imply lack of function in a specific area. It is therefore imperative to identify normal functional areas such as rolandic cortex for motor mapping and face motor cortex and speech areas for language

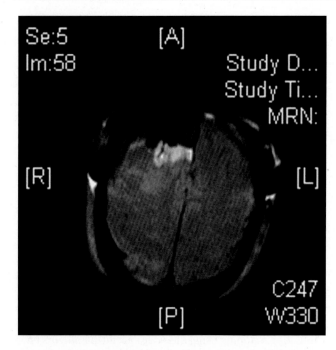

Fig. 12.5 Diffusion weighted MRI showing ischemic changes at the inferior portion of a tumor resection cavity.

mapping. The question however remains, "What do I do if I cannot localize functional cortex as a reference point?" In these situations, it is essential to consider all potential influences including anesthetic effects and appropriate stimulation levels. SSEP can be utilized as an indirect localizer of motor/sensory cortex; however, there is no equivalent for speech mapping. Utilizing functional imaging for localization carries a certain amount of risk as they do not exactly correlate with direct stimulation mapping, which obviously can be a significant issue in eloquent cortex, especially in the face of intraoperative brain shift. Therefore, in our opinion, functional mapping currently cannot be a complete substitute for direct stimulation mapping.

Even with precise intraoperative mapping, neurological deficits can still be elicited with resections near functional cortex. With the utilization of MRI diffusion weighted imaging, it is now apparent that some of these deficits are due to ischemia (**Fig. 12.5**). It is therefore imperative to practice extreme caution with the microvasculature near eloquent cortex. Utilizing subpial dissection techniques near the sulci provides a safer resection strategy. Finally, with cortical lesions that distort the surface anatomy, subcortical mapping may be necessary to avoid damage to the descending fibers.

References

1. Bartholow R. Experimental investigations into the function of the human brain. Am J Med Sci 1874;67:305–313
2. Cushing H. A note upon the faradic stimulation of the postcentral gyrus in conscious patients. Brain 1909;32:44–54
3. Penfield W, Rasmussen T. *The Cerebral Cortex of Man: A Clinical Study of Localization and Function.* New York: Macmillan; 1950
4. Penfield W, Jaspar H. *Epilepsy and the Functional Anatomy of the Human Brain.* Boston: Little, Brown 1954
5. Ojemann G, Ojemann J, Lettich E. Cortical language localization in left dominant hemisphere: an electrical stimulation mapping investigation in 117 patients. J Neurosurg 1989;71:316–326
6. Ojemann GA. Cortical organization of language. J Neurosci 1991;11: 2281–2287
7. Berger MS, Kincaid J, Ojemann GA, et al. Brain mapping techniques to maximize resection, safety, and seizure control in children with brain tumors. Neurosurgery 1989;25(5):786–792
8. Haglund MM, Berger MS, Shamseldin M, et al. Cortical localization of temporal lobe language sites in patients with gliomas. Neurosurgery 1994;34(4):567–576, discussion 576
9. Berger MS. Minimalism through intraoperative functional mapping. Clin Neurosurg 1996;43:324–337
10. Aoyama H, Kamada K, Shirato H, et al. Integration of functional brain information into stereotactic irradiation treatment planning using magnetoencephalography and magnetic resonance axonography. Int J Radiat Oncol Biol Phys 2004;58(4):1177–1183
11. Binder JR, Rao SM, Hammeke TA, et al. Lateralized human brain language systems demonstrated by task subtraction functional magnetic resonance imaging. Arch Neurol 1995;52(6):593–601
12. Kamada K, Houkin K, Takeuchi F, et al. Visualization of the eloquent motor system by integration of MEG, functional, and anisotropic diffusion-weighted MRI in functional neuronavigation. Surg Neurol 2003;59(5):352–361, discussion 361–2
13. Rabin ML, Narayan VM, Kimberg DY, et al. Functional MRI predicts post-surgical memory following temporal lobectomy. Brain 2004;127 (Pt 10):2286–2298
14. Rao SM, Binder JR, Hammeke TA, et al. Somatotopic mapping of the human primary motor cortex with functional magnetic resonance imaging. Neurology 1995;45(5):919–924
15. Witwer BP, Moftakhar R, Hasan KM, et al. Diffusion-tensor imaging of white matter tracts in patients with cerebral neoplasm. J Neurosurg 2002;97(3):568–575
16. Berger MS, Cohen WA, Ojemann GA. Correlation of motor cortex brain mapping data with magnetic resonance imaging. J Neurosurg 1990;72(3):383–387
17. Quinones-Hinojosa A, Ojemann SG, Sanai N, et al. Preoperative correlation of intraoperative cortical mapping with magnetic resonance imaging landmarks to predict localization of the Broca area. J Neurosurg 2003;99(2):311–318
18. Golaszewski SM, Siedentopf CM, Baldauf E, et al. Functional magnetic resonance imaging of the human sensorimotor cortex using a novel vibrotactile stimulator. Neuroimage 2002;17(1):421–430
19. Golaszewski SM, Siedentopf CM, Koppelstaetter F, et al. Human brain structures related to plantar vibrotactile stimulation: a functional magnetic resonance imaging study. Neuroimage 2006;29(3):923–929
20. Noll D, Vazquez A. Contrast mechanisms and acquisition methods in functional MRI. Conf Proc IEEE Eng Med Biol Soc 2004;7:219–5222
21. Kober H, Nimsky C, Moller M, et al. Correlation of sensorimotor activation with functional magnetic resonance imaging and magnetoencephalography in presurgical functional imaging: a spatial analysis. Neuroimage 2001;14(5):1214–1228
22. Korvenoja A, Kirveskari E, Aronen HJ, et al. Sensorimotor cortex localization: comparison of magnetoencephalography, functional MR imaging, and intraoperative cortical mapping. Radiology 2006;241(1): 213–222

23. Schiffbauer H, Berger MS, Ferrari P, et al. Preoperative magnetic source imaging for brain tumor surgery: a quantitative comparison with intraoperative sensory and motor mapping. Neurosurg Focus 2003; 15(1):E7

24. Kamada K, Houkin K, Iwasaki Y, et al. Rapid identification of the primary motor area by using magnetic resonance axonography. J Neurosurg 2002;97(3):558–567

25. Dodrill CB, Ojemann GA. An exploratory comparison of three methods of memory assessment with the intracarotid amobarbital procedure. Brain Cogn 1997;33(2):210–223

26. Snyder PJ, Harris LJ. The intracarotid amobarbital procedure: an historical perspective. Brain Cogn 1997;33(1):18–32

27. Wada J, Rasmussen T. Intracranial injection of amytal for the lateralization of cerebral speech dominance. J Neurosurg 1960;17:266–282

28. Ojemann JG, Neil JM, MacLeod AM, et al. Increased functional vascular response in the region of a glioma. J Cereb Blood Flow Metab 1998; 18(2):148–153

29. Bahn MM, Lin W, Silbergeld DL, et al. Localization of language cortices by functional MR imaging compared with intracarotid amobarbital hemispheric sedation. AJR Am J Roentgenol 1997;169(2):575–579

30. Yetkin FZ, Swanson S, Fischer M, et al. Functional MR of frontal lobe activation: comparison with Wada language results. AJNR Am J Neuroradiol 1998;19(6):1095–1098

31. Kamada K, Todo T, Masutani Y, et al. Visualization of the frontotemporal language fibers by tractography combined with functional magnetic resonance imaging and magnetoencephalography. J Neurosurg 2007;106(1):90–98

32. Kamada K, Sawamura Y, Takeuchi F, et al. Expressive and receptive language areas determined by a non-invasive reliable method using functional magnetic resonance imaging and magnetoencephalography. Neurosurgery 2007;60(2):296–305, discussion 305–6

33. Roux FE, Boulanouar K, Lotterie JA, et al. Language functional magnetic resonance imaging in preoperative assessment of language areas: correlation with direct cortical stimulation. Neurosurgery 2003;52(6):1335–1345, discussion 1345–7

34. Benson RR, FitzGerald DB, LeSueur LL, et al. Language dominance determined by whole brain functional MRI in patients with brain lesions. Neurology 1999;52(4):798–809

35. Ojemann SG, Berger MS, Lettich E, et al. Localization of language function in children: results of electrical stimulation mapping. J Neurosurg 2003;98(3):465–470

36. Davies KG, Risse GL, Gates JR. Naming ability after tailored left temporal resection with extraoperative language mapping: increased risk of decline with later epilepsy onset age. Epilepsy Behav 2005;7(2):273–278

37. Schaffler L, Luders HO, Beck GJ. Quantitative comparison of language deficits produced by extraoperative electrical stimulation of Broca's, Wernicke's, and basal temporal language areas. Epilepsia 1996;37(5):463–475

38. Liu EH, Wong HK, Chia CP, et al. Effects of isoflurane and propofol on cortical somatosensory evoked potentials during comparable depth of anaesthesia as guided by bispectral index. Br J Anaesth 2005; 94(2):193–197

39. Strahm C, Min K, Boos N, et al. Reliability of perioperative SSEP recordings in spine surgery. Spinal Cord 2003;41(9):483–489

40. Hermanns H, Lipfert P, Meier S, et al. Cortical somatosensory-evoked potentials during spine surgery in patients with neuromuscular and idiopathic scoliosis under propofol-remifentanil anaesthesia. Br J Anaesth 2007;98(3):362–365

41. Keifer JC, Dentchev D, Little K, et al. A retrospective analysis of a remifentanil/propofol general anesthetic for craniotomy before awake functional brain mapping. Anesth Analg 2005;101(2):502–508, table of contents

42. Hans P, Bonhomme V. Anesthetic management for neurosurgery in awake patients. Minerva Anesthesiol 2007;73:507–512

43. Hans P, Bonhomme V. Why we still use intravenous drugs as the basic regimen for neurosurgical anaesthesia. Curr Opin Anaesthesiol 2006;19(5):498–503

44. Sartorius CJ, Berger MS. Rapid termination of intraoperative stimulation-evoked seizures with application of cold Ringer's lactate to the cortex. Technical note. J Neurosurg 1998;88(2):349–351

45. Rowed DW, Houlden DA, Basavakumar DG. Somatosensory evoked potential identification of sensorimotor cortex in removal of intracranial neoplasms. Can J Neurol Sci 1997;24(2):116–120

46. Grant GA, Farrell D, Silbergeld DL. Continuous somatosensory evoked potential monitoring during brain tumor resection. Report of four cases and review of the literature. J Neurosurg 2002;97(3):709–713

47. Snyder AZ. Steady-state vibration evoked potentials: descriptions of technique and characterization of responses. Electroencephalogr Clin Neurophysiol 1992;84(3):257–268

48. Silbergeld DL, Miller JW. Intraoperative cerebral mapping and monitoring. Contemp Neurosurg 1996;18:1–6

49. Silbergeld DL. Intraoperative transdural functional mapping. Technical note. J Neurosurg 1994;80(4):756–758

50. Romstock J, Fahlbusch R, Ganslandt O, et al. Localisation of the sensorimotor cortex during surgery for brain tumours: feasibility and waveform patterns of somatosensory evoked potentials. J Neurol Neurosurg Psychiatry 2002;72(2):221–229

51. Berger MS, Ojemann GA. Intraoperative brain mapping techniques in neuro-oncology. Stereotact Funct Neurosurg 1992;58(1–4):153–161

52. Silbergeld DL, Ojemann GA. The tailored temporal lobectomy. Neurosurg Clin N Am 1993;4(2):273–281

53. Ojemann GA, Dodrill CB. Verbal memory deficits after left temporal lobectomy for epilepsy. Mechanism and intraoperative prediction. J Neurosurg 1985;62(1):101–107

54. Lucas TH II, McKhann GM II, Ojemann GA. Functional separation of languages in the bilingual brain: a comparison of electrical stimulation language mapping in 25 bilingual patients and 117 monolingual control patients. J Neurosurg 2004;101(3):449–457

55. Ojemann GA, Whitaker HA. The bilingual brain. Arch Neurol 1978; 35(7):409–412

13 Callosotomy

Jean-Pierre Farmer, Abdulrahman J. Sabbagh, and Jeffrey D. Atkinson

The goal of the majority of surgical and medical therapies for the treatment of epilepsy is the complete cessation of seizures with the preservation of maximal brain function. Despite this, there remain syndromes where curative procedures are not a relevant consideration and palliative approaches toward the control of symptoms or the reduction of seizure burden, with associated gains in the quality of life (QOL), are more appropriate goals. Increasing variety in the pharmacotherapy of epilepsy has reduced the role surgery plays in such cases. Division of the corpus callosum to limit the spread of ictal discharges and thus reduce generalized epileptic symptomatology remains a procedure of some utility. Newer palliative options such as vagal nerve stimulation (VNS) have attempted to provide a similar QOL gain with reductions in the potential neurological morbidity associated with the procedure. Nevertheless, in carefully selected patients callosotomy remains an effective tool to control atonic seizures specifically, with an acceptable incidence of significant neurological morbidity.

History

Surgical sectioning of the corpus callosum was first performed by Dandy, to access the third ventricle.[1] In 1940, Van Wagenen and Herren proposed that division of commissural pathways in the corpus callosum might be helpful to treat epilepsy.[2] They stated that this surgery "may serve to limit the spread of an epileptic wave to the opposite hemisphere." Several observations in patients with long-standing epilepsy that improved or resolved after neoplastic, ischemic, or traumatic damage to corpus callosum led them to propose this procedure. They described partial callosotomy from the genu and the body of the corpus callosum up to and/or including the splenium, in combination with sectioning the fornix. Eight out of 10 patients who underwent the procedure stopped having convulsive seizures impairing consciousness.[2] A decade later Kopeloff et al experimented with callosotomy on monkeys.[3] The surgery was reintroduced in the 1960s, by Bogen and colleagues. Their experience was detailed in several consecutive reports during the 1970s.[4-7] The procedure gained acceptance quickly and several institutes in the '80s and '90s reported on a large number of corpus callosotomies, including the Montreal Neurological Institute,[8,9] Yale University,[10-13] and Dartmouth-Hitchcock Medical Centre in New Hampshire,[14] with promising results. The advent of VNS, a less invasive procedure with similar indications (i.e., relief of atonic seizures), led to a reduction in callosotomy frequency in recent years. Incomplete seizure control following VNS insertion has led to a redefinition of the role of callosotomy in the management of refractory seizures.

Anatomy

Topographic Anatomy

The corpus callosum is the largest identifiable white matter fiber bundle in the brain. It interconnects the hemispheres, mostly contralateral homotopic structures, but there are also connections between heterotopic areas of brain. It contains more than 3×10^8 fibers.[15] The mean measurements of the callosum on magnetic resonance imaging (MRI) and cadaver dissection are as follows: length, 74.9 mm and 87.2 mm; maximum height, 25.5 mm and 19.7 mm, respectively.[16]

It is generally agreed upon that the corpus callosum, at its midsagittal plane, is comprised of five anatomical segments: the rostrum, genu, body, isthmus, and splenium. Forceps minor and major are large callosal fiber tracts arising from the genu and the splenium, respectively (**Fig. 13.1**). They are best identified in the axial plane. Several authors further classify the midsagittal plane regions of the corpus callosum from geometric, topographic, and morphometric perspectives. Witelson[17] subdivided the corpus callosum geometrically into (1) the anterior third (region I containing fibers projecting into prefrontal, premotor, and supplementary motor regions); (2) the anterior midbody (region II with callosal motor fiber bundles); (3) the posterior midbody (region III with somaesthetic, posterior parietal projections); (4) the isthmus (region IV with posterior parietal, superior temporal projections); and (5) the splenium (region V with occipital, inferior temporal projections).

Recently, diffusion tensor magnetic resonance imaging (dtMRI) fiber tractography has been used by Hofer and Frahm[15] to outline five regional partitions of the corpus callosum in live human subjects. Region I, the anterior sixth, includes fibers going to the prefrontal region. Region II, the rest of the anterior half, contains fibers projecting to premotor and supplementary motor cortical areas. This would be the largest subdivision of the corpus callosum. Region III is the posterior half without the posterior third, and it contains fibers crossing to the primary motor cortex (unlike the Witelson classification). Region IV is the posterior one-third minus the posterior one-fourth. It contains primary sensory fibers. Region V, is the posterior one-fourth, and its fibers cross to parietal, temporal, and occipital areas (**Fig. 13.2**).

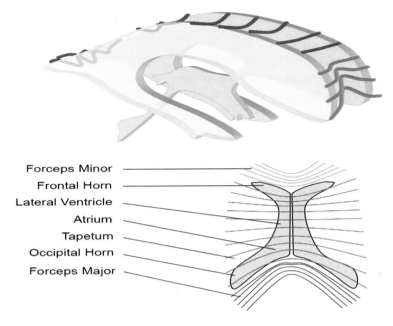

Fig. 13.1 Major pathways of corpus callosum in relation to periventricular anatomy.

Forceps Minor
Frontal Horn
Lateral Ventricle
Atrium
Tapetum
Occipital Horn
Forceps Major

Surgical and Vascular Anatomy

The corpus callosum represents the largest component of the ventricular lining.[18] The rostrum forms the floor of the frontal horn. Forceps minor forms the anterior wall of the frontal horn. The genu and body of the corpus callosum form the roof of the frontal horn and the body of the lateral ventricle. Forceps major produces a prominence called the bulb in the upper part of the medial wall of the atrium and occipital horn. Another fiber tract, the tapetum, which arises in the posterior part of the body and splenium, sweeps laterally and inferiorly to form the roof and lateral wall of the atrium and the temporal and occipital horns[18] (**Fig. 13.1**).

The arterial supply to the corpus callosum delivers blood from the outer surface in, whereas the venous drainage forms in the inner ependymal surface[19] and drains in the deep venous system.

Three main arteries contribute to the arterial supply of the corpus callosum, the anterior communicating artery, the pericallosal artery, and the posterior pericallosal artery. The anterior communicating artery contributes branches; the subcallosal and the median callosal arteries.[20] The former is present in 50% of cases and is a single dominant artery that supplies the rostrum and genu of the corpus callosum. It also supplies the anterior hypothalamus, the subcallosal area, the fornix, and the medial portion of the anterior commissure.[20] The median callosal artery is present in 30% of cases and may contribute to the blood supply of the body, and occasionally the splenium.[20]

Approximate location of cortical connections within the corpus callosum

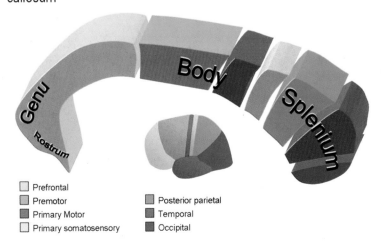

Prefrontal
Premotor
Primary Motor
Primary somatosensory

Posterior parietal
Temporal
Occipital

Fig. 13.2 Connecting fibers of major brain regions and their anatomical relationships within the corpus callosum.

The pericallosal artery runs in the callosal sulcus in ~60% of cases.[20] It branches into the short and long callosal arteries.[21] The short callosal arteries are present in 98% of hemispheres; they directly penetrate the corpus callosum and provide it with significant arterial supply.[21] There are around seven such arteries on either side. The long callosal arteries, on the other hand, are fewer in number and are less commonly present.[20,21] They contribute to the formation of the pericallosal pial plexus and provide a source of anastomoses with the posterior callosal artery.[20] Ture et al further subclassified the short arteries into the callosal, cingulocallosal, and long callosal arteries that form the pericallosal pial plexus and the recurrent cingulocallosal artery.[20]

The posterior pericallosal artery is present two-thirds of the time.[22] After branching off the posterior cerebral artery, at the level of the splenium, it splits into superior and inferior branches at this level.[20] The superior branch anastomoses with branches from the pericallosal artery. The anastomoses between the pericallosal artery and posterior callosal artery occur at the splenium in the majority of cases.[20,22–24] The posterior cerebral artery also indirectly supplies the corpus callosum through choroidal branches.[19]

Callosal and calloso-cingulate (also called transcallosal) veins drain blood from the corpus callosum and course in the direction of the lateral ventricles, to drain into the septal and atrial veins. The septal and atrial veins drain into the deep central cerebral veins.[19]

Indications

Prior to proposing corpus callosotomy for the control of refractory seizures in a given patient, several admissibility criteria must be met. First, the patient must clearly demonstrate medical intractability.[25] Several authors have attempted to define failure to antiepileptic medication.[25–31] Most agree that epilepsy spanning 18 months, failing two antiepileptic medications with an average seizure frequency of one seizure per month, and no period of freedom of seizures longer than 2 months is considered intractable epilepsy.[27]

Given that callosotomy is a palliative treatment aimed at seizure reduction rather than seizure cure, the team considering the patient for seizure surgery should ensure that there is no clearly defined focal onset for the seizure disorder based on imaging and electrographic data including single photon emission tomography (SPECT) scans, both ictal and interictal modes, as well as detailed MRI, and video electroencephalogram (EEG) telemetry. In children, in particular, even infantile spasms can occasionally be related to a focal anatomical or physiological anomaly of the brain.[32–34] In these cases resective surgery should be offered to a patient because of the higher incidence of cure of seizures, the ultimate "focal" resection being a complete hemispherectomy.

In cases where anatomical or electrographic damage appears to be clearly bilateral, in patients where the bilateral disorders are primarily frontal, and in patients who exhibit developmental difficulties as well as multiple seizure types with bilateral but initially focalized onset, callosotomy can be considered. The primary seizure type that responds to callosotomy is the atonic seizure, whereas repeated generalized tonic, tonic clonic, and myoclonic seizures tend to respond less well.[35–39] The chance of the procedure exhibiting a significant impact on the QOL of these patients is proportional to the extent of the disconnection.[36] Very severely involved children and adults with Lennox-Gastaut syndrome, in particular, are very unlikely to suffer from disconnection syndrome following an extensive callosotomy because of their baseline poor neurological development. It becomes clear in those patients that a more extensive callosotomy, preferably in one stage, is a good therapeutic option.

The advent of vagus nerve stimulation for the palliation of severe seizures disorders has put in question the traditional indications for callosotomy. Vagus nerve stimulation, although associated with less immediate morbidity (except, perhaps, in patients with pseudobulbar states) remains a "technology driven" treatment that is, therefore, expensive over a lifetime to maintain, and is not readily accessible in all areas of the globe. Given that it is less invasive than callosotomy, it is, however, likely to be the first line of treatment for patients with multiple seizure types, poor development, and no evidence of unilateral focality for resective surgery.

We have had the opportunity of offering callosotomy to two patients who had had prior VNS implantations but were still manifesting frequent atonic seizures. In both patients, an anterior two-thirds callosotomy was successful at controlling the atonic seizures after the VNS had led to a reduction of other seizure types, including generalized epilepsy.

Approaches

In most refractory epilepsy cases, with significant atonic seizures, callosotomy is performed over the anterior one-half to two-thirds. More rarely, for seizure spread in posterior brain areas, exclusively posterior sectioning is performed. Complete sectioning of the corpus has been performed as a multistaged operation, but some authors advocate performing callosotomy up to the splenium in a single position and single surgery.[39] Others have been able to completely section the corpus callosum including the splenium with one procedure.[35] This may be particularly useful in severe Lennox-Gastaut cases. Neuronavigation has been very helpful in confirming intraoperatively that the desired extent of callosal section has been attained.

Patients undergoing standard anterior corpus callosotomy will usually be positioned supine using head fixation, and appropriate padding for the body and extremities. Patient positioning for anterior callosotomy is most often performed such that the body of the corpus callosum is perpendicular to the floor, that is, with the head in a neutral position and with a 20-degree flexion of the head.[40] Some have advocated that the head be rotated toward the floor, either to have the falx parallel with the floor, or to a somewhat more limited extent, such that the frontal lobe on the dependent side

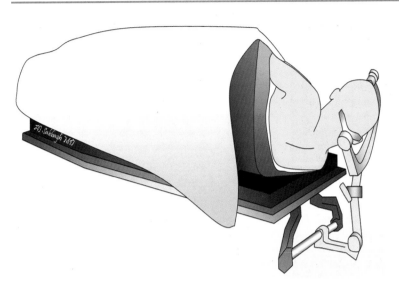

Fig. 13.3 Positioning of patient in a semilateral fashion to allow dependent hemisphere to fall away from falx by gravity.

would fall away from the falx with gravity rather than retraction (**Figs. 13.3 and 13.4**). On the other hand, the surgeon's orientation may be less "natural" in this position than if the head is placed in a neutral orientation. Neuronavigation systems can be quite helpful in the planning of the surgery, both to locate the actual craniotomy and to determine the side of the craniotomy, away from the predominance of cortical draining veins.[41]

With the patient positioned, incisions are made in either a curvilinear or "lazy S" fashion centered on the coronal suture. The standard craniotomy crosses the midline with a slight predominance on one side or the other (depending on the draining vein configuration as defined by neuronavigation). The craniotomy will be approximately two-thirds in front and one-third behind the coronal suture and may be

quite small, although the preoperative understanding of the cortical venous drainage will determine the extent of exposure required. Dural opening is based toward the midline to allow the interhemispheric fissure to be opened, and often, separate dural incisions around proximal located veins draining into the sinus may be necessary to allow adequate exposure of the midline. Again, proper preoperative planning and neuronavigation will be essential to allow access to the interhemispheric fissure to an adequate extent without stretching or injuring cortical draining veins or the cingulum (**Fig. 13.5**). Ideally no cortical veins should be divided, particularly those located posterior to the coronal suture.

The interhemispheric fissure is divided along the falx using standard microsurgical techniques until the callosum is identified between the pericallosal arteries. Occasionally,

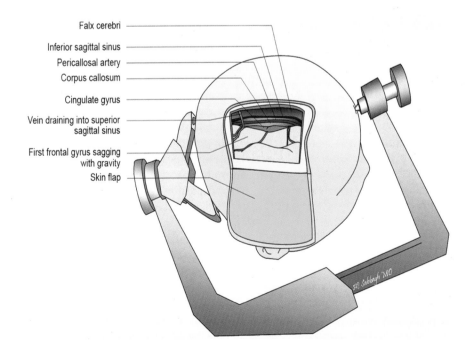

Falx cerebri
Inferior sagittal sinus
Pericallosal artery
Corpus callosum
Cingulate gyrus
Vein draining into superior sagittal sinus
First frontal gyrus sagging with gravity
Skin flap

Fig. 13.4 Closer view of lateral position showing the frontal lobe falling away from the flax by gravity thus providing an operative corridor to the corpus callosum.

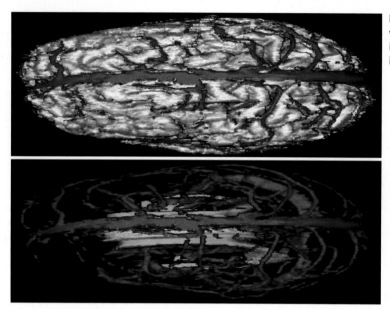

Fig. 13.5 Neuronavigation generated three-dimensional view of surface anatomy, corpus callosum, and major draining cortical veins into the sagittal sinus. Surgical approach is tailored to avoid the major bridging veins.

the falx is incomplete and interfrontal adhesions can mislead the surgeon toward the contralateral frontal lobe. Frequently, the two pericallosal arteries are not located at the same depth, the anatomy being distorted by a preexisting unilateral ventricular enlargement or by an orthostatic retractor, which iatrogenically raises one side over the other. It is important to avoid being lateral to one or the other pericallosal as most of the small arterial branches feeding the medial hemisphere are lateral to the parent vessel. Sectioning occurs using microsurgical instruments and suction/aspiration or the Cavitron through the callosum to the midline leaves of the septum pellucidum. Frequently, the width of the exposure initially only allows enough room for a microsuction or the Cavitron micro-tip adaptor. It may be advantageous, from a postoperative complication point of view, to preserve the ependymal lining beneath the corpus callosum. If this is not possible, cottonoid application within the ventricles to limit the risk of aseptic meningitis and/or postoperative hydrocephalus is a good practice. The posterior extent of the section can be determined by the callosal anatomy (see previously) and with neuronavigation.[42] Complete sectioning posteriorly will divide the splenium to the pia–arachnoid around the vein of Galen, a structure that needs to be preserved at all cost and, that, if injured, is at the deepest point of the surgical bed and will therefore result in a difficult hemostasis challenge. The extent of anterior callosal disconnection will reach the anterior commissure. Near-complete section to the splenium can occur from virtually the same incision and position,[39] whereas complete section has been described by making a larger craniotomy with extension posteriorly to almost the bregma.[35] If a second stage (splenial) section is necessary, the approach is similar to the occipital transtentorial approach to a pineal tumor (without the tentorial section) so as to effect retraction with the help of gravity on the occipital cortex as opposed to the central

area. Furthermore, there are very few bridging veins to the superior sagittal sinus in this area.

Less invasive techniques for callosal sectioning have also been described. There has been one technical report of a limited incision and endoscopic assisted anterior two-thirds callosotomy. These authors used an eyebrow incision and a rigid endoscope to section the corpus callosum in human cadavers. They determined that the operation was a safe and feasible way to achieve sectioning of a reasonable portion of the callosum and might be particularly useful in small children who have yet to aerate their frontal sinuses, which could potentially complicate the low-set craniotomy. These authors used the endoscope itself to section the callosum and admitted that the presence of active circulation in living patients might potentially result in venous bleeding that would be technically problematic. They felt that this might be partially offset by the presence of cerebrospinal fluid (CSF), which would make endoscopic visualization easier.[43] Injury to anterior communicating artery branches that also irrigate the frontal basal area and hypothalamus might be another consideration. As yet there are no reports of this technique being used in living human subjects.

Stereotactic radiosurgical techniques have been used for a variety of functional surgical procedures including epilepsy procedures. One group has used Gamma Knife to functionally section the corpus callosum. They reported their results in three patients.[44] Two of these patients had reasonable functional and seizure outcome results; however, both had previously undergone surgical functional hemispherectomy and the radiosurgical procedure was used in focal areas only to complete an incomplete disconnection. The third patient was diagnosed with Lennox-Gastaut syndrome and had previously undergone right anterior temporal resection without significant improvement in the seizures. He had no significant improvement in his epilepsy findings subsequent to an attempt at complete section of the corpus callosum using multiple radiosurgical isocentres. No acute complications were noted. Others have treated several patients with anterior callosotomy with relatively good results for atonic and generalized seizures and no significant complications apart from early headache.[45] In these reports, atonic seizures were abolished in 38% of patients and significantly reduced in 63%. Generalized seizures showed improvement in all patients with complete elimination in 50%.[45] Some improvement in partial seizures was also obtained in patients treated after failed hemispherectomy.[45] These results suggest that radiosurgery might be useful for focal injury to short segments of the corpus callosum but for exclusive treatment in nonsurgically treated patients it remains uncertain that this technique is of benefit. Long-term complications, particularly to nearby vascular structures and the cingulum, are also not known, though they appear to be minimal in up to 12 years of follow-up in one study.[45]

Results

Most patients being considered for callosotomy exhibit multiple, different seizure types that are refractory to several combinations of medical polytherapy. Callosotomy is a palliative procedure that does not necessarily aim to completely control all seizure types. As such the goals of surgery need to be adjusted to the population of patients being studied. Seizure freedom from specific disabling seizures types and worthwhile reduction in seizure frequency, with resultant improvement in QOL, are the common end points to studies of the procedure. Nevertheless, there are some groups of patients, with predominance of specific seizure types who can be expected to become seizure free after the procedure. Traditionally, atonic seizures have been thought of as showing the best response rate. A meta-analysis/systematic review of the literature for the results of all seizure surgery showed a 35% rate of seizure freedom for atonic seizures with corpus callosotomy.[46] Oguni et al, in 43 patients with anterior corpus callosotomy, found a reduction of the frequency of the predominant seizure pattern of more than 50% in 56% of patients and of more than 75% in 33% of patients.[36] They deemed greater than 50% seizure frequency reduction as a worthwhile improvement. The patients with atonic seizure patterns showed the best response and patients with generalized tonic clonic seizures showed the least impressive response. Wong et al followed 268 patients operated on over a long time period with different follow-up durations. They described that 50% of the patients in their overall series had a 50% reduction in seizure rate. Medication freedom was reported in only 9.3% of patients after a long follow-up.[38] Cukiert et al described their experience in 76 patients with extended callosotomy with sparing of the splenium. Overall, they had 91% of patients with a greater than 50% reduction of seizures. The response rate was 92% for atonic seizures, 82% for atypical absence, 57% for tonic clonic seizures, 51% for tonic, and 27% for myoclonic sei-

zures. Sixty-eight percent of all patients had at least a 90% reduction in seizures.[39]

The optimal age for patients to undergo the procedure has not been studied clearly. However, this procedure is often performed in children with severely disabling, medically refractory epilepsies and the results appear to be at least as good as those reported in adults. Several series have reported the results of corpus callosal section in children specifically. In a series of 76 children operated on by Shimizu, a 90% seizure free rate was noted in 35 children with complete callostomy and a 67% seizure free rate in six patients with partial sectioning.[47] In 16 patients with anterior two-thirds callosotomy 69% of children had Engel class II or better outcomes, which the authors defined as worthwhile outcome. The best response was with atonic seizures. The worst response was seen in tonic seizures and 13% of patients had new tonic seizures after surgery.[37]

Many other factors have been looked at to predict patient response to callosotomy. In the 43 patients of Oguni et al there was an attempt to stratify outcome by EEG pattern, intraoperative factors, and preoperative clinical factors.[36] In this series, EEG patterns, which were lateralized, were more likely to be associated with good outcome and frontal lobe epilepsies had the best clinical response. Greater extent of callosotomy was associated with better results with anterior two-thirds callosotomy faring better than anterior one-half callosotomy. Lateralized structural abnormalities on MRI, age at operation, or full scale IQ did not show significant effects on outcome. Others have found that callosotomy may be effective with certain preoperative imaging findings. Kawai et al reported excellent results in terms of bihemispheric malformations of cortical development. In their series almost all of their nine patients had a significant improvement in atonic seizures and a good response for all other seizure types.[35]

QOL has not been studied extensively. Shimizu et al reported that QOL improved in 77% of 76 children operated on for corpus callosotomy with a family satisfaction rate of 97%.[47] Good seizure control rates with callosotomy translated into 27% of patients with considerably improved QOL scores, in a recent study by Larysz et al.[48] Other studies have looked at attention levels in a nonspecific marker for QOL and found an improvement of 90% of operated patients.[39] Fifty percent of patients in a study of 16 children by Turanli et al showed improvement of activities of daily living after corpus callosotomy and 50% were able to attend classes that were previously impossible for them.[37]

As the indications for corpus callosotomy overlap somewhat with those for VNS, outcomes must be compared. Both procedures are considered palliative and outcomes are generally reported in terms of seizure frequency reduction[49] rather than freedom from seizures. In one study comparing the two techniques in two retrospective cohorts, for generalized seizures, callosotomy provides a slightly better control rate (79% vs. 50% reduction of seizures by 50% or more) with similar rates of control of atonic seizures. Complications of callosotomy were higher: 21% versus 8% compared with VNS.[50] Although others have reported lower permanent morbidity rates for callosotomy (see below), a differential in the incidence and severity of complications likely exists between the two procedures. There have been attempts at both VNS insertion after failed callosotomy[51] and callosotomy after inadequate response to VNS. We favor the second approach. Given the above response data and complication rates, it would appear more useful to perform the least invasive procedure first if both procedures may ultimately be indicated in a given patient.[38]

Complications

Callosotomy is a relatively safe procedure, although acute neurological effects are not uncommon and these can be attributed often to injury to neighboring vascular or cortical structures. For example, a frontal venous infarct from bridging vein damage, a cingular contusion, an occipital contusion, for a posterior approach, ischemia in the pericallosal territory, in the anterior communicating artery territory, and bilateral mesiofrontal damage will all have associated transient or permanent sequelae. Understanding of the anatomy and careful use of navigation to position and guide the section will help minimize such sequelae. Also, attempting a complete section in a patient where the reach for the splenium becomes more difficult than anticipated should be avoided. It is better to prepare the family for the possibility of a second-stage procedure preoperatively.

Lesions damaging the corpus callosum in a left hemispheric dominant person do not generally preclude activities of daily living but may result in a syndrome of (1) inability to name objects presented briefly to the left hemifield; (2) left hemi alexia; (3) left hemianomia; (4) difficulty imitating the hidden other hand; (5) unilateral tactile anomia; (6) unilateral left agraphia; and (7) right-hand constructional apraxia, that is, inability to copy a complex design with the right hand but ability to outperform this by using the left hand.[52] As mentioned previously, in severely handicapped individuals with developmental delay, a disconnection syndrome may go unnoticed and be offset by the QOL gains associated with reduced atonic seizure frequency.

Mortality is relatively rare and epilepsy-associated deaths may be avoided by successful surgery. Morbidity is often reported only in terms of surgical complications without taking into account the fairly common acute disconnection syndromes. Shimizu reported a mortality rate of 1.3% and a morbidity rate of 5.6% in 76 operated children with complications including epidural bleeds, subdural collections, and hydrocephalus.[47] Oguni et al described early surgical morbidity in 37% of patients.[36] Not including transient mutism and transient increase in seizures, Wong et al reported a 3.6% rate of complications.[38] Kawai et al experienced a 20% rate of transient neurological complications, and a 10% rate of other

morbidity in a small series of 10 patients.[35] Acute callosal disconnection symptoms with a mean duration of 16 days were reported by Cukiert et al in 89% of operated patients, with 3% having prolonged disconnection symptomatology.[39] Six percent of patients in a study of 16 children by Turanli et al suffered operative complications with a 6% rate of temporary disconnection symptoms.[37]

Mortality for all patients with epilepsy is higher than the general population, but for surgeries where seizure control is complete, mortality returns close to the baseline. Consistent with this is the view that callosotomy patients with incompletely resolved seizures present with an extremely high mortality, higher than the average of operated patients and among the highest of any studied group.[53]

Conclusion

Callosotomy is a "relatively" safe intracranial procedure available for surgical palliation in patients with medically intractable epilepsy who do not show any imaging or electrographic admissibility criteria for resective epilepsy surgery. The epilepsy is therefore usually bilateral in origin, and the manifestations are those of multiple seizure types in patients usually exhibiting developmental delay. The best outcomes on QOL have come when the epilepsy appears to be bifrontal or is associated with bifrontal anomalies on imaging, and the success rate of the procedure is proportional to the extent of the callosal resection.[9,36,37,39,47,48] The morbidity associated with a full callosotomy is higher, particularly with respect to the disconnection syndrome, but this is a relatively small price to pay in patients with severe debilitating epilepsy and developmental disorders. Even if the preoperative plan was for a complete section, if the intraoperative conditions do not appear favorable a planned "second-stage" posterior section might be more advisable.

The advent of VNS for the palliative treatment of patients with similar clinical epilepsy profiles makes the use of callosotomy, in countries where VNS is available, even more selective. As the learning curve and cost issues are analyzed with respect to the implantable devices, the relative role of the two procedures in the palliation of severe seizure disorders will clarify itself. Currently, both procedures carry similar indications. Callosotomy has been used in patients having undergone VNS implantation who continue to manifest a significant problem with the atonic seizures with a very significant success rate. In such patients, if the stimulator implantation led first to a reduction of other seizure types, with a persistence of debilitating atonic seizures, a more restrictive, usually anterior callosotomy (associated with less morbidity) appears to be quite successful at alleviating the atonic seizures. Unless clear distinct indications emerge for each of these two procedures in the future, a staged combination treatment could ultimately be defined as the treatment of choice for patients not meeting criteria for resective surgery.

References

1. Dandy W. Diagnosis, localization and removal of tumors of the third ventricle. Johns Hopkins Hospital Bulletin 1922;33:188–189

2. Van Wagenen W, Herren R. Surgical division of commissural pathways and the corpus callsoum: relation to spread of an epileptic attack. Arch Neurol Psychiatry 1940;44:740–759

3. Kopeloff N, Kennard MA, Pacella BL, et al. Section of corpus callosum in experimental epilepsy in the monkey. Arch Neurol Psychiatry 1950;63(5):719–727

4. Mann L, Bogen JE, Vogel PJ, et al. Cerebral commissurotomy in man: EEG findings. Electroencephalogr Clin Neurophysiol 1969;27: 660

5. Bogen JE. The other side of the brain, I: dysgraphia and dyscopia following cerebral commissurotomy. Bull Los Angeles Neurol Soc 1969; 34(2):73–105

6. Bogen JE, Fisher ED, Vogel PJ. Cerebral commissurotomy. A second case report. JAMA 1965;194(12):1328–1329

7. Bogen JE, Vogel PJ. Treatment of generalized seizures by cerebral commissurotomy. Surg Forum 1963;14:431–433

8. Olivier A. Surgery of epilepsy: methods. Acta Neurol Scand Suppl 1988; 117:103–113

9. Oguni H, Andermann F, Gotman J, et al. Effect of anterior callosotomy on bilaterally synchronous spike and wave and other EEG discharges. Epilepsia 1994;35(3):505–513

10. Spencer SS, Spencer DD, Williamson PD, et al. Corpus callosotomy for epilepsy, I: Seizure effects. Neurology 1988;38(1):19–24

11. Sass KJ, Spencer DD, Spencer SS, et al. Corpus callosotomy for epilepsy. II. neurologic and neuropsychological outcome. Neurology 1988;38(1):24–28

12. Spencer SS, Spencer DD, Sass K, et al. Anterior, total, and two-stage corpus callosum section: Differential and incremental seizure responses. Epilepsia 1993;34(3):561–567

13. Spencer SS, Katz A, Ebersole J, et al. Ictal EEG changes with corpus callosum section. Epilepsia 1993;34(3):568–573

14. McInerney J, Siegel AM, Nordgren RE, et al. Long-term seizure outcome following corpus callosotomy in children. Stereotact Funct Neurosurg 1999;73(1–4):79–83

15. Hofer S, Frahm J. Topography of the human corpus callosum revisited—comprehensive fiber tractography using diffusion tensor magnetic resonance imaging. Neuroimage 2006;32(3):989–994

16. Goncalves-Ferreira AJ, Herculano C, Melancia JP, et al. Corpus callosum: microsurgical anatomy and MRI. Surg Radiol Anat 2001;23(6): 409–414

17. Witelson SF. Hand and sex differences in the isthmus and genu of the human corpus callosum. A postmortem morphological study. Brain 1989;112:799–835

18. Rhoton AL, ed. *The Cerebrum*. Rhoton's Anatomy, Part 2. Vol. 53. CNS, Lippincot, Williams & Wilkins; 2003:29–79

19. Wolfram-Gabel R, Maillot C. The venous vascularization of the corpus callosum in man. Surg Radiol Anat 1992;14(1):17–21

20. Ture U, Yasargil MG, Krisht AF. The arteries of the corpus callosum: a microsurgical anatomic study. Neurosurgery 1996;39(6):1075–1084

21. Perlmutter D, Rhoton AL. Microsurgical anatomy of the distal anterior cerebral artery. J Neurosurg 1978;49:204–228

22. Yamamoto I, Kageyama N. Microsurgical anatomy of the pineal region. J Neurosurg 1980;53:205–221

23. Milisavljević M, Marinković S, Lolić-Draganić V, Djordjević L. Anastomoses in the territory of the posterior cerebral arteries. Acta Anat (Basel) 1986;127:221–225

24. Zeal AA, Rhoton AL. Microsurgical anatomy of the posterior cerebral artery. J Neurosurg 1978;48:534–559

25. Berg AT, Kelly MM. Defining intractability. Epilepsia 2006;47:431–436

26. Arts WF, Geerts AT, Brouwer OF, et al. The early prognosis of epilepsy in childhood: the prediction of a poor outcome. The Dutch study of epilepsy in childhood. Epilepsia 1999;40:726–734

27. Berg AT, Vickrey BG, Testa FM, et al. How long does it take for epilepsy to become intractable? A prospective investigation. Ann Neurol 2006;60:73–79

28. Camfield PR, Camfield CS. Antiepileptic drug therapy: when is epilepsy truly intractable? Epilepsia 1996;37(Suppl 1):S60–S65

29. Dlugos DJ, Sammel MD, Strom BL, et al. Response to first drug trial predicts outcome in childhood temporal lobe epilepsy. Neurology 2001;57:2259–2264

30. Kwan P, Brodie MJ. Drug treatment of epilepsy: when does it fail and how to optimize its use? CNS Spectr 2004;9:110–119

31. Wilensky A. History of focal epilepsy and criteria for medical intractability. Neurosurg Clin N Am 1993;4(2):193–198

32. Chugani HT, Shields WD, Shewmon DA, et al. Infantile spasms, I: PET identifies focal cortical dysgenesis in cryptogenic cases for surgical treatment. Ann Neurol 1990;27(4):406–413

33. Chugani HT, Shewmon DA, Shields WD, et al. Surgery for intractable infantile spasms: Neuroimaging perpectives. Epilepsia 1993;34(4): 764–771

34. Asano E, Juhasz C, Shah A, et al. Origin and propagation of epileptic spasms delineated on electrocorticography. Epilepsia 2005;46(7): 1086–1097

35. Kawai K, Shimizu H, Yagishita A, et al. Clinical outcomes after corpus callosotomy in patients with bihemispheric malformations of cortical development. J Neurosurg 2004;101(1, Suppl)7–15

36. Oguni H, Olivier A, Andermann F, et al. Anterior callosotomy in the treatment of medically intractable epilepsies: A study of 43 patients with a mean follow-up of 39 months. Ann Neurol 1991;30(3):357–364

37. Turanli G, Yalnizoglu D, Genc-Acikgoz D, et al. Outcome and long term follow-up after corpus callosotomy in childhood onset intractable epilepsy. Childs Nerv Syst 2006;22(10):1322–1327

38. Wong TT, Kwan SY, Chang KP, et al. Corpus callosotomy in children. Childs Nerv Syst 2006;22(8):999–1011

39. Cukiert A, Burattini JA, Mariani PP, et al. Extended, one-stage callosal section for treatment of refractory secondarily generalized epilepsy in patients with Lennox-Gastaut and Lennox-like syndromes. Epilepsia 2006;47(2):371–374

40. Apuzzo ML, Giannotta SL. Transcallosal interforniceal approach. In: Apuzzo ML, ed. *Surgery of the Third Ventricle*. Baltimore: Williams & Wilkins; 1987:354–380

41. Hodaie M, Musharbash A, Otsubo H, et al. Image-guided, frameless stereotactic sectioning of the corpus callosum in children with intractable epilepsy. Pediatr Neurosurg 2001;34(6):286–294

42. Awad IA, Wyllie E, Luders H, et al. Intraoperative determination of the extent of corpus callosotomy for epilepsy: two simple techniques. Neurosurgery 1990;26(1):102–105

43. Tubbs RS, Smyth MD, Salter G, et al. Eyebrow incision with supraorbital trephination for endoscopic corpus callosotomy: a feasibility study. Childs Nerv Syst 2004;20(3):188–191

44. Eder HG, Feichtinger M, Pieper T, et al. Gamma knife radiosurgery for callosotomy in children with drug-resistant epilepsy. Childs Nerv Syst 2006;22(8):1012–1017

45. Feichtinger M, Schrottner O, Eder H, et al. Efficacy and safety of radiosurgical callosotomy: a retrospective analysis. Epilepsia 2006;47(7): 1184–1191

46. Tellez-Zenteno JF, Dhar R, Wiebe S. Long-term seizure outcomes following epilepsy surgery: a systematic review and meta-analysis. Brain 2005;128(Pt 5):1188–1198

47. Shimizu H. Our experience with pediatric epilepsy surgery focusing on corpus callosotomy and hemispherotomy. Epilepsia 2005;46 (Suppl 1):30–31

48. Larysz D, Larysz P, Mandera M. Evaluation of quality of life and clinical status of children operated on for intractable epilepsy. Childs Nerv Syst 2007;23(1):91–97

49. DeGiorgio CM, Schachter SC, Handforth A, et al. Prospective long-term study of vagus nerve stimulation for the treatment of refractory seizures. Epilepsia 2000;41(9):1195–1200

50. Nei M, O'Connor M, Liporace J, et al. Refractory generalized seizures: response to corpus callosotomy and vagal nerve stimulation. Epilepsia 2006;47(1):115–122

51. Amar AP, Apuzzo ML, Liu CY. Vagus nerve stimulation therapy after failed cranial surgery for intractable epilepsy: results from the vagus nerve stimulation therapy patient outcome registry. Neurosurgery 2004;55(5):1086–1093

52. Brazis PW, Masdeu JC, Biller J. *Localization in Clinical Neurology.* 4th ed., Philadelphia: Lippincott, Williams & Wilkins; 2001:507–508

53. Sperling MR, Saykin AJ, Roberts FD, et al. Mortality after epilepsy surgery. Epilepsia 2005;46(Suppl 11):49–53

14 Anatomical Hemispherectomy

Gregory G. Heuer and Phillip B. Storm

The general principle of surgery for intractable epilepsy is the removal or isolation of the region of brain that is generating the seizures from the normal brain. Anatomical hemispherectomy is epilepsy surgery in its most radical form, namely the surgical removal of the entire hemisphere.

Background

Walter Dandy is credited with performing the first hemispherectomy.[1] In 1929, Dandy performed a resection of the entire hemisphere in a patient with a diffuse right-sided glioma. The patient survived the procedure, and Dandy felt the patient did have some clinical benefit. Despite the early clinical benefit, the patient eventually died as the glioma recurred. The first hemispherectomy for epilepsy was performed by McKenzie in 1938.[2] The patient was cured of the epilepsy after the procedure. The first clinical series of the use of hemispherectomy to treat epilepsy was published by Krynauw in 1950.[3] He described a series of 12 patients, mostly with infantile hemiplegia syndrome, and found most of the patients, 10 of 12, had a significant reduction in seizures after surgery.

Anatomical hemispherectomy is most often performed in the young pediatric population. Indications for hemispherectomy include conditions in which the pathological process wholly or in large part affects one entire cerebral hemisphere. These conditions include Sturge-Weber syndrome, Rusmussen's encephalitis, porencephaly syndromes, schizencephaly, trauma, hemimegalencephaly, and cortical dysplasia involving a significant area of a single cerebral hemisphere.

The seizure control obtained in these early studies was encouraging, and the technique was widely employed in the 1960s. After a large number of the surgeries were performed, some common complications were found to be associated with the procedure. These complications included late postoperative hydrocephalus and superficial cerebral hemosiderosis.[4] These complications have been described to occur in up to a third of patients in the early studies.[5–7] Some technical modifications of the procedure have led to decreased complications and maintained the seizure reduction seen in the early studies.[8–12] More recent series have demonstrated seizure control in 60 to 94% of patients after hemispherectomy.[12,13] The seizure control rates are partial dependant on the age of the patient at the time of surgery, the specific disease pathology, and the length of time that seizures have been occurring.

Operative Technique

The availability of a specialized pediatric anesthesiologist familiar with the hemispherectomy procedure and the unique associated risks is imperative. A major risk of an anatomical hemispherectomy is blood loss. Prior to beginning the procedure it is imperative to have excellent intravenous (IV) access and blood products available. A pulmonary artery catheter in not routinely used, but central lines and arterial lines are placed in all patients. Frequent dialogue between the neurosurgeon and the anesthesiologist is imperative to accurately record and follow blood loss. When blood loss reaches one blood volume, we seriously consider aborting the procedure, especially if there is a substantial amount of brain that needs to be resected along the sagittal or transverse sinus where there is potential for brisk bleeding.

After the patient is anesthetized and adequate monitoring and venous access is obtained, the patient is positioned in the supine position with a gel roll under the ipsilateral shoulder and hip. The head is supported in a Mayfield horseshoe headholder (Integra Lifesciences Corp., Plainsboro, NJ) and rotated so that the nose is parallel with the floor. If the neck is not supple or there is a concern of decreased venous drainage, the bed is rotated until the head position is ideal. The head of the bed is raised to ~30 degrees. The hair is minimally shaved with electric clippers. Prior to making the incision, the patient is given antibiotics and dexamethasone. However, unlike tumor resections or other epilepsy surgeries, mannitol is not given.

A T-shaped incision is used. The first incision is made in the sagittal plane, starting in the midline behind the hairline and extending posteriorly until the inion. A second incision is made in the coronal plane, starting at the level of the zygoma in front of the ear and extending so that it intersects the initial incision in the midline at a right angle (**Fig. 14.1A**). The scalp is then reflected to give excellent exposure of the skull (**Fig. 14.1B**). During the exposure, steps are taken to reduce blood loss including infiltrating the wound with a solution of bupivicaine and epinephrine and the placement of Raney clips on the wound edges.

A series of bur holes are placed in the midline directly over the sagittal sinus. Multiple bur holes are placed to decrease the risk of injuring the transverse and sagittal sinuses. In children <18 months of age, the dura is often difficult to free from the overlying bone. Therefore, bur holes are placed within 2.5 cm of each other along the sagittal suture. Additional bur holes are placed in the keyhole and above the

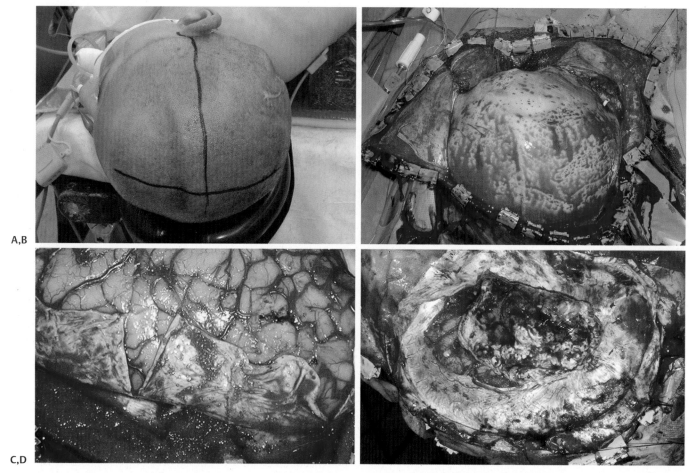

Fig. 14.1 Serial surgical photographs from a representative left hemispherectomy. (Note: in all figures medial is at the bottom and anterior is at the left.) **(A)** Representative incision. **(B)** Surgical field after the skin incision. **(C)** Radial cuts made toward the sagittal sinus. **(D)** Postresection surgical field.

zygoma in the squamous temporal bone. A craniotome is used between the bur holes. If necessary, the bone flap is extended with a Leksell rongeur and Kerirson punches so that the sagittal sinus and the torcular can be adequately visualized. It should be noted that occasionally the craniotomy can result in copious blood loss to a degree that necessitates aborting the procedure. This is more common in very young patients. In those instances in which a significant blood loss occurred with the craniotomy and the procedure had to be aborted, the patient returns to the operating room in 1 to 2 weeks and the hemispherectomy is performed.

Once the bone is removed, the dura is opened in a C-shaped fashion based on the sphenoid bone. The opening should be at least 4 cm lateral of the sagittal and transverse sinuses to avoid bridging veins. Approximately four to eight radial cuts are made toward the sagittal and transverse sinuses (**Fig. 14.1C**). The cuts are easily tailored anteriorly or posteriorly to avoid bridging veins. If the bridging veins cannot be spared, the portion of dura attached to the vein is left intact and the vein is coagulated after arterial feeders are removed along with adjacent brain.

Prior to beginning the resection, some specialized devices and materials are added to the surgical field. The simultaneous use of two bipolar setups enables two surgeons to work independently and can help to reduce the total blood loss. The use of Isocool Bipolar Forceps (Codman, Raynham, MA), designed to reduce tissue sticking to the bipolar tips, may be helpful in large resections. Other adjuncts, such as thrombin-soaked cotton balls or Floseal (Baxter, Deerfield, IL) can minimize blood loss.

The resection is performed in a step-wise fashion based on anatomical regions. First the middle temporal gyrus is entered and the dissection is carried down to the temporal horn of the ventricle. Next, the dissection is continued in the middle temporal gyrus approximately 2 cm deep to the gray-white junction, and continued posteriorly in a C-shaped fashion around the sylvian fissure. This dissection plane is then carried anteriorly along the inferior frontal gyrus. During this part of the dissection, the branches of the middle cerebral artery (MCA) are coagulated. The result of this dissection is an extended C-shaped trough from the temporal lobe, behind the sylvian fissure, and along the inferior frontal lobe. The trough is packed with thrombin-soaked cotton balls. After meticulous hemostasis is achieved, the temporal lobe and the frontal lobes are removed simultaneously.

The temporal lobectomy is performed in the standard fashion with the following exceptions. After the standard anterior lobectomy, the entire superior gyrus is removed starting at the most proximal portion of the sylvian fissure and moving posteriorly until the initial trough is encountered. The vein of Labbé is spared at this point unless it is very small or is under tension and therefore at risk for inadvertent rupture. The distal MCA branches are coagulated and cut as they are encountered. Weck clips and aneurysm clips are available but are normally unnecessary if the arteries are adequately coagulated. An amygdalohippocampectomy is then performed.

After the temporal lobe is resected, the frontal lobe dissection is performed. If two surgeons are available, it is possible to perform the dissection of the frontal lobe simultaneously with the removal of the temporal lobe. The dissection is begun in the motor strip at the level of the initial trough, and it is carried around the sylvian fissure and then medially toward the sagittal sinus. The dissection is continued anteriorly in the superior frontal gyrus until the orbital ridge is encountered. Bridging veins from the superior frontal gyrus are left intact. As before, the trough is packed with thrombin-soaked cotton balls. After meticulous hemostasis is achieved, the superior, middle, and inferior frontal gyri are undermined approximately 1 cm deep to the gray-white junction and removed in one large piece.

Next, the bridging veins are coagulated that arise from the remaining superior frontal gyrus, moving in an anterior to posterior direction. Because it is difficult to control bleeding adjacent to the sagittal sinus, these veins should be cut close to the cortex and not close to the sinus. After coagulating and cutting the bridging veins the remaining portion of the superior frontal gyrus is retracted laterally off of the falx. The cingulate gyrus, anterior cerebral arteries (ACA), and corpus callosum are identified. It is very important to remember that the branches of the ACA are often stacked in a superior inferior orientation and not right and left. Great care must be taken not to incorrectly identify these arteries and accidentally sacrifice the contralateral artery. Preoperative imaging, such as an angiogram or magnetic resonance imaging (MRI), may be useful in defining the relationship of the vessels. Using a subpial dissection technique to remove the cingulate gyrus, using gentle suction, and refraining from the use of the bipolar cautery can reduced the risk of damaging the ACA branches. Staying lateral to the pial layer, the corpus callosum is entered and split with the bipolar on a setting of 20 J and with gentle suction. This dissection is then carried posteriorly to complete the callostomy. During the dissection, once the ipsilateral ACA is correctly identified, it may be clipped proximal to the origin of the callosomarginal.

The parietal lobe is then removed similarly to the frontal lobe, by starting laterally at the level of the initial trough around the sylvian fissure and working posteromedially in the parietal gyrus adjacent to the parietooccipital sulcus. The dissection is then continued anteriorly, parallel to the sagittal sinus, again avoiding bridging veins. The parietal lobe is then undermined apporoximately 1 cm below the gray-white junction. As before, the bridging veins going into the sagittal sinus are coagulated. The remaining portion of the parietal lobe is gently lifted off of the falx, coagulating any bridging veins as it is lifted. The splenium of the corpus callosum is identified along with the pericallosal artery. The remaining portion of the parietal lobe is removed above the cingulated gyrus. We again perform a subpial removal of the cingulate gyrus with suction and avoid the use of the bipolar.

The last lobe removed is the occipital lobe. Before removing the occipital lobe, examine the bridging veins going into the transverse sinus with particular attention to the location of the vein of Labbé. The occipital lobe at this point is quite mobile, and the surgeon must be careful not to avulse a bridging vein out of the sagittal, transverse, or sigmoid sinus. We typically coagulate these veins prior to removing the occipital lobe. Once the veins are cut, the occipital lobe can easily be manipulated. However, the bridging veins along the tentorium must be coagulated prior to lifting up the occipital lobe. This is started at the most posterior location of the temporal lobectomy in the lateral ventricle. We then bipolar and aspirate inferiorly to the tentorium. The brainstem is located medially, traversing the incisura. Care should be taken to stay in the subpial plane to avoid coagulating perforators in the ambien cistern. The posterior cerebral artery (PCA) can be safely coagulated after it exits the ambien cistern. Next, the dissection is continued posterior-medially, lifting the occipital lobe off the tentorium and coagulating bridging veins. A useful anatomical reference is the occipital horn of the ventricle, as it serves as a marker for the appropriate depth of resection. The dissection is continued just superficial to the ependyma as the falx is approached. Prior to the final disconnection, the area along the falx is examined by retracting the occipital lobe laterally, to assure that there are no veins or arteries that have not been coagulated. The occipital pole usually lifts out very easily. However, during the process of removing the occipital lobe, one should be aware of any veins that are tethering this tissue to a venous sinus or the tentorium.

If adequate hemostasis is achieved when removing the individual lobes, the final inspection of the surgical cavity normally demonstrates very little residual bleeding (**Fig. 14.1D**). The exception is in cases were the total blood loss was excessive or where the surgery took an excessive amount of time. In these instances, peri- and postoperative coagulopathies can occur, resulting in life-threatening bleeding.[14,15] Prior to closing, the MCA, PCA, and ACA should be inspected to assure that these vessels are adequately coagulated.

After meticulous hemostasis is obtained, the surgical cavity is copiously irrigated to remove debris. The removal of this debris possibly reduces the development of the postoperative fever that has been associated with this material.[16] The dura is closed in a water-tight fashion and the closure is augmented with an onlay dural substitute such as DuraGen (Integra Lifesciences Corp., Plainsboro NJ). The placement of dural tacking sutures may be useful in preventing the development of epidural collections. The bone is attached with Synthes absorbable plates and screws (Synthes, West Chester, PA), and the incision is closed in the standard layered fashion. A comparison of preoperative (**Fig. 14.2A**) and postoperative (**Fig. 14.2B**) imaging can confirm a proper resection.

Postoperatively, patients are observed in the intensive care unit. For the first 48 hours, we keep the patient positioned with the craniotomy side up to give the newly created cavity time to fill up with CSF. This allows the pressure to equalize in the two hemispheric compartments and may reduce the risk of life-threatening brain shift.[17] After the 48 hours, patients begin rigorous physical therapy and occupational therapy. The patients are watched carefully for signs and symptoms of hydrocephalus. Within the first 2 to 3 weeks after surgery the diagnosis can easily be confirmed by the prescence of a large, firm pseudomeningocele. After a few weeks, the diagnosis may be more subtle, therefore, we obtain a baseline computed tomography (CT) prior to discharge. An important technical point is to place the proximal catheter in the contralateral ventricle, not the resection cavity. This substan-tially decreases the formation of a pseudomenigocele and a cerebrospinal (CSF) leak because the brain on the contralateral side will seal the tract around the catheter.

Complications

The postoperative complications that occur with any neurosurgical procedure, such as wound infections and strokes, can occur after hemipherectomies. However, there are some postoperative complications that are unique to this procedure. Although extremely rare, significant brain shift can occur and result in sudden death after a hemispherectomy.[17] Aspetic meningitis can occur in the postoperative period and is often effectively treated with a short course of steroids.[18,19] As stated earlier, irrigation of the surgical cavity and removal of any debris may reduce the incidence of this complication. Hydrocephalus can develop in patients at two time periods: in the immediate postoperative period and in a delayed fashion in some patients.[19,20–25] This must be recognized and treated with standard shunt placement.

Conclusion

Anatomical hemispherectomy is an important and useful surgical technique in selected patients with intractable epilepsy. A complete understanding of the surgical anatomy is needed to safely perform this procedure and care must be taken to monitor and minimize blood loss. When performed carefully in the correct patients at an institution capable of handling the unique surgical and postoperative needs of these patients, hemispherectomy can result in significant control of a patient's seizures.

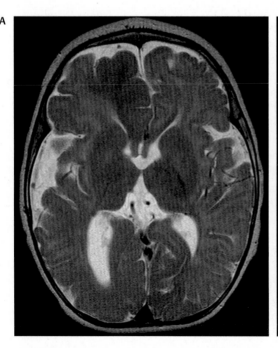
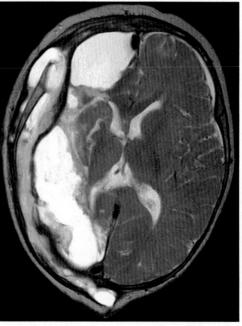

Fig. 14.2 Representative hemispherectomy of a patient with hemimegencephaly. **(A)** Preoperative MRI demonstrating right-sided hemimenencephaly. **(B)** Immediate postoperative MRI after right-sided hemispherectomy.

References

1. Dandy W. Physiological studies following extirpation of the right cerebral hemisphere in man. Bull Johns Hopkins Hosp 1933;53:31–51

2. McKenzie KG. The present status of a patient who had the right cerebral hemisphere removed. JAMA 1938;111:168–183

3. Krynauw RA. Infantile hemiplegia treated by removing one cerebral hemisphere. J Neurol Neurosurg Psychiatry 1950;13(4):243–267

4. Almeida AN, Marino R. The early years of hemispherectomy. Pediatr Neurosurg 2005;41:137–140

5. Taylor DC, Falconer MA, Bruton CJ, et al. Focal dysplasia of the cerebral cortex in epilepsy. J Neurol Neurosurg Psychiatry 1971;34(4):369–387

6. Rasmussen T. Postoperative superficial hemosiderosis of the brain, its diagnosis, treatment and prevention. Trans Am Neurol Assoc 1973;98:133–137

7. Kaufman S, Poupyrev I, Miller E, et al. New interface metaphors for complex information space visualization: an ECG monitor object prototype. Stud Health Technol Inform 1997;39:131–140

8. Adams HP Jr, Putman SF, Corbett JJ, et al. Amaurosis fugax: the results of arteriography in 59 patients. Stroke 1983;14(5):742–744

9. Winston KR, Welch K, Adler JR, et al. Cerebral hemicorticectomy for epilepsy. J Neurosurg 1992;77(6):889–895

10. Carson BS, Javedan SP, Freeman JM, et al. Hemispherectomy: a hemidecortication approach and review of 52 cases. J Neurosurg 1996;84(6):903–911

11. Carson BS, Lauer JA, Guarnieri M, et al. Hemispherectomy: a review. Neurosurg Q 1996;6:155–175

12. Kossoff EH, Vining EP, Pyzik PL, et al. The postoperative course and management of 106 hemidecortications. Pediatr Neurosurg 2002;37(6):298–303

13. Ellenbogen RG, Cline MJ. Hemispherectomy. In: Miller JW, Silbergeld DL, eds. *Historical Perspective and Current Surgical Overview. Epilepsy Surgery: Principles and Controversies.* New York: Taylor and Francis; 2006:563–576

14. Brian JE Jr, Deshpande JK, McPherson RW. Management of cerebral hemispherectomy in children. J Clin Anesth 1990;2(2):91–95

15. Piastra M, Pietrini D, Caresta E, et al. Hemispherectomy procedures in children: haematological issues. Childs Nerv Syst 2004;20(7):453–458

16. Peacock WJ, Wehby-Grant MC, Shields WD, et al. Hemispherectomy for intractable seizures in children: a report of 58 cases. Childs Nerv Syst 1996;12:376–384

17. Cabieses F, Jeri R, Landa R. Fatal brain-stem shift following hemispherectomy. J Neurosurg 1957;14(1):74–91

18. Fountas KN, Smith JR, Robinson JS, et al. Anatomical hemispherectomy. Childs Nerv Syst 2006;22:982–991

19. Basheer SN, Connolly MB, Lautzenhiser A, et al. Hemispheric surgery in children with refractory epilepsy: seizure outcome, complications, and adaptive function. Epilepsia 2007;48(1):133–140

20. McKissock W. The operative technique for cerebral hemispherectomy in the treatment of infantile hemiplegia. Zentralbl Neurochir 1954;14(1–2):42–48

21. White HH. Cerebral hemispherectomy in the treatment of infantile hemiplegia: review of the literature and report of two cases. Confin Neurol 1961;21:1–50

22. Davies KG, Maxwell RE, French LA. Hemispherectomy for intractable seizures: long-term results in 17 patients followed for up to 38 years. J Neurosurg 1993;78:733–740

23. Kalkanis SN, Blumenfeld H, Sherman JC, et al. Delayed complications thirty-six years after hemispherectomy: a case report. Epilepsia 1996;37(8):758–762

24. Di Rocco C, Iannelli A. Hemimegalencephaly and intractable epilepsy: complications of hemispherectomy and their correlations with the surgical technique. A report on 15 cases. Pediatr Neurosurg 2000;33(4):198–207

25. de Almeida AN, Marino R Jr, Marie SK, et al. Factors of morbidity in hemispherectomies: surgical technique x pathology. Brain Dev 2006;28(4):215–222

15 Functional Hemispherectomy and Periinsular Hemispherotomy

Jean-Guy Villemure and Roy Thomas Daniel

The introduction of functional techniques in surgery for hemispheric epilepsy has generated renewed interest in this small subgroup of epilepsy surgery. Although anatomical hemispherectomy for the treatment of intractable epilepsy secondary to widespread hemispheric damage provided excellent seizure control, this technique introduced by Dandy,[1] but first used by McKenzie to control seizures,[2] and later on popularized by Krynauw,[3] was abandoned following the observations of many complications, some occurring late, namely superficial cerebral hemosiderosis.[4] The observation that subtotal hemispheric removal led to fewer postoperative complications, although at the expense of reduced seizure control, led Rasmussen to introduce functional hemispherectomy, consisting in subtotal hemispheric removal, but complete disconnection; the aim was to lower complications while providing seizure control similar to anatomical hemispherectomy.[5,6] The objectives of functional hemispherectomy were met as demonstrated since its introduction more than 30 years ago; actually, functional hemispherectomy has been associated with fewer complications and good to excellent seizure outcome.[7] The technique of functional hemispherectomy evolved over time to less brain resection in favor of a greater ratio of disconnection, leading to the technique of periinsular hemispherotomy (PIH) first reported in 1993.[8] These disconnection techniques that minimize brain resection and maximize disconnection are essentially of two types. The lateral approaches include functional hemispherectomy first described by Rasmussen[5] and PIH described in details in 1995[9]; variants of this approach have also been described.[10,11] The other approach is the vertical hemispherotomy described by Delalande et al.[12] All these techniques aim at reducing perioperative morbidity and long-term complications, while maintaining the same seizure outcome that would be otherwise obtained with anatomical hemispherectomy.

Indications

The indications for surgery in the setting of hemispheric epilepsy have similarities to that of epilepsy in general, but have a few specific differences.[13] Because most patients with hemispheric epilepsy are in the pediatric age group, the noxious effects of seizures and multiple drugs on the developing brain need to be considered and weighed against the risks associated with surgery at a young age. Patients considered for hemispheric epilepsy should fulfill certain absolute criteria: intractable epilepsy usually established early and contralateral loss of voluntary distal motor function. Neuropsychological examination to establish baseline functioning and the integrity of the normal hemisphere to support most cerebral functions is essential. The preoperative investigations should include magnetic resonance imaging (MRI) and electroencephalographic (EEG) studies that should be concordant and demonstrate widespread abnormalities involving the whole hemisphere contralateral to the hemiplegia. EEG abnormalities ipsilateral to the good hemisphere, which are quite frequent findings in this population, are not an absolute contraindication to surgery.[14]

Hemispherectomy patients are subdivided into certain distinct surgically remediable hemispheric epilepsy syndromes. The congenital syndromes include infantile hemiplegia seizure syndrome, hemimegalencephaly, Sturge-Weber syndrome and nonhypertrophic migrational disorders. The most common and well-recognized acquired syndrome is Rasmussen's encephalitis; other acquired causes also include sequelae of trauma, hemorrhagic lesions, and meningoencephalitis. The timing of surgery is a matter of debate. Although the presence of a complete hemispheric syndrome, that is, hemiplegia, hemianopsia, and brain hemiatrophy, are considered necessary for the indication of hemispherectomy, we are of the opinion that, at least in children, earlier surgery is preferable because the window of opportunity offered while the plasticity of the brain remains high should not be lost. Furthermore we strongly believe that, in certain hemispheric epilepsy syndromes that are progressive and invariably lead to a complete hemispheric deficit (Rasmussen's encephalitis and extensive Sturge-Weber syndrome), hemispherectomy should be performed prior to maximal deficit. It remains that each clinical situation should be individualized.

Operative Techniques

General anesthesia is used for the procedure. The patient is placed in the supine position, a soft cushion under the ipsilateral shoulder, with the head fixed on a three-pin fixation system, or taped, turned 90 degrees to the contralateral side, and minimally extended.

Functional Hemispherectomy

A large "U"-shaped skin incision and flap are used with the anterior limb originating at the zygoma, overlapping the coronal suture and extending medially to reach the midline; it goes posteriorly along the midline to the lambdoid suture and extends inferiorly toward the transverse sinus 2 cm behind the level of the ear. The bone flap should stop at 1 cm lateral to the midline to avoid the sagittal sinus; in cases of severe atrophy, the midline may be shifted to the ipsilateral side and thus, the landmarks may be different. The dura is reflected toward the midline.

Inspection of the brain is essential to recognize a large atrophic lesion with porencephaly or cystic replacement of portions of white matter, shift of structures due to atrophy and consequent bone remodelling, and venous and arterial structures to be preserved. Palpation should indicate whether the resection-disconnection will be performed with the manual suction-aspiration technique or with the ultrasonic aspirator.

The aim of surgery consists in anatomical subtotal removal, but complete disconnection of the hemisphere. There are four main surgical steps to functional hemispherectomy: (1) excision of the temporal lobe (including amygdala and hippocampus); (2) excision of the frontoparietal region (cortex and white matter), including the parasagittal tissue down to the corpus callosum (CC); (3) interrupting the frontal and parietooccipital fibers left entering the CC at their junction with the CC; and (4) resecting the insular cortex.

Temporal Lobectomy

The anterior temporal lobectomy should reach posteriorly to a plane corresponding to the anterior portion of the ventricular atrium. This will facilitate the posterior disconnection of the parietooccipital lobe in a later step (**Fig. 15.1A**).

The resection is performed according to standard subpial resection technique. The pia overlying the first temporal gyrus (T1) is coagulated and incised. T1 is excised with aspiration until the circular sulcus is encountered; the inferior portion of the insula is thus exposed. A posterior incision is created with similar technique, going from the posterior T1 to reach the floor of the middle fossa. The collateral sulcus is exposed from this lateral approach, and the white matter between the inferior insula and the top of the collateral sulcus is resected until the temporal horn is entered. The resection of the temporal lobe is continued by section of the infrainsular white matter, using the bipolar coagulation, with one limb in the ventricle and the other just inferior to the insula. The anterior temporal lobe is freed by subpial aspiration, prolonging more anteriorly and medially the subpial resection of T1, until the free edge of the tentorium is identified. The incision is prolonged lateral to the hippocampus and parahippocampal gyrus to reach the posterior section; the temporal neocortex is excised. The medial structures

are then excised, starting with the uncus and amygdala; the amygdala should be resected rostrally until a plane corresponding to the roof of the temporal horn, and medially as long as there is pia visualized. The hippocampus is resected using suction, with great care to preserve the medial pia.

During this step, large sylvian veins as well as the vein of Labbé should be preserved. Passing arteries going to the posterior temporal and anterior occipital lobes should also be preserved.

Resection of the Frontoparietal Region

The central region volume to resect extends anteriorly from the level of sphenoid wing toward the midline in a plane underlying the coronal suture; posteriorly the incision level will extend from the posterior temporal resection site to the midline just anterior to the lamda.

There are four stages for the central region removal. Initially, the frontoparietal opercular cortices are resected according to the subpial aspiration technique. In the frontal region, this starts at the level opposite the sphenoid wing, and extends posteriorly to a level corresponding to the most posterior T1 resection. The suprasylvian portion of the insula is exposed until the circular sulcus is reached. The white matter of the corona radiata is transected perpendicularly, from front to back, to reach the lateral ventricle.

In a second stage, a cortical incision reaching the ventricle is made in the parietal lobe corresponding to the posterior margin of the frontoparietal slab to be removed; it extends from the most posterior part of T1 resection, to the falx, just anterior to the lambda, and reaches the CC parasagittally (**Fig. 15.1B**).

In a third stage, a frontal incision is performed from the pterional area through the whole thickness of the frontal lobe reaching slightly posterior to the sphenoid wing, entering the frontal horn of the ventricle and extending also along the falx to reach the CC. Identification of the cingulate sulcus, as well as the parasagittal pia and the A2 segment of the anterior cerebral artery are good anatomical landmarks for orientation.

Finally, the central resection is completed with dissection of the parasagittal tissue, either subpially or extrapially, until the fibers entering in the boby of the CC are transected. The central region brain volume can be resected (**Fig. 15.1C**).

Frontal and Parietooccipital Disconnection

Despite a large resection of the frontoparietal tissue extending to the CC, the medial portions of the frontal and parietal lobes are left attached to the CC. The callosotomy has to be completed by sectioning all fibers entering the CC at the level of the genu and rostrum anteriorly, as well posteriorly at the level of the splenium. This is accomplished from within the ventricle, transecting tissue on the medial wall, as it reaches the CC; visualization of the medial pia and peri-

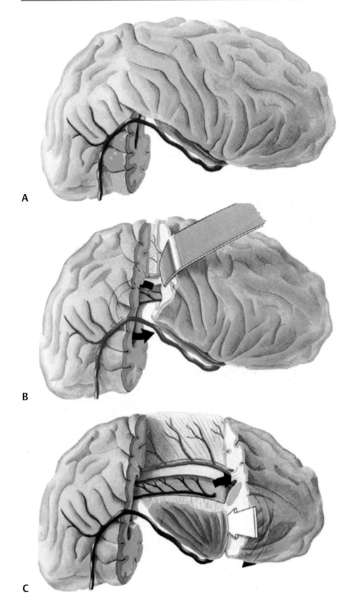

Fig. 15.1 Artistic representation of right functional hemispherectomy. **(A)** Temporal lobectomy. **(B)** Parietal incision for central removal (*arrows* indicate the ventricle). **(C)** Status after frontoparietotemporal removal (*black arrow* indicates site of callosotomy; *white arrow* indicates frontobasal disconnection).

callosal vessels are good landmarks to guarantee the disconnection (**Fig. 15.2A**).

Insula

At this stage of functional hemispherectomy, the only cortex still functional is the insula. Exclusion of the insula is no longer a matter of debate, and the insular cortex should be resected with aspiration in between vessels, or subpially, all around, from the circular sulcus.[15,16] At this stage, the residual hemisphere rostral to the diencephalon is completely isolated from ipsi- and contralateral structures (**Fig. 15.2B**).

A "U"-shaped skin flap (**Fig. 15.3A**) is designed with the anterior limb originating at the zygoma and overlapping the coronal suture; the medial limb of the incision reaches the mid convexity level and the posterior limb extends down behind the ear, but does not have to reach the transverse sinus. The bone flap (**Fig. 15.3B**), centered over the insular region, is longer in the anteroposterior direction to give good access to the insula and circular cistern. A dural flap is turned, based anteriorly or inferiorly to provide good exposure of the sylvian vessels and the opercular cortices. The intradural part of the surgery, performed under magnification, is best described in different stages and steps as detailed below. There are three major stages: supra-insular window, infra-insular window, and insula (**Figs. 15.4A and 15.4B**).

Suprainsular Window Stage

1. *Cortico-Subcortical Step* (**Fig. 15.5A**). A linear cortical incision is placed 5 mm above the sylvian fissure over the frontal and parietal opercular cortices. This is deepened, in between vessels to be protected through the white matter, and the opercular cortex is resected until the superior limb of the circular cistern is reached. This exposes the superior half of the insula, which can be viewed through two layers of pia and in between middle cerebral artery (MCA) branches. Along the entire length of the circular cistern, the incision is made into the white matter perpendicular to the insular surface toward the body of the lateral ventricle, which is opened along its whole length. Large cottonoids are placed in the ventricle to avoid seepage of blood. During this stage of the surgery, the approach can be confounded by the presence of large and multiple perisylvian cysts, which are often encountered in patients with large atrophic lesions. Recognition of intraventricular structures such as choroid plexus and foramen of Monroe directs the surgeon to the correct opening of the ventricle to complete the suprainsular window. During the creation of this window, it is important to preserve as many arteries and veins that irrigate the brain; this is accomplished by making pial incisions in a discontinuous fashion, thereby creating multiple windows to the ventricle.

    On a functional level, the approach to the ventricle disconnects at the level of the corona radiata–internal capsule transition, the afferent and efferent fibers passing through the anterior and posterior limb of the internal capsule.

2. *Intraventricular Step* (**Fig. 15.5B**). It begins with the identification of the position of the CC in a slightly parasagittal plane. The ideal site for starting the incision for the transventricular parasagittal callosotomy would be at the junction of the septum pellucidum and the roof of the lateral ventricle. Occasionally, this demarcation can be difficult to ascertain. We have found that the best way to begin is

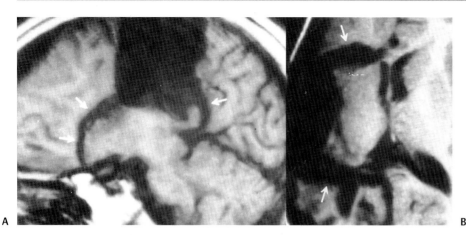

Fig. 15.2   Postoperative MRI. **(A)** T1, parasagittal, illustrating the anterior (frontal) and posterior (parietooccipital) callosal disconnection (*arrows*). **(B)** T1, axial, illustrating the frontobasal disconnection.

Fig. 15.3   (A) Skin incision for right periinsular hemispherotomy (PIH). **(B)** Postoperative skull x-ray demonstrating the bone flap for PIH.

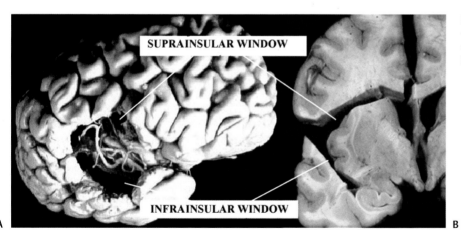

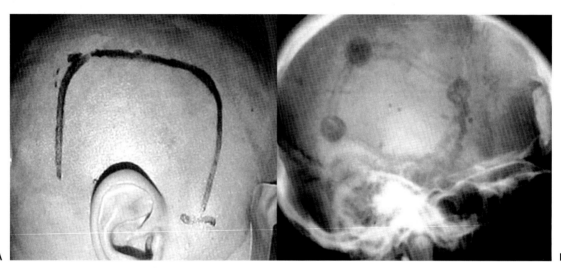

Fig. 15.4   Right periinsular hemispherotomy —anatomical preparation. **(A)** Right lateral view. **(B)** Coronal section (level of mamillary bodies).

by a vertical incision (perpendicular to the intended callosal incision) at an estimated midpoint of the callosum. Visualization of the choroid plexus in the lateral ventricle and the foramen of Monroe are good landmarks for this step. By deepening the vertical incision along the medial wall, through the cingulate gyrus, the pericallosal cistern will be entered into and the pericallosal arteries visualized. These arteries are the definite markers for the cal-

losum, which is recognized under them. The midpoint of the callosum (where the initial vertical incision is placed) may be more anterior than in a normal-sized ventricle due to the relative anterior shift of the deep ganglionic structures secondary to the atrophy or maldevelopment of the corona radiata and internal capsule. Injudicious placement of the vertical incision can therefore direct the incision toward the splenium where the white matter to

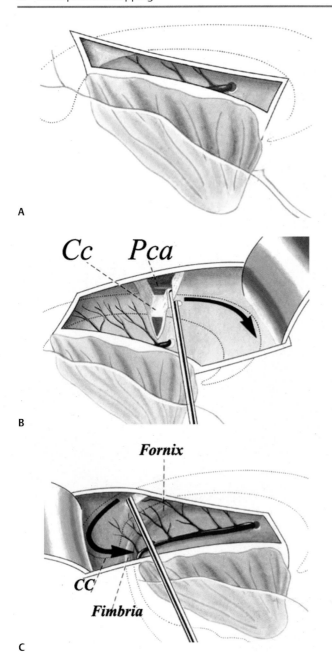

Fig. 15.5   Artistic representation of right periinsular hemispherotomy, suprasylvian window. **(A)** Cortico-subcortical step. **(B)** Intraventricular step (Cc, corpus callosum; Pca, pericallosal artery). **(C)** Posterior hippocampotomy (CC, corpus callosum).

be sectioned is much thicker and the pericallosal arteries much smaller; this may be confounding.

The callosotomy incision in this plane is performed from within the lateral ventricle, interrupting all parasagittal fibers entering the CC. This is accomplished using the bipolar coagulation and suction. The completeness of anterior and posterior extent of the callosotomy is best ascertained by the recognition of the pericallosal vessels, and callosum curvature that characterizes the genu and the splenium.

Posteriorly it is directed to reach the splenium; during this phase of the CC section, the hippocampal outflow into the fornix is dealt with, by section of the posterior hippocampus (posterior hippocampotomy) at the level of the trigone (**Fig. 15.5C**). This is accomplished by continuation of the posterior end of the callosotomy, going around the splenium, onto the medial wall of the ventricle, to reach the choroidal fissure anteroinferiorly, thus interrupting the fornix. Anteriorly, the callosotomy will go around the genu and reach the rostrum (**Fig. 15.6A and B**).

3. *Frontobasal Disconnection.* This represents the final portion in the suprainsular window stage. The frontobasal cortex is disconnected in a coronal plane, which is parallel and slightly posterior to the sphenoid ridge. This incision is started subpially from the lateral convexity after inspection of the sphenoid ridge subdurally. It is carried through the frontal lobe, reaching the frontobasal pia inferiorly, identifying the gyrus rectus medially, until the parasagittal pia. This leads to reaching the most frontal and inferior portion of the suprainsular window. From within the ventricular cavity, the incision is started at the rostral end of the callosal incision, exposing the pericallosal arteries around the genu, until the rostrum and the frontobasal incisions are reached.

The intraventricular part of the suprainsular window sections interhemispheric connections through the CC. The frontobasal disconnection interrupts the fibers of the frontobasal cortex through the anterior commissure, anterior sublenticular projections, uncinate fasciculus, short and long arcuate fibers, and anatomical continuity with the insular periallocortical cortex. The posterior hippocampotomy interrupts the major output of the temporal lobe that projects through the fornix.

Infrainsular Window Stage

1. *Cortico-Subcortical Step.* This window is created through T1 gyrus in a discontinuous fashion similar to the suprainsular window, thereby preserving as many superficial veins and arteries. T1 subpial resection extends anteriorly and medially to include the uncus. The inferior half of the insula and the circular cistern are exposed. From the depth of the circular cistern, the white matter incision is carried toward the ventricle. The recognition of possible perisylvian cysts and identification of the intraventricular structures such as the hippocampus and choroid plexus are crucial to a good orientation. This window is then joined posteriorly to the suprainsular window; viewing intraventricular anatomy guides the surgeon in completing the window across the atrium of the ventricle and prevents injudicious entry into the deep ganglionic structures (**Fig. 15.7**).

This part of the surgery disconnects the projections of the temporal and occipital lobes through the sub- and retrolenticular portions of the internal capsule.

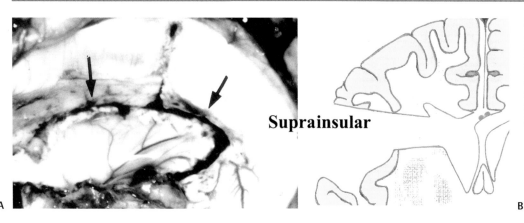

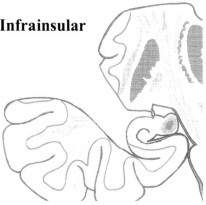

A

Fig. 15.6 Transventricular parasagittal callosotomy (TvPsC). **(A)** Per-operative photomicrograph illustrating the TvPsC (*arrows*). **(B)** Schematic coronal representation of the suprainsular window illustrating the site of callosotomy.

B

2. *Intraventricular Step.* The infrainsular intraventricular part begins with the identification of the amygdala and the hippocampus. The estimation of the extent of amygdalar resection should be of concern to avoid inadvertent entry into the basal ganglia; the amygdala resection should be limited to a plane corresponding to the roof of the temporal horn rostrally, and medially to the pial bank. The anterior part of the hippocampus is resected until the choroid fissure is reached. The rest of the hippocampus has already been de-efferented with the posterior hippocampotomy in the suprainsular window.

The intraventricular portion of the infrainsular window removes the structures that still have connections through the posterior limb of the anterior commissure, stria terminalis, and projections to the basal ganglia, hypothalamus, and brainstem.

Insula Stage

The insular cortex could be a source for residual seizures if left untreated, though the necessity for its removal remains debatable[15,16] (**Fig. 15.8A**). In cases where the insula is firm, the resection of this structure can be cumbersome when performed between the preserved middle cerebral vessels lying on its surface. We recommend a disconnection at the level of the external capsule or the claustrum (**Fig. 15.8B**). This can

be easily done introducing the bipolar forceps through the two windows on either side of the insula, at a plane deep to the insular cortex, thereby performing a subcortical disconnection.

Postoperative Management

During the entire intraventricular phase of the surgery, care should be taken to adequately fill the ventricles with cottonoids, and to irrigate the ventricles with saline. This would wash out blood and brain debris and help prevent early and delayed hydrocephalus. It should also prevent excessive brain shift consequent to removal of large volume of cerebrospinal fluid (CSF). A drain is left into the ventricle, and leveled at slightly positive pressure. The dura is closed watertight and the bone flap anchored. The scalp is closed in layers over a subgaleal drain. The patient is transferred to the intensive care for monitoring.

Particular attention should be paid to the intraventricular drainage. This is kept for 2 to 3 days so that blood and brain debris are drained, which should reduce early morbidity and the incidence of hydrocephalus. However, the drainage should be carefully regulated to make sure that excess CSF is not drained.

It is quite frequent to have low-grade fever and mild meningeal signs in the early postoperative period, and antibiotics are not given routinely. Corticosteroids are not used

A

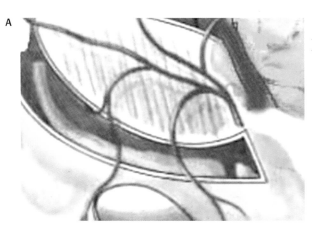

B

Infrainsular

Fig. 15.7 Artistic representation of right Infrainsular window. **(A)** Lateral projection, with preservation of sylvian vessels. **(B)** Coronal projection.

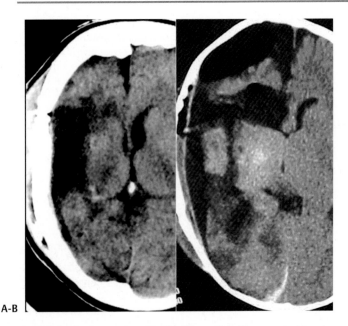

A-B

Fig. 15.8   Postoperative CT. **(A)** Illustrating the resected insula. **(B)** Illustrating insular disconnection.

routinely. The antiepileptic drugs are continued and are only reduced at follow-up visits, unless there are drug-induced problems.

Early postoperative radiological imaging is only done if clinically indicated.

Complications and Their Avoidance

Complications of different nature following hemisherectomy have been reported. They vary according to the hemispherectomy technique utilized.[17]

- In the pediatric population, great care relative to blood loss and replacement is mandatory to avoid complications related to hypovolemia and coagulopathy.[18]
- In disconnective hemispherectomy, a large volume of vascularized brain may be left in the cranium. It is thus essential that as many arteries and veins be preserved to lower the risk of hemorrhagic infarct and brain swelling, which in some instances no or minimal atrophy may lead to increased intracranial pressure and its consequences (**Fig. 15.7**).[19]

- Excessive ventricular drainage of CSF may lead to hemorrhages that are distant from the operative site. This can be avoided by meticulous measurement of CSF drainage in the postoperative period.[20]
- The incidence of early and late hydrocephalus should be lowered by reducing spillage of blood in the ventricles, using cottonoids to fill the ventricles as soon as possible; copious irrigation of the ventricular cavities and operative field will also contribute to prevention of hydrocephalus.[21]
- In instances of small ventricle, such as in early Rasmussen's encephalitis, extensive Sturge-Weber, hemimegalencephaly, and nonhypertrophic diffuse hemispheric dysplasia, a clear understanding of the surgical anatomy of PIH is mandatory to avoid complications and assure complete hemispheric disconnection.
- Before one is familiar with the surgical anatomy of PIH, we recommend that this technique be used only in patients with an enlarged ventricle.
- It is to be kept in mind that the volume of tissue resected in PIH may be modulated according to needs and that this technique may, per-operatively, need to be traded for larger resection (functional hemispherectomy) at the benefit of a good understanding of the surgical anatomy.

Conclusion

Functional hemispherectomy and Peri-insular hemisphere-rotomy share, with other forms of hemispherectomy, two major goals. While seizure control remains the primary aim, removing the deleterious effects of uncontrolled seizures on the developing brain assumes great importance in pediatric patients who form the majority in this group of patients with hemispheric epilepsy. When compared to anatomical hemispherectomy and hemidecortication, functional techniques of hemispherectomy have lesser complications, while maintaining excellent seizure outcomes.

Acknowledgments

We thank Dr. C. R. Mascott for the anatomical preparation (**Fig. 15.4A**) and Dr. Zoltan Bodor for the artistic representations.

References

1. Dandy W. Removal of right cerebral hemisphere for certain tumors with hemiplegia: preliminary report. JAMA 1928;90:823–825

2. McKenzie K. The present status of a patient who had the right cerebral hemisphere removed. JAMA 1938;111:168–183

3. Krynauw RA. Infantile hemiplegia treated by removing one cerebral; hemisphere. J Neurol Neurosurg Psychiatry 1950;13:243–267

4. Oppenheimer DR, Griffith HB. Persistent intracranial bleeding as a complication of hemispherectomy. J Neurol Neurosurg Psychiatry 1966;29:229–240

5. Rasmussen T. Hemispherectomy revisited. Can J Neurol Sci 1983;10: 71–78

6. Villemure JG, Rasmussen T. Functional hemispherectomy: methodology. J Epilepsy 1990;3(suppl):177–182

7. Villemure JG. Functional hemispherectomy: evolution of technique and results in 65 cases. In: Luders HO, Comair YG, eds. *Epilepsy Surgery*. Philadelphia: Lippincott, Williams & Wilkins; 2001:733–738

8. Villemure JG, Mascott CR. Hemispherotomy: The peri-insular approach—technical aspects. Epilepsia 1993;34(suppl 6):48

9. Villemure JG, Mascott CR. Peri-insular hemispherotomy: surgical principles and anatomy. Neurosurgery 1995;37:975–981

10. Schramm J, Kral T, Clusmann H. Transsylvian keyhole functional hemispherectomy. Neurosurgery 2001;49:891–900

11. Shimizu H, Maehara T. Modification of peri insular hemispherotomy and surgical results. Neurosurgery 2000;47:367–376

12. Delalande O, Fohlen M, Jalin C, Pinard JM. From hemispherectomy to hemispherotomy. In: Luders HO, Comair YG, eds. *Epilepsy Surgery*. Philadelphia: Lippincott, Williams & Wilkins; 2001:741–746

13. Villemure JG. Hemispherectomy: indications. In: Resor Jr SR, Hutt K, eds. *The Medical Treatment of Epilepsy*. New York: Marcel Dekker Inc.; 1992:243–249

14. Smith SJM, Andermann F, Villemure JG, Rasmussen TB, Quesney LF. Functional hemispherectomy: EEG findings, spiking from isolated brain postoperatively, and prediction of outcome. Neurology 1991;41: 1790–1794

15. Freeman JM, Arroyo S, Vining EP, et al. Insular seizures: a study in Sutton's Law. Epilepsia 1994;35(suppl 8):49

16. Villemure JG, Mascott C, Andermann F, Rasmussen TB. Is removal of the insular cortex in hemispherectomy necessary? Epilepsia 1989;30(5):728

17. Villemure JG. Hemispherectomy techniques and complications. In: Wyllie E, ed. *The Treatment of Epilepsy: Principles and Practice*. 2nd ed. Baltimore: Williams & Wilkins; 1996:1081–1086

18. Brian JE, Deshpande JK, McPherson RW. Management of cerebral hemispherectomy in children. J Clin Anesth 1990;2:91–95

19. Daniel RT, Villemure JG. Peri-insular hemispherotomy: Potential pitfalls and complication avoidance. Stereotact Funct Neurosurg 2003; 80:22–27

20. De Ribaupierre S, Villemure JG, Chalaron M, Cotting J, Pollo C. Contralateral frontal and cerebellar haemorrhages after peri-insular hemispherotomy. Acta Neurochir (Wien) 2004;146:743–744

21. Villemure J-G, Adams CBT, Hoffman HJ, Peacock WJ. Hemispherectomy. In: Engel Jr J, ed. *Surgical Treatment of the Epilepsies*. New York: Raven Press Ltd.; 1993:511–518

IV Neuromodulation

16 Vagus Nerve Stimulation

Uzma Samadani and Gordon H. Baltuch

Vagal nerve stimulation was first reported as potentially having efficacy in three out of four seizure patients in 1990,[1] and it was approved by the Food and Drug Administration for the treatment of medically refractory epilepsy in 1997. As of November 2006, 45,000 patients have received the VNS Therapy System (Cyberonics*, Inc., Houston, TX) pulse generator attached to silicon-coated leads with contact electrodes on the vagus nerve.[2] This chapter reviews the history of vagus nervous system stimulation for the treatment of epilepsy, our limited understanding of its mechanism of action, and the indications, surgical technique, management, and outcomes of vagus nerve stimulation for epilepsy.

Seizures are episodes of disturbed brain function that cause changes in attention or behavior due to abnormal electrical excitation in the brain. Seizures as a clinical entity were described in Indian, Chinese, and Mesopotamian literature ~3000 years ago. Hippocrates of Galen subsequently postulated that such activity might be due to an excess of phlegm caused by abnormal brain consistency. Epilepsy, defined as two or more seizures, afflicts nearly 3% of the population at some point in their lifetime, though only one-tenth of this number has epilepsy that is active. The consequences of uncontrolled epilepsy are vast and range from physical injury such as contusions, fractures, lacerations, and burns to psychosocial disorders resulting from depression, social withdrawal, embarrassment, decreased independence, and limited employment opportunities.[3] Mortality rates are four to seven times greater than in the general population and sudden death can result directly from seizures, or occur as an indirect consequence of severe depression and suicide.[3] Of the 0.3% of the population that are active epileptics, two-thirds are controlled by medical therapy, and one-third are refractory even after 18 months of aggressive therapy with two standard antiepileptic agents.[4] A percentage of the medically refractory patients will have seizures arising from a focal area that is not in eloquent cortex and thus are candidates for surgical resection of their seizure focus. The remainder of these active epileptics are possible candidates for alternative surgical therapy, such as stimulation.

History

Electrical stimulation of the nervous system as a mechanism for reduction of epilepsy has been practiced for at least 2000 years. In 76 A.D., the Greek herbalist and physician Pedanius Discorides advocated seizure treatment with the electric torpedo ray (*Torpedo nobiliana*).[5] During the 11th century, the Persian physician Ali Abu Ibn-Sina (Latinized by translators to Avicenna) noted efficacy against epilepsy with placement of an electric catfish on the brow of the afflicted.[5] The 18th century clergyman and electrotherapist John Wesley, described a patient with a 7-year history of twice daily drop attack seizures he was able to cure with a single electric shock.[6] The invention of the Leyden jar, a protoype capacitor, in 1745 by German Ewald Georg van Kleist further enabled the use of electric shock as a means for treating seizures. The Leyden jar was named after the hometown of its second independent inventor in the Netherlands, Pieter van Musschenbroek.[7]

Altered brain electricity in epilepsy was hypothesized by the 19th century British physician Robert Bentley Todd, perhaps best known for his eponymous post-ictal paralysis, and his contemporary, electroscientist Michael Faraday.[8] John Hughlings Jackson further popularized belief in the electrical basis of epilepsy beginning in 1873.[9]

British neurophysiologist Richard Caton invented the electroencephalogram (EEG) in 1875, and German psychiatrist Hans Burger performed the first human EEG via scalp recordings in 1924, ultimately enabling visualization of seizure activity.[7] The discovery of EEG served as further proof for the electrical basis of nerve conduction, which was confirmed with the Nobel-winning squid action potential work of neurophysiologists Alan Hodgkin and Andrew Huxley in 1952.[10]

In 1938, stimulation of the severed proximal end of vagus nerve in cats was found to cause cortical EEG changes by Percival Bailey and Frederic Bremer in Chicago.[11] Dell and Olson further demonstrated in 1951 that such stimulation of the proximal end of the severed vagus projected to forebrain, thalamus, midbrain, and cerebellum[12,13]; these projections were found to be extinguished by a tight ligature on the vagus nerve by Zanchetti et al in 1952.[14]

The mechanism of action of Pranayama, and other yogas postulated to be efficacious against epilepsy, is hypothesized as partially due to respiratory stimulation of the vagus nerve.[15] Such respiratory stimulation, also advocated in classes for childbearing women in labor, was allegedly the inspiration for development of the vagal nerve stimulator.

The Philadelphia neurophysiologist Jacob Zabara attended such a class with his wife in 1971[16] and postulated that if mild stimulation of vagal nerve afferents was sufficient to decrease labor pain, then greater stimulation could further suppress the nervous system for other potentially clinical applications. Zabara first applied vagal nerve stimulation to cats to reduce xylazine-induced emesis.[17] The second application for his vagal nerve stimulator was to reduce strychnine-induced seizures in dogs.[17] Zabara's experiments were duplicated in other species; vagal nerve stimulation was found to reduce experimentally induced seizures in monkeys[18] and rats.[19,20] Recognizing the clinical relevance of his work, he partnered with pacemaker designer S. Reese Terry to found Cyberonics, Inc., the manufacturer of vagal nerve stimulators.

The first human vagal nerve stimulator was placed by pediatric neurosurgeon William Bell on November 16, 1988. Neurologists J. Kiffin Penry and Christine Dean presented the results from Bell's patient at a special conference on vagal nerve stimulation at the American Epilepsy Society meeting in Boston in December 1989 where seven other related articles were presented.[1] By then a total of 14 patients had been implanted at three centers, and of the nine of these who had been followed for at least 6 weeks, seven had seen a reduction in the number of seizures.[1,21] Two patients were seizure free at 1 year and there were only minor complications such as temporary hoarseness from the stimulation, and one case of lead breakage.

Clinical trials with the vagal nerve stimulator have been performed as crossover trials with the stimulator on or off and as randomized prospective trials with low versus high levels of stimulation.[22] Based on the results of clinical trials, the Food and Drug Administration approved the vagal nerve stimulator for the treatment of epilepsy in 1997.

Mechanism of Action

Seizures on EEG are represented by abnormal synchronization of neuronal activity. Desynchronization, then, should diminish seizure activity. Vagal nerve stimulation was first hypothesized to work via desynchronization of the EEG.[23] Michael Chase at UCLA and colleagues demonstrated in cats that the frequency dependent effect of vagus nerve stimulation on EEG was due to activation of particular fibers at varying frequencies. Vagus stimulation at frequencies above 70 Hz and intensities >3 V were shown to be desynchronizing. If the intensity was dropped to <3 V and only myelinated fibers were stimulated, the EEG would be synchronized. Lower frequencies (20 to 50 Hz) and higher voltages were also shown to be desynchronizing. Desynchronization was shown to be the result of stimulation of vagal fibers that conduct at 1 to 15 m/s.[24]

Early studies suggested that unlike in animals, vagal nerve stimulation did not affect human EEG regardless of level of alertness.[25] On longer follow-up, however, at a mean of 16.8 months after implantation, EEG changes were seen after vagal nerve stimulation with desynchronization dominating over synchronization and diminished interictal spikes.[26] In children, a decrease in the number of interictal epileptiform discharges has been seen as early as 3 months after stimulator implantation.[27]

The vagus nerve, so named for its "wandering" course (Latin), has special visceral efferent fibers that project to the nucleus ambiguus from the pharyngeal and laryngeal muscles. Its general visceral efferent fibers arising from the dorsal motor nucleus innervate the heart, lungs, and viscera. The vagus also has sensory afferent projections, notably from the concha of the ear. The vagus' visceral afferents travel via the tractus solitarius to the thalamus, amygdale, and forebrain, and via the medullary reticular formation to other cortical areas[28] (reviewed in Rutecki[23]). The vagus' diffuse projections mediate several visceral reflexes including the baroreceptive response, coughing, vomiting, and swallowing. Projections to the hypothalamus affect appetite, blood pressure, and volume homeostasis.

Projections via the tractus solitarius and medullary reticular formation may be responsible for the antiepileptic impact of vagus nerve stimulation. In rat studies, the hippocampus and striatum are among the epilepsy-mediating areas that have altered metabolism after vagal nerve stimulation.[29] Projections to the frontal cortex and cingulate gyrus are highlighted on positron emission studies of patients receiving the vagal nerve stimulator for depression.[30]

Given the diffuse projections of the vagus nerve and despite understanding some of the properties of stimulation that are most likely to result in EEG desynchronization, we still do not have a clear understanding of the mechanism of vagal nerve stimulation. Decreased excitatory and increased inhibitory neurotransmission[31] and changes in cerebral blood flow are observed after both acute and chronic vagal nerve stimulation.[32–34] In a rat model, neuronal activity in the locus ceruleus is directly modified by vagal nerve stimulation.[35] Chronic stimulation may alter limbic circuitry to reduce epileptogenesis.[33]

Indications

Selim Benbadis and colleagues have generated an algorithm for the management of epilepsy.[36] Patients with seizures for 9 months or greater who are refractory to medical treatment by a neurologist should be referred for EEG video monitoring, magnetic resonance imaging (MRI), and confirmation of the diagnosis and type of intractable epilepsy. After this confirmation, patients with nonlocalizable seizures should be considered for vagal nerve stimulation either directly, or after consideration of the ketogenic diet, depending on clinical circumstances. Among patients with localizable lesions resulting in seizures, vagal nerve stimulation should be considered for those who fail surgical resection, or who have bilateral cortical localization.[36]

Evidence exists to support the use of vagal nerve stimulation earlier rather than later after the onset of epilepsy to maximize its benefit. Epilepsy patients who had tried four or fewer seizure medications or who were implanted with the vagal nerve stimulator within 5 years of onset of the seizure disorder were three times more likely to report no seizures after 3 months of treatment than those who had received the device after failing more medications or waiting longer than 5 years.[37]

A randomized clinical trial comparing vagal nerve stimulation to standard of care antiepileptic drugs (AEDs) has not been performed. Comparisons in cost accounting for extra hospitalizations due to seizures suggests that the savings of vagal nerve stimulation versus medical management are significant.[38–40] An additional advantage of vagal nerve stimulation over medical therapy regards compliance and side-effect profiles. Approximately 75% of patients receiving AEDs discontinue therapy within 5 years,[41] whereas only ~20% of vagal nerve stimulation patients discontinue therapy.[42]

The safety of vagal nerve stimulation for epilepsy at the extremes of age and during pregnancy has not been fully explored. Patients <5 years of age appear to tolerate the stimulation well, and have had excellent reductions in seizures.[43] One patient has been reported to have a normal pregnancy outcome after vagal nerve stimulation for depression.[44]

Vagal nerve stimulator patients appear to tolerate MRI and functional MRI (fMRI) scans without incident; the manufacturer recommends that a transmit and receive head coil be used with a 1.5 T scanner. MRIs have been performed with the stimulator turned on to evaluate the impact of the stimulation.[45–51] In one study, the patient had a seizure on the table and diffusion-weighted imaging demonstrated transient ischemia at the focus, which returned to normal at seizure completion.[52] Most of the MRI data were obtained on 1.5 T scanners.

Operative Technique

The technique for vagal nerve stimulation is straightforward for a surgeon experienced in exposure of the cervical carotid artery. We use the technique provided by the device manufacturer, which has minor modifications from the technique originally described by Steven Reid.[53]

The device components are purchasable as kits from Cyberonics and consist of a titanium-housed pulse generator with a lithium carbon monofluoride battery, and a 43 cm lead wire with two platinum/iridium helical electrodes and a tethering anchor (**Figs. 16.1 and 16.2**).[54] The electrode and anchor are available in either 2 or 3 mm diameters, and we have always used the smaller of the two; both are associated with a 2-mm lead. There are four models of pulse generator, the most recent of these measures 5.2 × 5.2 × 0.7 cm and uses a single-pin lead. The battery life is estimated at 6 years, but it is affected by stimulation parameters. The VNS lead we currently implant is the model 302–20, which has a single pin for the generator. Earlier generator models were slightly larger and used a double-pin lead. A newer model double-pin pulse generator is still available for replacement in patients with the older lead.

Vagus nerve stimulators are implanted on the left side because studies in dogs have demonstrated that stimulation of the right vagus slowed heart rate more than stimulation of the left vagus.[55] The right vagus innervates the sinoatrial node and the left, via cardiac branches to the recurrent laryngeal nerve, the atrioventricular node. The right vagus also mediates the tonic inhibitory effect on sympathetic outflow in dogs.[56] It is important to place the stimulator inferior to the branch points for the cardiac branches of the vagus nerve to avoid potential bradycardia or asystole upon stimulation (**Fig. 16.3**). Right-sided vagal nerve stimulation has been performed in three children who had previous vagal nerve

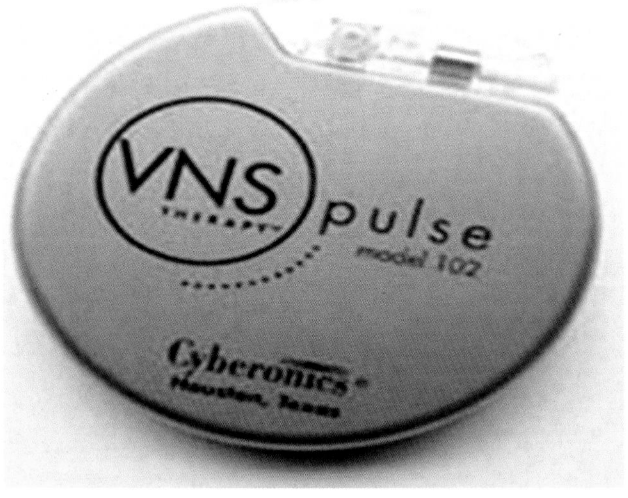

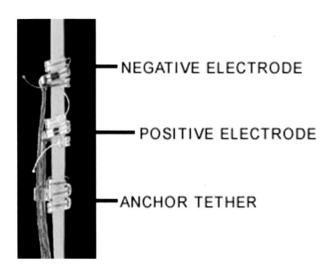

Fig. 16.1   The model 102 VNS pulse generator. (Reprinted with permission from Cyberonics.)

Fig. 16.2   The electrodes and anchor tether are seen on a model of the vagus nerve. (Reprinted with permission from Cyberonics.)

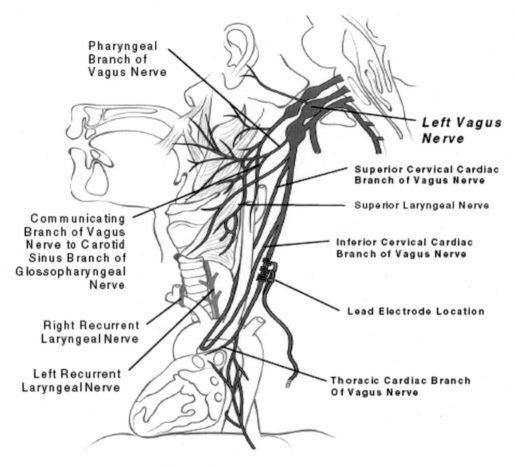

Fig. 16.3 Anatomy of the left vagus nerve demonstrating placement of the electrodes distal to cardiac branches of the nerve. (Reprinted with permission from Cyberonics.)

Pharyngeal Branch of Vagus Nerve

Communicating Branch of Vagus Nerve to Carotid Sinus Branch of Glossopharyngeal Nerve

Right Recurrent Laryngeal Nerve

Left Recurrent Laryngeal Nerve

Left Vagus Nerve

Superior Cervical Cardiac Branch of Vagus Nerve

Superior Laryngeal Nerve

Inferior Cervical Cardiac Branch of Vagus Nerve

Lead Electrode Location

Thoracic Cardiac Branch Of Vagus Nerve

stimulator placements and removals on the left side. Efficacy was similar to left-sided implantation, but two of the three children had respiratory side effects.[57] It is also possible to remove completely and re-implant the generator and lead on the left side.[58]

The patient is advised to continue epilepsy medications throughout the perioperative period. After administration of general endotracheal anesthesia and antibiotics, the patient is positioned supine on the operating room table with the head level on a donut pillow and turned slightly to the right side. The left neck and chest are prepared and draped after marking a 3- to 4-cm horizontal incision in a neck crease extending from the medial aspect of the sternocleidomastoid muscle to the midline, as described by Cloward for the performance of anterior cervical discectomy.[59] The incision is roughly halfway between the mastoid and clavicle. For the generator we mark an ~5-cm incision either parallel to and about 5 cm below the clavicle in men, or linear and just medial to the axilla and superior to the breast in women (**Fig. 16.4**). The incision sites are infiltrated with lidocaine prior to incision. The platysma is divided using bipolar cautery as needed; monopolar cautery is not used for the duration of the procedure. We bluntly generate a subcutaneous pocket the size of the generator (5.2 cm in length and height) and then perform tunneling for the stimulator lead using the smaller of the two tunneling devices provided by the manu-

facturer. We tunnel from the cervical to the infraclavicular incision, taking care to pass over the clavicle (**Fig. 16.5**). The lead is pulled through with the tunneling device and attached to the generator using the hex screwdriver provided by the manufacturer (**Fig. 16.6**). The generator is then tucked into the infraclavicular pocket to avoid movement during the

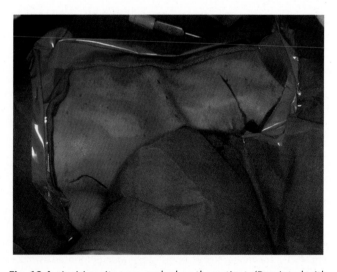

Fig. 16.4 Incision sites are marked on the patient. (Reprinted with permission from Cyberonics.)

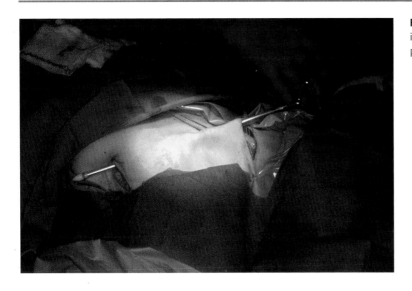

Fig. 16.5   The tunneling device is passed over the clavicle from neck to pulse generator site. (Reprinted with permission from Cyberonics.)

duration of the procedure, but leaving sufficient slack on the lead to allow easy manipulation and placement (**Fig. 16.7**).

Attention is then returned to the cervical incision. Following the fascial plane along the medial aspect of the sternocleidomastoid muscle, the carotid sheath is identified medial to the internal jugular vein. Weitlaner self-containing retractors provide sufficient visualization of the cervical anatomy.

The vagus nerve is usually nestled in between the common carotid artery and internal jugular vein, and a 3-cm length of it represents sufficient exposure for the implantation. We temporarily place a 3 × 3 cm square of plastic sheeting cut from an impermeable drape behind the exposed vagus to enhance visualization and prevent the electrodes from adhering to adjacent structures. The operative microscope can be used if necessary. The two vagal nerve stimulator helical electrodes and the third anchor tether coil

are then applied in a cranial to caudal fashion using vascular forceps (**Figs. 16.8 and 16.9**). It is sometimes helpful to have the surgical assistant gently hold the electrodes behind the nerve to facilitate application. After the electrodes and anchor tether have been attached, we create a strain relief bend of lead to provide slack during future movement of the neck (**Fig. 16.10**). Distal to this, a tacking suture is placed on a silicon lead holder supplied by the manufacturer and secured to the fascia adjacent to the sternocleidomastoid muscle (**Fig. 16.11**). The wounds are closed in anatomical layers using absorbable suture. The device is checked with a system diagnostic performed with the wand and programming computer prior to removal of drapes and reversal of anesthesia. Lead impedance is checked to ensure that the helical electrodes are in good contact with the nerve. The test will also be abnormal if the lead is not inserted into the

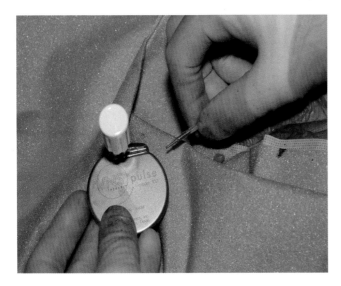

Fig. 16.6   The lead is connected to the pulse generator and secured with a hex screwdriver. (Reprinted with permission from Cyberonics.)

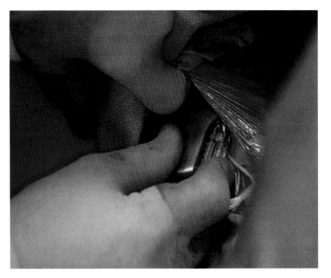

Fig. 16.7   The pulse generator is inserted into the subclavicular pocket. (Reprinted with permission from Cyberonics.)

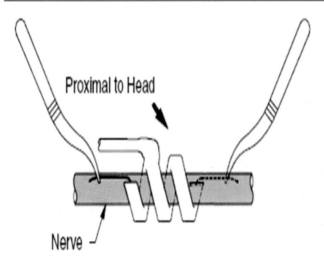

Fig. 16.8   Schema demonstrating application of an individual lead to the vagus nerve. The free suture ends are grasped with vascular forceps to guide the electrodes into place. (Reprinted with permission from Cyberonics.)

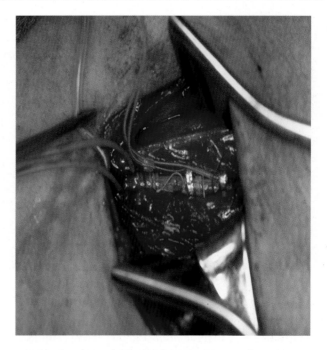

Fig. 16.9   The electrodes and tether in position on the vagus nerve. (Reprinted with permission from Cyberonics.)

generator correctly. The system diagnostic is performed for 1 minute passing 1 mA of output current with a pulse width of 500 microseconds at a pulsing rate of 20 Hz. While the system diagnostic lasts approximately 1 minute, the actual stimulation time is only ~14 seconds. The anesthesiologist is advised that bradycardia or even asystole[60] may occur during testing. The patient is generally discharged to home after recovery from anesthesia. A schema of the implanted device is illustrated in (**Fig. 16.12**).

Management

Human vagus nerve stimulators are usually programmed to be on 24 hours a day with pulsing stimulation starting about 2 weeks after the implantation surgery. Typical settings are 1.0 to 2.0 mA, 0.5 millisecond pulsewidth, 20 to 30 Hz for 30 seconds, then off for 5 to 10 minutes. However, the range of possible settings for the pulse generator is 0 to 3.5 mA, 0.13 to 1.0 milliseconds pulsewidth, 1 to 130 Hz, 7 to 60 seconds on, 12 seconds to 180 minutes off, allowing other stimulation strategies to be utilized.[61]

Patients are also discharged from the hospital with a magnet. When this is held over the pulse generator, it prevents any stimulation from occurring. When the magnet is

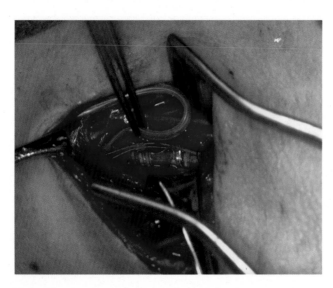

Fig. 16.10   A loop of lead provides slack for neck movement. (Reprinted with permission from Cyberonics.)

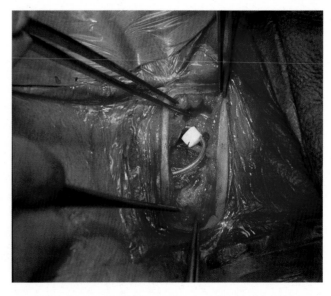

Fig. 16.11   Superficially, the lead is secured to the fascia on the sternocleidomastoid muscle. (Reprinted with permission from Cyberonics.)

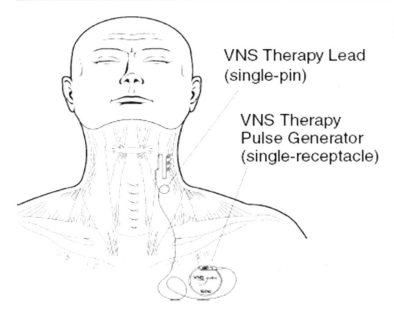

Fig. 16.12 Schema for the implanted VNS lead and generator. (Reprinted with permission from Cyberonics.)

passed over the pulse generator, pulses of stimulation can be administered at a preprogrammed frequency and amplitude. Battery life is variable depending on stimulation parameters, and patients who report an increase in the frequency or severity of seizures after experiencing efficacious treatment should be evaluated for the necessity of changing the pulse generator.[62]

Results

Unlike most of the medications that are efficacious against epilepsy, vagal nerve stimulation may have increasing benefit after a greater period of time. Five-year follow-up of 26 patients revealed that although seizure frequency decreased from baseline by 28% at 1 year, it further dropped to 72% less than baseline at 5 years.[63] The sudden unexplained death in epilepsy rate in vagal nerve stimulation patients drops from 5.5 per 1000 over the first 2 years, a rate comparable to that of other epilepsy cohorts, to 1.7 per 1000 thereafter.[64]

The number and dosage of AEDs were able to be reduced in 76% of 21 patients at 13 months after vagal nerve stimulator implantation.[65]

Vagal nerve stimulation has benefits beyond seizure reductions. Patients report enhanced mood,[66] reduced daytime sleepiness,[67] independent of seizure control, increased slow wave sleep,[68] and improved cognition,[69] memory,[70] and quality of life.[71] Children with vagal nerve stimulators are noted to have enhanced verbal communication and school performance.[72] The impact of vagal nerve stimulation on affect has led to its recent approval for treatment resistant depression. Recent studies with vagal nerve stimulation in Alzheimer's patients demonstrate that many either improve or do not decline after device implantation.[73]

Side effects and risks of vagal nerve stimulation include voice alteration or hoarseness, coughing during stimulation, and exacerbation of sleep apnea.[74,75] In children, increased drooling and hyperactivity have also been reported.[72] Twenty percent of epilepsy patients are ultimately explanted with the device due to poor efficacy or inability to tolerate side effects.

Conclusion

Electrical stimulation of the nervous system has been practiced for 2000 years and appears to have myriad benefits, though its mechanism remains elusive. Vagal nerve stimulation is one modern treatment modality for medically refractory epilepsy that has a tolerable side-effect profile, quantifiable efficacy, and other advantages beyond seizure reduction.

References

1. Penry JK, Dean JC. Prevention of intractable partial seizures by intermittent vagal stimulation in humans: preliminary results. Epilepsia 1990;31(Suppl 2):S40–S43
2. Cyberonics Revises Sale Guidance for the First Half of Fiscal Year 07, Houston, TX edition, 2006
3. Sperling MR. The consequences of uncontrolled epilepsy. CNS Spectr 2004;9:98–109
4. Kwan P, Brodie MJ. Early identification of refractory epilepsy. N Engl J Med 2000;342:314–319
5. Kellaway P. The part played by electric fish in the early history of bioelectricity and electrotherapy. Bull Hist Med 1946;20:112–137
6. Malony H. *Perspectives on Science and Christian Faith.* Pasadena, CA: American Scientific Affiliation; 1995
7. Malmivuo J, Plonsley R. *Bioelctromagnetism: Principles and Applica-*

tion of Bioelectric and Biomagnetic Fields. New York: Oxford University Press; 1995

8. Reynolds EH. Todd, Faraday, and the electrical basis of epilepsy. Epilepsia 2004;45:985–992

9. Reynolds E. Todd, Hughlings Jackson, and the electrical basis of epilepsy. Lancet 2001;358:575–577

10. Hodgkin AL, Huxley AF. Propagation of electrical signals along giant nerve fibers. Proc R Soc Lond B Biol Sci 1952;140:177–183

11. Bailey P, Bremer F. Sensory cortical representation of the vagus nerve. J Neurophysiol 1938;1:4405–4412

12. Dell P, Olson R. [Secondary mesencephalic, diencephalic and amygdalian projections of vagal visceral afferences.] C R Seances Soc Biol Fil 1951;145:1088–1091

13. Dell P, Olson R. [Thalamic, cortical and cerebellar projections of vagal visceral afferences.] C R Seances Soc Biol Fil 1951;145:1084–1088

14. Zanchetti A, Wang SC, Moruzzi G. The effect of vagal afferent stimulation on the EEG pattern of the cat. Electroencephalogr Clin Neurophysiol 1952;4:357–361

15. Yardi N. Yoga for control of epilepsy. Seizure 2001;10:7–12

16. Fuller A. An electronic victory against epilepsy. Am Herit Invent Technol 2001;17(2):40

17. Zabara J. Neuroinhibition of xylazine induced emesis. Pharmacol Toxicol 1988;63:70–74

18. Lockard JS, Congdon WC, DuCharme LL. Feasibility and safety of vagal stimulation in monkey model. Epilepsia 1990;31(Suppl 2):S20–S26

19. Woodbury DM, Woodbury JW. Effects of vagal stimulation on experimentally induced seizures in rats. Epilepsia 1990;31(Suppl 2):S7–S19

20. Woodbury JW, Woodbury DM. Vagal stimulation reduces the severity of maximal electroshock seizures in intact rats: use of a cuff electrode for stimulating and recording. Pacing Clin Electrophysiol 1991;14:94–107

21. Uthman BM, Wilder BJ, Hammond EJ, Reid SA. Efficacy and safety of vagus nerve stimulation in patients with complex partial seizures. Epilepsia 1990;31(Suppl 2):S44–S50

22. DeGiorgio CM, Schachter SC, Handforth A, et al. Prospective long-term study of vagus nerve stimulation for the treatment of refractory seizures. Epilepsia 2000;41:1195–1200

23. Rutecki P. Anatomical, physiological, and theoretical basis for the antiepileptic effect of vagus nerve stimulation. Epilepsia 1990;31(Suppl 2):S1–S6

24. Chase MH, Nakamura Y, Clemente CD, Sterman MB. Afferent vagal stimulation: neurographic correlates of induced EEG synchronization and desynchronization. Brain Res 1967;5:236–249

25. Hammond EJ, Uthman BM, Reid SA, Wilder BJ, Ramsay RE. Vagus nerve stimulation in humans: neurophysiological studies and electrophysiological monitoring. Epilepsia 1990;31(Suppl 2):S51–S59

26. Koo B. EEG changes with vagus nerve stimulation. J Clin Neurophysiol 2001;18:434–441

27. Hallbook T, Lundgren J, Blennow G, Stromblad LG, Rosen I. Long term effects on epileptiform activity with vagus nerve stimulation in children. Seizure 2005;14:527–533

28. Vonck K, Van Laere K, Dedeurwaerdere S, Caemaert J, De Reuck J, Boon P. The mechanism of action of vagus nerve stimulation for refractory epilepsy: the current status. J Clin Neurophysiol 2001;18:394–401

29. Dedeurwaerdere S, Cornelissen B, Van Laere K, et al. Small animal positron emission tomography during vagus nerve stimulation in rats: a pilot study. Epilepsy Res 2005;67:133–141

30. Conway CR, Sheline YI, Chibnall JT, George MS, Fletcher JW, Mintun MA. Cerebral blood flow changes during vagus nerve stimulation for depression. Psychiatry Res 2006;146:179–184

31. Ben-Menachem E, Hamberger A, Hedner T, et al. Effects of vagus nerve stimulation on amino acids and other metabolites in the CSF of patients with partial seizures. Epilepsy Res 1995;20:221–227

32. Henry TR, Bakay RA, Pennell PB, Epstein CM, Votaw JR. Brain blood-flow alterations induced by therapeutic vagus nerve stimulation in partial epilepsy, II: prolonged effects at high and low levels of stimulation. Epilepsia 2004;45:1064–1070

33. Henry TR, Bakay RA, Votaw JR, et al. Brain blood flow alterations induced by therapeutic vagus nerve stimulation in partial epilepsy, I: acute effects at high and low levels of stimulation. Epilepsia 1998;39:983–990

34. Henry TR, Votaw JR, Pennell PB, et al. Acute blood flow changes and efficacy of vagus nerve stimulation in partial epilepsy. Neurology 1999;52:1166–1173

35. Groves DA, Bowman EM, Brown VJ. Recordings from the rat locus coeruleus during acute vagal nerve stimulation in the anaesthetised rat. Neurosci Lett 2005;379:174–179

36. Benbadis SR, Tatum WO, Vale FL. When drugs don't work: an algorithmic approach to medically intractable epilepsy. Neurology 2000;55:1780–1784

37. Renfroe JB, Wheless JW. Earlier use of adjunctive vagus nerve stimulation therapy for refractory epilepsy. Neurology 2002;59:S26–S30

38. Boon P, D'Have M, Van Walleghem P, et al. Direct medical costs of refractory epilepsy incurred by three different treatment modalities: a prospective assessment. Epilepsia 2002;43:96–102

39. Ben-Menachem E, French J. VNS Therapy versus the latest antiepileptic drug. Epileptic Disord 2005;7(Suppl 1):22–26

40. Ben-Menachem E, Hellstrom K, Verstappen D. Analysis of direct hospital costs before and 18 months after treatment with vagus nerve stimulation therapy in 43 patients. Neurology 2002;59:S44–S47

41. Lhatoo SD, Wong IC, Polizzi G, Sander JW. Long-term retention rates of lamotrigine, gabapentin, and topiramate in chronic epilepsy. Epilepsia 2000;41:1592–1596

42. Alexopoulos AV, Kotagal P, Loddenkemper T, Hammel J, Bingaman WE. Long-term results with vagus nerve stimulation in children with pharmacoresistant epilepsy. Seizure 2006;15:491–503

43. Blount JP, Tubbs RS, Kankirawatana P, et al. Vagus nerve stimulation in children less than 5 years old. Childs Nerv Syst 2006;22:1167–1169

44. Husain MM, Stegman D, Trevino K. Pregnancy and delivery while receiving vagus nerve stimulation for the treatment of major depression: a case report. Ann Gen Psychiatry 2005;4:16

45. Benbadis SR, Nyhenhuis J, Tatum WO, Murtagh FR, Gieron M, Vale FL. MRI of the brain is safe in patients implanted with the vagus nerve stimulator. Seizure 2001;10:512–515

46. Mu Q, Bohning DE, Nahas Z, et al. Acute vagus nerve stimulation using different pulse widths produces varying brain effects. Biol Psychiatry 2004;55:816–825

47. Chae JH, Nahas Z, Lomarev M, et al. A review of functional neuroimaging studies of vagus nerve stimulation (VNS). J Psychiatr Res 2003;37:443–455

48. Narayanan JT, Watts R, Haddad N, Labar DR, Li PM, Filippi CG. Cerebral activation during vagus nerve stimulation: a functional MR study. Epilepsia 2002;43:1509–1514

49. Bohning DE, Lomarev MP, Denslow S, Nahas Z, Shastri A, George MS. Feasibility of vagus nerve stimulation-synchronized blood oxygenation level-dependent functional MRI. Invest Radiol 2001;36:470–479

50. Lomarev M, Denslow S, Nahas Z, Chae JH, George MS, Bohning DE.

Vagus nerve stimulation (VNS) synchronized BOLD fMRI suggests that VNS in depressed adults has frequency/dose dependent effects. J Psychiatr Res 2002;36:219–227

51. Sucholeiki R, Alsaadi TM, Morris GL III, Ulmer JL, Biswal B, Mueller WM. fMRI in patients implanted with a vagal nerve stimulator. Seizure 2002;11:157–162

52. Tatum WO, Malek A, Recio M, Orlowski J, Murtagh R. Diffusion-weighted imaging and status epilepticus during vagus nerve stimulation. Epilepsy Behav 2004;5:411–415

53. Reid SA. Surgical technique for implantation of the neurocybernetic prosthesis. Epilepsia 1990;31(Suppl 2):S38–S39

54. Woldag H, Atanasova R, Renner C, Hummelsheim H. [Functional outcome after decompressive craniectomy: a retrospective and prospective clinical study.] Fortschr Neurol Psychiatr 2006;74:367–370

55. Randall WC, Ardell JL, Becker DM. Differential responses accompanying sequential stimulation and ablation of vagal branches to dog heart. Am J Physiol 1985;249:H133–H140

56. Barron KW, Bishop VS. Roles of right versus left vagal sensory nerves in cardiopulmonary reflexes of conscious dogs. Am J Physiol 1985;249:R301–R307

57. McGregor A, Wheless J, Baumgartner J, Bettis D. Right-sided vagus nerve stimulation as a treatment for refractory epilepsy in humans. Epilepsia 2005;46:91–96

58. Espinosa J, Aiello MT, Naritoku DK. Revision and removal of stimulating electrodes following long-term therapy with the vagus nerve stimulator. Surg Neurol 1999;51:659–664

59. Cloward RB. The anterior approach for removal of ruptured cervical discs. J Neurosurg 1958;15:602–617

60. Tatum WO, Moore DB, Stecker MM, et al. Ventricular asystole during vagus nerve stimulation for epilepsy in humans. Neurology 1999;52:1267–1269

61. Physician's Manual, NeuroCybernetic Prosthesis Programming Software Model 250 Version 4.6. Houston, TX: Cyberonics, Inc.; 2002

62. Tatum WO, Ferreira JA, Benbadis SR, et al. Vagus nerve stimulation for pharmacoresistant epilepsy: clinical symptoms with end of service. Epilepsy Behav 2004;5:128–132

63. Spanaki MV, Allen LS, Mueller WM, Morris GL III. Vagus nerve stimulation therapy: 5-year or greater outcome at a university-based epilepsy center. Seizure 2004;13:587–590

64. Annegers JF, Coan SP, Hauser WA, Leestma J. Epilepsy, vagal nerve stimulation by the NCP system, all-cause mortality, and sudden, unexpected, unexplained death. Epilepsia 2000;41:549–553

65. Tatum WO, Johnson KD, Goff S, Ferreira JA, Vale FL. Vagus nerve stimulation and drug reduction. Neurology 2001;56:561–563

66. Hallbook T, Lundgren J, Stjernqvist K, Blennow G, Stromblad LG, Rosen I. Vagus nerve stimulation in 15 children with therapy resistant epilepsy; its impact on cognition, quality of life, behaviour and mood. Seizure 2005;14:504–513

67. Malow BA, Edwards J, Marzec M, Sagher O, Ross D, Fromes G. Vagus nerve stimulation reduces daytime sleepiness in epilepsy patients. Neurology 2001;57:879–884

68. Hallbook T, Lundgren J, Kohler S, Blennow G, Stromblad LG, Rosen I. Beneficial effects on sleep of vagus nerve stimulation in children with therapy resistant epilepsy. Eur J Paediatr Neurol 2005;9:399–407

69. Dodrill CB, Morris GL. Effects of vagal nerve stimulation on cognition and quality of life in epilepsy. Epilepsy Behav 2001;2:46–53

70. Ghacibeh GA, Shenker JI, Shenal B, Uthman BM, Heilman KM. The influence of vagus nerve stimulation on memory. Cogn Behav Neurol 2006;19:119–122

71. Sirven JI, Sperling M, Naritoku D, et al. Vagus nerve stimulation therapy for epilepsy in older adults. Neurology 2000;54:1179–1182

72. Helmers SL, Wheless JW, Frost M, et al. Vagus nerve stimulation therapy in pediatric patients with refractory epilepsy: retrospective study. J Child Neurol 2001;16:843–848

73. Merrill CA, Jonsson MA, Minthon L, et al. Vagus nerve stimulation in patients with Alzheimer's disease: additional follow-up results of a pilot study through 1 year. J Clin Psychiatry 2006;67:1171–1178

74. Malow BA, Edwards J, Marzec M, Sagher O, Fromes G. Effects of vagus nerve stimulation on respiration during sleep: a pilot study. Neurology 2000;55:1450–1454

75. Marzec M, Edwards J, Sagher O, Fromes G, Malow BA. Effects of vagus nerve stimulation on sleep-related breathing in epilepsy patients. Epilepsia 2003;44:930–935

17 Stimulation of Amygdala and Hippocampus

Claudio Pollo and Jean-Guy Villemure

Despite considerable advances in pharmacological therapy for epilepsy, 25 to 30% of medically treated epileptic patients continue to have seizures and are considered as pharmacoresistant.[1] Resective surgery has shown its efficacy in the control of intractable seizures if presurgical evaluation clearly demonstrates a focal epileptogenic zone (EZ) that can be removed without causing unacceptable neurological deficit. Higher success has been achieved with temporal lobe epilepsy (TLE).[2] However, up to 30% of TLE cases are unsuitable for surgery either because of the involvement of eloquent areas or the bilateral or multifocal nature of the ictal onset or because they show an unsatisfactory response to previous surgical treatment.[3] Moreover, some patients may not have access to surgical therapy because of the limitation of human or technical resources or the high technical complexity and cost.

Electrical stimulation of the brain has been proposed as an additional option to resective surgery. The first trial of epilepsy treatment by brain stimulation was made by Cooper et al in 1973,[4] who reported reduction of seizure frequency by cerebellar subdural stimulation. Since the 1980s, other preliminary studies have suggested some effect on seizure frequency by stimulation of several targets among deep brain structures including the anterior thalamus,[5–7] the centromedian thalamic nucleus,[8–17] the caudate nucleus,[18,19] the mamillary body,[20,21] the subthalmic nucleus,[22–24] and more recently, the amygdalohippocampal (AH) complex.[25,26] Velasco et al[17,25] have observed improvement over time in interictal spike as well as in seizure frequency with subacute AH high-frequency stimulation during invasive recording with depth electrodes or subdural grids. Similar effects have been reported with long-term stimulation using quadripolar electrode and implantable device.[26] More recently, a prospective randomized study conducted on four patients has confirmed some long-term benefits and absence of adverse effects of hippocampal electrical stimulation in mesial TLE, although the effects were smaller than those reported earlier.[27] Finally, as the mechanisms of AH stimulation have not clearly been elucidated and as this recent therapeutic issue has been proposed to a low number of patients, there are no definitive data concerning either the optimal site of implantation or the optimal implantable device properties, or even the ideal stimulation parameters. Electrical stimulation of the brain needs further, large, controlled and completed clinical trials to be definitely validated as a therapy for intractable epilepsy. However, it is an attractive and promising new treatment modality.

Indications

Typical candidates for AH electrical stimulation should include intractable epileptic patients presenting with either unilateral or bilateral mesial temporal lobe epilepsy (MTLE) with one predominant side. Noninvasive tools of the presurgical evaluation (history of childhood onset epilepsy, clinical symptoms, scalp and sphenoidal electroencephalogram [EEG], video EEG, positron emission tomography [PET], single photon emission tomography [SPECT]) should clearly identify the EZ in the mesial portion of the temporal lobe.[28–30] When bilateral onset is suspected, depth electrodes recording may be needed for identification of the dominant side and to rule out independent co-dominant foci. Neuropsychological testing should typically show normal interictal speech (dominant side) or spatial (nondominant side) memory function associated with severe postictal dysfunction and should be correlated with the absence of clearly identifiable hippocampal sclerosis (HS), atrophy, or hypertrophy on MRI sequences. In these patients, seizure outcome after surgery is known to be less favorable compared with patients with structural lesions such as mesial temporal sclerosis.[31] Moreover, resection of mesial temporal lobe structures in these cases may be associated with a higher risk of memory impairment. When HS is visible, selective Wada test should be performed to assess the functional integrity of the hippocampus and predict memory deficits in case of hippocampal removal. Other criteria such as preexisting psychiatric illness, professional and/or psychosocial impact of memory dysfunction on patient life, and operability should be taken in consideration for the selection of the therapeutic strategy (**Table 17.1**).

Operative Technique

In our institution, a three-dimensional (3-D) T1-weighted MRI is performed under stereotactic conditions (we use a CRW frame, Integra Radionics, Inc., Burlington, MA) to allow computed 3-D surgical planning (FrameLink stereotactic software, Medtronic Inc., Minneapolis, MN). The approach trajectory is selected along the main axis of the hippocam-

Table 17.1 Typical Findings in Candidates Eligible for Amygdala and Hippocampus Electrical Stimulation

History of the Epilepsy	Adult Onset
Noninvasive presurgical evaluation	MTLE
Depth electrodes (when needed)	One predominant side with contralateral propagation
	Absence of bilateral independant EZ
MRI	No hippocampal sclerosis and/or atrophy
Neuropsychological evaluation	
Interictal	Normal or discrete memory dysfunction
Postictal	Severe memory dysfunction
Wada test (when needed)	Severe memory dysfunction homolateral to the EZ
Psychiatric evaluation	No associated illness
Professional and psychosocial impact of memory dysfunction	Severe

Abbreviations: MTLE, mesial temporal lobe epilepsy; EZ, epileptogenic zone.

pus to place the contacts of the DBS electrode at the junction between the hippocampus and the parahippocampal gyrus with the distal contact located within the inferior aspect of the amygdala to avoid intraventricular trajectory (**Fig. 17.1**).

In the operating room, the patient under general anesthesia is placed in a semi-sitting position. A U-shaped skin incision is performed in the occipital region precisely determined by the entry point of the planned trajectory (**Fig. 17.2**). The skull is opened with a 3-mm twist-drill.

The dura is carefully perforated with coagulation to avoid significant cerebrospinal fluid (CSF) leakage and the quadripolar DBS electrode (we have used so far the Pisces-Quad,

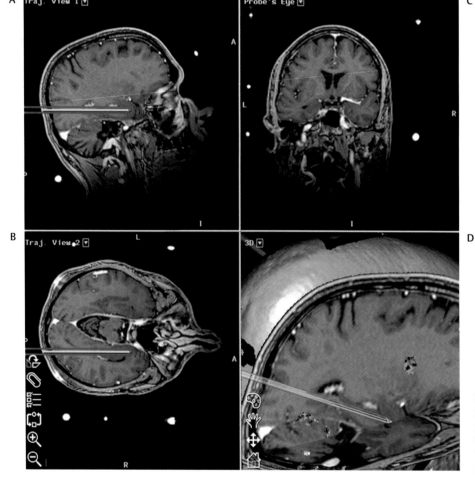

Fig. 17.1 Trajectory views of the surgical planning (**A**, vertical plane; **B**, horizontal plane; **C**, perpendicular; **D**, 3-D) along the main axis of the hippocampus at the junction between the hippocampus and the parahippocampal gyrus (**C**).

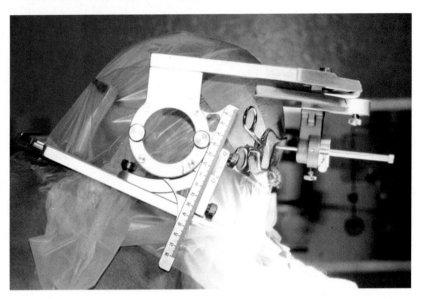

Fig. 17.2 View of the patient in the operating room with the stereotactic frame and the occipital approach.

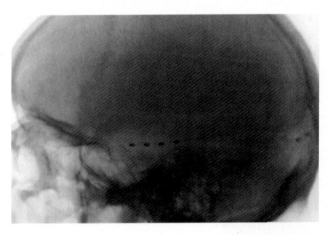

Fig. 17.3 Fluoroscopic lateral view of the implanted electrode with the distal end in an upward direction.

Medtronic, Inc.) is implanted under lateral fluoroscopic control with the distal end in an upward direction into the amygdala (**Fig. 17.3**=radio).

The electrode is then fixed to the skull with a titanium miniplate and external extension is performed to provide deep recordings (stereo-electro-encephalography; SEEG) for 3 to 4 days in an attempt to localize more precisely the EZ (**Fig. 17.4**). The day after the implantation procedure, a postoperative 3D T1 weighted MRI is performed to control the position of the electrode contacts (**Fig. 17.5**). The stimulator (Soletra 7426, Medtronic, Inc.) is finally implanted in the ipsilateral subclavicular space under general anesthesia.

Monopolar stimulation is delivered simultaneously through the four contacts up to 2 V. Electrical current is delivered at a frequency of 130 Hz and a pulse width of 450 microseconds.

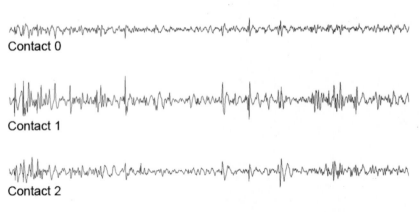

Contact 0

Contact 1

Contact 2

Contact 3

Fig. 17.4 Monopolar recording through the four contacts of the implanted electrode (contact 0=distal to contact 3=proximal) showing interictal spikes predominant on contact 1.

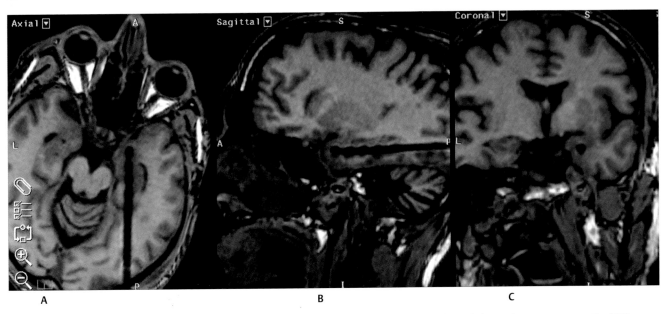

Fig. 17.5   Trajectory views (**A**, horizontal plane; **B**, vertical plane; **C**, perpendicular) of the implanted electrode on a postoperative MRI.

Discussion

Although limited studies have been conducted on DBS in animal models of epilepsies, high-frequency stimulation of the amygdala and hippocampus has been evaluated in rat models of partial seizures.[32,33] The author observed a long-lasting increase in the afterdischarge threshold as well as decrease in seizure frequency, suggesting a possible effect of DBS in cortico-subcortical network excitability. Animal studies have also been supported by the observation of improvement over time in interictal spike frequency and seizure frequency in patients evaluated for possible mesial temporal epilepsy with implanted hippocampal stimulating electrodes.[25] These patients had implantation of depth electrodes into hippocampus or the parahippocampal gyrus via a posterior approach, and electrical current was delivered at high frequency and low intensity (130 Hz, 0.2 to 0.4 mA) for up to 3 weeks. As the electrodes used in this study were not suitable for long-term stimulation, Vonck et al[26] evaluated the efficacy of long-term recording and stimulation through DBS quadripolar electrodes (Activa 3387, Medtronic, Inc.) in three patients. They reported a significant reduction in seizure frequency (>50%). However, the short follow-up of these patients (3 to 6 months) may not necessarily be correlated with a long-term efficacy of AH DBS.

Success of ablative surgery in MTLE has been shown to be correlated with the posterior extent of hippocampal removal.[34,35] This is the rationale justifying the use of the Pisces-Quad electrodes. Each contact of the quadripolar electrode is 3 mm long with 6 mm spacing. With a total span of 30 mm, the position of the proximal contact provides current delivery in the posterior portion of the hippocampus, whereas the position and the upward direction

of the distal contact provide stimulation of the amygdala, located rostral and cranial to the ventricular wall. Based on experimental data obtained from finite element model of DBS, monopolar stimulation with a pulse width of 450 microseconds in duration may increase charge delivery around each electrode contact and, consequently, the volume of tissue activated by stimulation within the amygdala and hippocampus.[36,37]

Hippocampus is part of the limbic network, and it is closely connected via the fornix to the mammillary bodies, then to the anterior thalamus, the cingulate gyrus, and finally—via the cingulum bundle—to the entorhinal cortex and back to the hippocampus. Neither the exact role of hippocampus in the pathogenesis of seizure propagation and generalization nor the precise mechanisms by which high-frequency electrical stimulation (typically 130 Hz) leads to reduced epileptogenicity is clearly understood. According to the concepts of inhibition-induced effects of subthalamic nucleus DBS for Parkinson's disease,[38,39] the antiepileptogenic action of DBS in TLE may be obtained through an inhibitory action of the stimulation on the targeted tissue, possibly located in specific cortical layers or cerebral pathways.[33] This inhibitory hypothesis is supported by Velasco et al,[16] who showed on SPECT studies hippocampal hypoperfusion induced by high-frequency electrical stimulation of hippocampus in human and autoradiographic studies performed on removed specimens where increased hippocampal benzodiazepine receptor binding was observed. However, stimulation at low frequencies (around 1 Hz) have been reported to have an inhibitory effect on epileptogenic focus or limbic structures on animals,[40,41] suggesting that activation of limbic networks at low frequency may interfere with ictal synchronization observed in epileptogenesis.

Conclusions

High-frequency AH DBS has been demonstated to improve the control of epileptogenicity in carefully selected patients with intractable TLE of mesial origin who are not candidates for resective surgery. However, only a few controlled clinical trials have been completed to definitely validate this as a standard therapy. The complex physiopathology of seizure onset and propagation justifies further electrophysiological and clinical research for the understanding of the precise correlations existing between clinical manifestations, epileptogenic brain pathologies, and networks involved in the control of epileptogenicity. Furthermore, a refined comprehension of the mechanisms of action of deep brain simulation at cortico-subcortical levels will certainly be helpful for the refinement of patient selection criteria, anatomical targets, and ideal stimulation parameters. For these reasons, we believe that electrode geometry and placement should provide current delivery in the amygdala as well as the posterior portion of the hippocampus. Based on experimental data, we prefer monopolar stimulation with a pulse width of 450 microseconds in duration to increase charge delivery around each electrode contact and, consequently, the volume of tissue activated by stimulation within the amygdala and hippocampus.

References

1. Hauser WA, Hesdorffer DC. Incidence and prevalence. In: Hauser WA, Hesdorffer DC, eds. Epilepsy: Frequency, Causes and Consequences. New York: Demos; 1990
2. Tellez-Zenteno JF, Dhar R, Wiebe S. Long-term seizure outcomes following epilepsy surgery: a systematic review and meta-analysis. Brain 2005;128:1188–1198
3. Kwan P, Brodie MJ. Early identification of refractory epilepsy. N Engl J Med 2000;342(5):314–319
4. Cooper IS, Amin I, Gilman S. The effect of chronic cerebellar stimulation upon epilepsy in man. Trans Am Neurol Assoc 1973;98:192–196
5. Hamani C, Ewerton FI, Bonilha SM, Ballester G, Mello LE, Lozano AM. Bilateral anterior thalamic nucleus lesions and high-frequency stimulation are protective against pilocarpine-induced seizures and status epilepticus. Neurosurgery 2004;54(1):191–195
6. Hodaie M, Wennberg RA, Dostrovsky JO, Lozano AM. Chronic anterior thalamus stimulation for intractable epilepsy. Epilepsia 2002; 43(6):603–608
7. Kerrigan JF, Litt B, Fisher RS, et al. Electrical stimulation of the anterior nucleus of the thalamus for the treatment of intractable epilepsy. Epilepsia 2004;45(4):346–354
8. Fisher RS, Uematsu S, Krauss GL, et al. Placebo-controlled pilot study of centromedian thalamic stimulation in treatment of intractable seizures. Epilepsia 1992;33:841–851
9. Velasco F, Velasco M, Jimenez F, et al. Predictors in the treatment of difficult-to-control seizures by electrical stimulation of the centromedian thalamic nucleus. Neurosurgery 2000;47(2):295–304
10. Velasco F, Velasco M, Jimenez F, Velasco AL, Marquez I. Stimulation of the central median thalamic nucleus for epilepsy. Stereotact Funct Neurosurg 2001;77(1–4):228–232
11. Velasco F, Velasco M, Marquez I, Velasco G. Role of the centromedian thalamic nucleus in the genesis, propagation and arrest of epileptic activity. An electrophysiological study in man. Acta Neurochir Suppl (Wien) 1993;58:201–204
12. Velasco F, Velasco M, Ogarrio C, Fanghanel G. Electrical stimulation of the centromedian thalamic nucleus in the treatment of convulsive seizures: a preliminary report. Epilepsia 1987;28(4):421–430
13. Velasco F, Velasco M, Velasco AL, Jimenez F. Effect of chronic electrical stimulation of the centromedian thalamic nuclei on various intractable seizure patterns, I: clinical seizures and paroxysmal EEG activity. Epilepsia 1993;34:1052–1064
14. Velasco F, Velasco M, Velasco AL, Jimenez F, Marquez I, Rise M. Electrical stimulation of the centromedian thalamic nucleus in control of seizures: long-term studies. Epilepsia 1995;36(1):63–71
15. Velasco M, Velasco F, Velasco AL, et al. Electrocortical and behavioral responses produced by acute electrical stimulation of the human centromedian thalamic nucleus. Electroencephalogr Clin Neurophysiol 1997;102(6):461–471
16. Velasco M, Velasco F, Velasco AL, Jimenez F, Brito F, Marquez I. Acute and chronic electrical stimulation of the centromedian thalamic nucleus: modulation of reticulo-cortical systems and predictor factors for generalized seizure control. Arch Med Res 2000;31(3):304–315
17. Velasco M, Velasco F, Velasco AL. Centromedian-thalamic and hippocampal electrical stimulation for the control of intractable epileptic seizures. J Clin Neurophysiol 2001;18(6):495–513
18. Chkhenkeli SA, Chkhenkeli IS. Effects of therapeutic stimulation of nucleus caudatus on epileptic electrical activity of brain in patients with intractable epilepsy. Stereotact Funct Neurosurg 1997;69(1–4, Pt 2):221–224
19. Chkhenkeli SA, Sramka M, Lortkipanidze GS, et al. Electrophysiological effects and clinical results of direct brain stimulation for intractable epilepsy. Clin Neurol Neurosurg 2004;106(4):318–329
20. Raftopoulos C, van Rijckevorsel K, Abu Serieh B, de Tourtchaninoff M, Ivanoiu A, Grandin C. Preliminary results of deep brain stimulation of the mammillary bodies and mammillothalamic tracts in chronic refractory epilepsy. Acta Neurochir (Wien) 2004;146:885
21. Van Rijckevorsel K, Abu Serieh B, de Tourtchaninoff M, Raftopoulos C. Deep EEG recordings of the mammillary body in epilepsy patients. Epilepsia 2005;46(5):781–785
22. Benabid AL, Minotti L, Koudsie A, de Saint Martin A, Hirsch E. Antiepileptic effect of high-frequency stimulation of the subthalamic nucleus (corpus luysi) in a case of medically intractable epilepsy caused by focal dysplasia: a 30-month follow-up:technical case report. Neurosurgery 2002;50(6):1385–1391
23. Chabardès S, Kahane P, Minotti L, Koudsie A, Hirsch E, Benabid AL. Deep brain stimulation in epilepsy with particular reference to the subthalamic nucleus. Epileptic Disord 2002;4(Suppl 3):S83–S93
24. Shon YM, Lee KJ, Kin HJ, et al. Effect of chronic deep brain stimulation of the subthalamic nucleus for frontal lobe epilepsy: subtraction SPECT analysis. Stereotact Funct Neurosurg 2005;83(2–3):84–90
25. Velasco M, Velasco F, Velasco AL, et al. Subacute electrical stimulation of the hippocampus blocks intractable temporal lobe seizures and paroxysmal EEG activities. Epilepsia 2000;41:158–169
26. Vonck K, Boon P, Achten E, De Reuck J, Caemaert J. Long-term amygdalohippocampal stimulation for refractory temporal lobe epilepsy. Ann Neurol 2002;52:556–565

27. Tellez-Zenteno JF, McLachlan RS, Parrent A, Kubu CS, Wiebe S. Hippocampal electrical stimulation in mesial temporal lobe epilepsy. Neurology 2006;66(10):1490–1494

28. Chen J, Larionov S, Pitsch J, et al. Expression analysis of metabotropic glutamate receptors I and III in mouse strains with different susceptibility to experimental temporal lobe epilepsy. Neurosci Lett 2005;375(3):192–197

29. Gu W, Gibert Y, Wirth T, et al. Using gene-history and expression analyses to assess the involvement of LGI genes in human disorders. Mol Biol Evol 2005;22(11):2209–2216

30. Volk HA, Burkhardt K, Potschka H, Chen J, Becker A, Loscher W. Neuronal expression of the drug efflux transporter P-glycoprotein in the rat hippocampus after limbic seizures. Neuroscience 2004;123(3):751–759

31. Radhakrishnan K, So EL, Silbert PL, et al. Predictors of outcome of anterior temporal lobectomy for intractable epilepsy: a multivariate study. Neurology 1998;51(2):465–471

32. Bragin A, Wilson CL, Engel J Jr. Rate of interictal events and spontaneous eizures in epileptic rats after electrical stimulation of hippocampus and its afferents. Epilepsia 2002;43(Suppl 5):81–85

33. Weiss SR, Eidsath A, Li XL, Heynen T, Post RM. Quenching revisited: low level direct current inhibits amygdala-kindled seizures. Exp Neurol 1998;154(1):185–192

34. Joo EY, Han HJ, Lee EK, et al. Resection extent versus postoperative outcomes of seizure and memory in mesial temporal lobe epilepsy. Seizure 2005;14(8):541–551

35. Hennessy MJ, Elwes RD, Binnie CD, Polkey CE. Failed surgery for epilepsy. A study of persistence and recurrence of seizures following temporal resection. Brain 2000;123:2445–2466

36. McIntyre CC, Savasta M, Walter BL, Vitek JL. How does deep brain stimulation work? Present understanding and future questions. J Clin Neurophysiol 2004;21(1):40–50

37. Kuncel AM, Grill WM. Selection of stimulus parameters for deep brain stimulation. Clin Neurophysiol 2004;115(11):2431–2441

38. Filali M, Hutchison WD, Palter VN, Lozano AM, Dostrovsky JO. Stimulation-induced inhibition of neuronal firing in human subthalamic nucleus. Exp Brain Res 2004;156(3):274–281

39. Meissner W, Leblois A, Hansel D, et al. Subthalamic high frequency stimulation resets subthalamic firing and reduces abnormal oscillations. Brain 2005;128:2372–2382

40. Yamamoto J, Ikeda A, Satow T, et al. Low-frequency electric cortical stimulation has an inhibitory effect on epileptic focus in mesial temporal lobe epilepsy. Epilepsia 2002;43(5):491–495

41. D'Arcangelo G, Panuccio G, Tancredi V, Avoli M. Repetitive low-frequency stimulation reduces epileptiform synchronization in limbic neuronal networks. Neurobiol Dis 2005;19:119–128

18 Deep Brain Stimulation

Casey Halpern, Uzma Samadani, Jurg L. Jaggi, and Gordon Baltuch

Approximately one-third of patients with epilepsy will have persistent seizures despite maximal antiepileptic drug (AED) therapy.[1–3] Resective brain surgery is typically indicated for patients with refractory partial seizures and can result in at least a 90% reduction in seizure frequency, though permanent neurological deficits or death can occur in nearly 4% of cases.[4] At least 50% of patients are not candidates for resection or choose not to undergo such an invasive procedure. Some of these patients opt to have a vagus nerve stimulator (VNS) placed as an adjunct to medical therapy, which is associated with up to a 50% reduction in seizure frequency.[5] However, most of these patients will not be seizure free. Thus, due to the success of deep brain stimulation (DBS) for movement disorders,[6,7] combined with its advantages of adjustability, reversibility, and less risk of permanent neurological deficits then surgical ablation,[8] there has been an explosion of research into implantable devices for treating pharmacoresistant epilepsy.[9,10]

The mechanism by which DBS may diminish seizures is not completely understood. However, stimulation-induced disruption of unopposed network activity is one hypothesis that appears to be consistent with available data.[11,12] Evidence from subthalamic nucleus (STN) DBS suggests that high-frequency stimulation may block epileptiform activity in the cortex,[13–15] whereas low-frequency stimulation may drive or synchronize cortical activity.

Deep Brain Stimulation for Epilepsy: Evidence from Animal Studies

Seizure suppression with electrical stimulation of deep brain structures is effective in animal models using various neural targets, including the cerebellum, hippocampus, caudate nucleus, thalamus, STN, and mammillary nuclei.[16–20] We will focus on animal studies of DBS of the anterior nucleus of the thalamic (ANT), which is currently being studied in an ongoing double-blind randomized trial (SANTE), evaluating its efficacy for epilepsy treatment.[21] As of March 27 2006, 58 patients at 15 centers had been implanted with deep brain stimulators in ANT.

Animal studies investigating efficacy of ANT DBS for epilepsy primarily reflect the work of Mirski and colleagues. Bilateral electrolytic lesions of the tracts connecting the mammillary bodies to the ANT in guinea pigs resulted in essentially complete protection from pentylenetetrazol-induced seizure activity.[22] This finding was supported by observations of enhanced glucose metabolism in ANT following administration of both pentylenetetrazole and ethosuximide to guinea pigs.[23] Recently, high-frequency DBS (100 Hz) of the ANT has been shown to increase the clonic seizure threshold in a pentylenetetrazole-induced seizure model.[24] Interestingly, low-frequency (8 Hz) DBS was proconvulsant as found in earlier studies.[15,25] In addition, bilateral ANT DBS may prolong the latency of onset of status epilepticus following administration of pilocarpine, whereas seizures were eliminated by bilateral anterior nuclear thalamotomy.[26] Efficacy of ANT DBS for epilepsy in animal models is still unclear given reports of lack of effect, as well as exacerbation of seizure frequency by chronic ANT DBS.[26,27]

Deep Brain Stimulation of the Anterior Nucleus of the Thalamus

Rationale

In 1937, James W. Papez described a circuit linking hippocampal output via the fornix and mammillary nuclei in the posterior hypothalamus to ANT.[28] ANT projects to the cingulum bundle deep to the cingulate gyrus, which travels around the wall of the lateral ventricle to the parahippocampal cortex, then completes the circuit by returning to the hippocampus.[29] Atrophy, magnetic resonance imaging (MRI) signal change, or sclerosis of structures within the classic circuit of Papez has been noted in mesial temporal sclerosis, as well as other forms of epilepsy.[30] Stimulation of targets within this circuit is hypothesized to result in direct anterograde cortical stimulation.

ANT is a preferred target for DBS because of its relatively small size and projections to limbic structures ultimately affecting wide regions of neocortex. Furthermore, it is not as deep or close to basal vascular structures as the mammillary nuclei. ANT has been lesioned stereotactically resulting in improved seizure control in humans.[31] These anatomical connections and precursor ablative techniques have motivated investigation of ANT DBS for epilepsy.

Indications[32–35]

ANT DBS is indicated for partial onset epilepsy with or without secondary generalization associated with frequent seizures, resulting in falls, injuries, and impaired quality of life, refractory to 12 to 18 months of at least two therapeutically dosed antiepileptic agents. Patients should be without evidence of progressive neurological or systemic disease and have failed surgical resection and/or vagal nerve stimulation. Scalp video electroencephalogram (EEG) monitoring is necessary to characterize seizure types and demonstrate bilateral or nonlocalizing findings. Preoperative imaging should rule out any lateralizing structural abnormalities. Subjects, family, or the legal guardian must be capable of recognizing the patient's seizures and maintaining an accurate seizure diary.

Targeting and Surgical Procedure[32-37]

General endotracheal anesthesia or local anesthesia is administered prior to placement of the Leksell frame. Frame tilt should be parallel to the lateral canthal-external auditory meatal line, which is itself approximately parallel to the anterior commissure–posterior commissure (AC-PC) line. After attachment of the MRI localizer, a 1.5 T MRI is obtained with both fast spin echo inversion recovery and standard T2 images. Computed tomography (CT) can also be used.

Target sites were selected from MRI by using 1-mm thick axial, coronal, and sagittal spoiled gradient echo pulse sequences. Indirect localization of ANT is performed with reference to a standard stereotactic atlas[38] by identifying the AC-PC line on the sagittal image. AC and PC coordinates relative to the center of the frame are obtained to calculate the midcommissural point (MCP). ANT is 5 mm lateral and 12 mm superior to MCP.[38] Because ANT is visible in the floor of the lateral ventricle on MRI, direct localization is possible and frame coordinates are calculated.

Simulation of the planned trajectory from entry point to ANT is performed using a surgical navigation system (Medtronic Stealth navigation, Medtronic, Inc., Louisville, CO) to confirm avoidance of sulcal vessels (**Fig. 18.1**). The MRI is downloaded into the StealthStation computer. Inputting the entry point at or anterior to the coronal suture plots the trajectory, as well as the anterior-posterior and lateral arc coordinates for the Leksell frame.

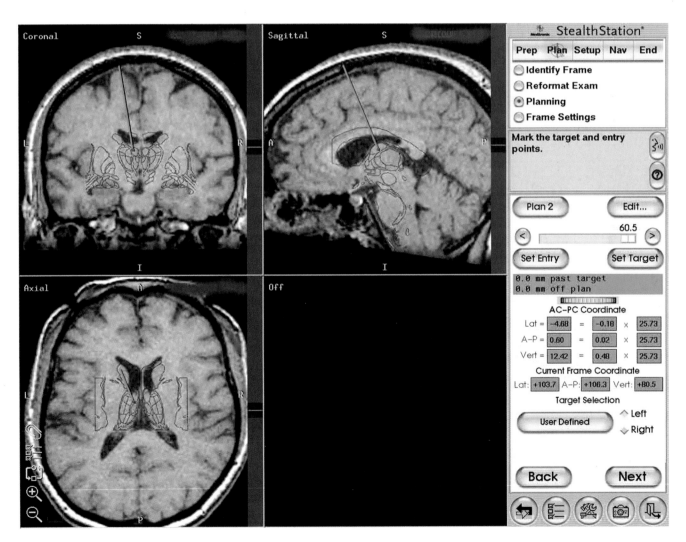

Fig. 18.1   Diagram demonstrating simulation of the planned trajectory to the anterior nucleus of the thalamus for deep brain stimulation using a surgical navigation system (Medtronic Stealth navigation, Medtronic, Inc. Louisville, CO) with a superimposed standard stereotactic atlas.

The patient is placed in a supine or semi-sitting position, and after sterile preparation of the unshaven head, and local infiltration with 1% Xylocaine (lidocaine) 1:100,000 epinephrine, an incision is made overlying the coronal suture. Bur holes are placed, and the dura and pia are sharply incised and cauterized. A guide cannula is inserted through the bur hole and advanced deep into the brain to a point 10 mm from the desired target under direct fluoroscopic and Leksell frame guidance. Under local anesthesia, a monopolar single-unit recording electrode (Advanced Research Systems, Atlanta, GA, or FHC, Inc., Bowdoinham, ME) can be introduced to confirm anatomical depth for entry into thalamic tissue after traversing the lateral ventricle. No units are recorded while positioned in the ventricle, but the electrode tip is advanced until recordings are first heard (ANT superficial surface) and then until units cease (intralaminar region) and recommence (dorsomedian nucleus of the thalamus) (**Fig. 18.2**). Extracellular action potentials are amplified with a GS3000 (Axon Instruments, Sunnyvale, CA) or Leadpoint (Medtronic, Inc., Minneapolis, MN) amplifier and simultaneously recorded using standard recording techniques (300 to 10,000 Hz), together with a descriptive voice channel. ANT neurons are identified based on (1) regional characteristics;

(2) a firing rate previously described for human recordings[33]; and (3) and a characteristic burst firing pattern.

After removing the single-unit recording electrode, a stimulation lead (Radionics Stimulation/Lesioning Probe, Burlington, MA) is introduced to elicit the driving response, suggestive of ANT placement (**Fig. 18.3**). ANT DBS has been associated with recruiting rhythms on cortical EEG in patients with the most pronounced seizure frequency reduction.[34] These changes in EEG signal morphology, however, can be elicited from several other thalamic nuclei.[25] Once this lead is removed, the DBS lead is advanced to ANT, ensuring that all contacts of the lead are within thalamic parenchyma. The cannula and lead stylet are withdrawn under fluoroscopy, after test stimulation demonstrates no adverse effects. Another fluoroscopic image is done to show that the electrode is secure. The stimulation leads we use are Medtronic 3387 (Medtronic, Inc.) DBS depth electrodes with four platinum-iridium stimulation contacts 1.5 mm wide with 1.5 mm edge-to-edge separation because ANT is relatively larger than other DBS targets. The lead is secured to a bur hole cap, and the skin incision is closed. The Leksell frame is removed, and the head, neck, and infraclavicular regions are sterilized in preparation for placement of the internal pulse gen-

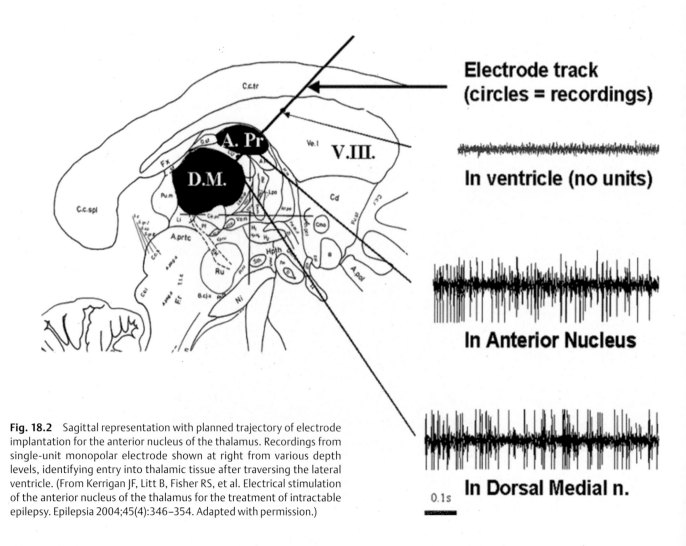

Fig. 18.2 Sagittal representation with planned trajectory of electrode implantation for the anterior nucleus of the thalamus. Recordings from single-unit monopolar electrode shown at right from various depth levels, identifying entry into thalamic tissue after traversing the lateral ventricle. (From Kerrigan JF, Litt B, Fisher RS, et al. Electrical stimulation of the anterior nucleus of the thalamus for the treatment of intractable epilepsy. Epilepsia 2004;45(4):346–354. Adapted with permission.)

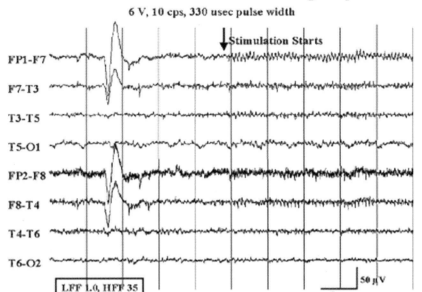

Stimulation L Anterior Nucleus: Driving Response

6 V, 10 cps, 330 usec pulse width

↓ Stimulation Starts

FP1-F7

F7-T3

T3-T5

T5-O1

FP2-F8

F8-T4

T4-T6

T6-O2

LFF 1.0, HFF 35

50 μV

1 sec

Fig. 18.3 Scalp EEG driving response to left-sided anterior nucleus of the thalamus stimulation. (From Kerrigan JF, Litt B, Fisher RS, et al. Electrical stimulation of the anterior nucleus of the thalamus for the treatment of intractable epilepsy. Epilepsia 2004;45(4):346–354. Adapted with permission.)

erator (IPG) (model Itrel II, Soletra, or Kinetra; Medtronic, Inc.) in a subclavicular pocket bilaterally. The scalp incision is reopened for connection of the lead to an extension wire (Medtronic 7495 Lead Extension, Medtronic, Inc.), which is tunneled subcutaneously to an IPG.

After reversal and recovery from anesthesia, placement location of the DBS leads is confirmed by MRI or CT (**Fig. 18.4**). Generally, patients should undergo postoperative monitoring in the epilepsy-monitoring unit, where simultaneous scalp and thalamic EEGs through the implanted leads can be recorded. Patients are discharged to home 2 days postoperatively, but multiple outpatient visits are usually necessary to optimize stimulation parameters. Stimulators are turned on approximately 10 to 14 days postoperatively. For initial stimulation, frequency is set at 90 to 130 Hz, pulse width at 60 to 90 microseconds, and pulse amplitude at 4 to 5 V; and the contact inducing the optimal clinical effect at minimal voltage and with the fewest side effects is identified. The benefits of bipolar versus monopolar stimulation remain to be determined as do "cycling" versus "continuous" stimulation. A recent study of bilateral ANT DBS in four patients with refractory epilepsy showed no significant difference in seizure frequency between cycling and continuous stimulation period using within-group comparisons.[32] One proposed method of cycling or intermittent stimulation using an "open-loop" device (discussed below) is through a "duty cycle" of 1 minute on and 5 minutes off.[9] Intermittent stimulation may increase the battery life of the IPG; is theoretically safer for neural tissue than chronic, continuous stimulation; and has been successful in clinical trials for vagus nerve stimulation for epilepsy.[34]

Pilot Studies

Unfortunately, we are limited to small-sample human pilot studies in evaluating ANT DBS as a treatment for pharmacoresistant epilepsies, though a multicenter random-

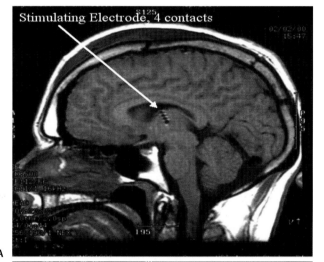

Stimulating Electrode, 4 contacts

A

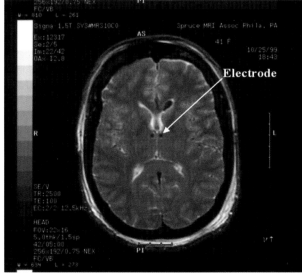

Electrode

B

Fig. 18.4 A T1-weighted sagittal (**A**) and T2-weighted axial (**B**) magnetic resonance image demonstrating lead placement for deep brain stimulation of the anterior thalamic nucleus.

ized clinical trial of intermittent bilateral ANT DBS for medically intractable seizures is currently underway.[21] Despite significant individual variation in outcome, overall bilateral high-frequency ANT DBS appears to be safe, well-tolerated, and effective in some subjects with inoperable, refractory epilepsy. **Table 18.1** summarizes the results of seven pilot studies of ANT DBS.

Upton et al (1987)[39] reported on 4 of 6 patients with intractable epilepsy who experienced a significant reduction in seizure frequency, one of whom was completely seizure free at follow-up.[39] This may be due to microthalamotomy or lesioning of the ANT, an effect that has been noted previously.[40] In fact, electrode implantation appears to decrease seizure frequency itself, and activation of the IPG and multiple subsequent adjustments to stimulatory parameters or contacts stimulated may not be linked to any further benefit in seizure control.[32,37] However, in one patient, the IPGs were turned off after 3 years of DBS with maintenance of improved seizure control for more than 1 year. Thus, it is difficult to distinguish the relative effects of electrode insertion and stimulation to the reduction in seizure frequency. The effect of microthalamotomy on seizure propagation, however, remains to be debated as a recent study was unable to detect a lesion effect during the immediate postoperative period.[35]

Other pilot studies of intermittent ANT DBS have reported significant reduction in frequency and propagation of generalized tonic-clonic seizures (GTCSs) and complex partial seizures in 4 of 5 patients.[33] However, only 1 of the 5 patients showed a statistically significant reduction in total seizure frequency. Importantly, discontinuation of DBS resulted in an immediate increase in seizure frequency and intensity that improved when stimulation was resumed. This suggests that ANT DBS–induced inhibition is at least in part implicated in reducing seizure frequency.[32,33,35] The beneficial response to closed-loop stimulation (described below) provides further support for a beneficial role of electrical stimulation.

A recent study reporting long-term follow-up noted that electrode implantation and stimulation in ANT was followed by more than a 50% seizure reduction in 5 of 6 patients. However, significant benefit in two patients was not seen until years 5 and 6, respectively, with the addition of further adjuvant AEDs.[37] There is evidence for a long-term effect of ANT DBS on the propensity to develop seizures,[37] and indeed, ongoing clinical benefit after cessation of DBS has been noted in tremor.[41] Bitemporal mesial epilepsy, as opposed to extratemporal or poorly localized seizures,[33,34,37] may be most responsive to ANT DBS given a recent report of more than a 75% reduction in seizure frequency.[35] Seizure frequency decreased by 93% in one patient, which is the most dramatic response reported in the literature. Alternatively, a higher mean frequency (157 Hz) may at least in part explain this impressive response.

Complications

ANT DBS appears to be a safe, well-tolerated treatment of refractory seizures with all of the reported complications and stimulation-induced adverse effects being mild and transient. Reported adverse effects due to stimulation are paranoid ideation, intermittent nystagmus with cycling stimulation, auditory hallucinations, anorexia, and lethargy.[35,37] Complications due to the surgical procedure or hardware include a small, right frontal hemorrhage without any permanent neurological deficit, scalp erosion necessitating removal of the implanted system, infection of the right anterior chest, and accidental turning-off of the stimulator.[32,34,42]

Other Anatomical Targets for Deep Brain Stimulation for Epilepsy

Although the SANTE trial will only be evaluating ATN DBS, other neural targets are worth discussing to provide a more thorough review of the potential for DBS in epilepsy. Some open-label clinical trials have reported on DBS of various

Table 18.1 Clinical Outcome Following ANT DBS in Six Pilot Studies in Humans

Series	N	Average Postoperative Follow-up	Stimulation type	Percent Seizure Frequency/ Month Reduction
Osorio et al (2007)[35]	4	36	Cycling	76*
Lee et al (2006)[42]	3	13	Cycling	75
Lim et al (2007)[32]	4	44	Continuous†	51
Hodaie et al (2002)[34]	5	15	Cycling	54‡
Kerrigan et al (2004)[33]	5	12	Cycing	14§
Andrade et al (2006)[37]	6	48	Cycling¶	51‖

* $p < 0.01$.

† Intermittent stimulation was later used to prolong battery life although the timescale was not reported.

‡ $p < 0.05$.

§ This study noted >50% reduction in serious seizure (generalized tonic-clonic seizures and complex partial seizures) frequency.

‖ Four of 6 patients had a significant decrease in the frequency of seizures/month ($p < 0.05$), but significance for overall mean reduction was not reported.

¶ Multiple changes in stimulation parameters, including continuous versus cycling, were performed in this study.

targets to treat pharmacoresistant seizures, demonstrating marginal efficacy in stimulating the centromedian nucleus of the thalamus (CMT), caudate nucleus, cerebellum, and STN.

Centromedian Nucleus of the Thalamus

Velasco and colleagues have contributed to the majority of work addressing CMT DBS. As first hypothesized by Penfield,[43] the CMT is an integral part of an ascending subcortical system, arising from the brainstem and diencephalons and projecting diffusely to cerebral cortex, supporting a role for the CMT in the pathophysiology of generalized seizures.[44] The beneficial effect of CMT DBS on seizure control may be due to desynchronization and hyperpolarization of the ascending reticular and cortical neurons.[44] A very recent open-label trial in 13 patients with Lennox-Gastaut syndrome reported overall seizure reduction of 80% with significant improvement in quality of life.[45] Although CMT DBS may be effective in controlling frequency of generalized seizures, results in patients with complex partial seizures are unclear.[46–49] In contrast to the results of these open-label studies, a trial of CMT DBS in seven patients using a double-blind, crossover design revealed no significant difference in seizure frequency,[50] and a recent report showed no short-term benefit in two patients, one of whom was subsequently implanted with electrodes in the ANT.[37]

Subthalamic Nucleus

Extensive experience of STN DBS for the treatment of movement disorders makes the STN an appealing target.[7] The substantia nigra pars reticulata (SNr) is known to play a role in gating and control of seizures through its γ-aminobutyric acid (GABA)ergic nigrotectal projections to the superior colliculus.[51] Inhibition of GABAergic SNr neurons results in suppression of partial and generalized epileptic seizures in animal models of epilepsy.[52] The STN exerts excitatory control on the nigral system. Indeed, pharmacological or electrical inhibition of STN leads to seizure suppression.[16] A case study of high-frequency bilateral STN DBS for a child with inoperable epilepsy due to focal centroparietal dysplasia observed an 81% improvement in seizure frequency at 30 months follow-up.[53] An 80% improvement in 2 of 5 patients with partial-onset seizures treated with STN DBS for 16 months has been reported.[54] Another open-label study of STN DBS demonstrated significant improvement of seizures in 4 of 5 patients (mean reduction of seizure frequency 64.2%).[55] Most recently, two case patients with refractory partial-onset seizures were treated with bilateral STN DBS.[56] The first patient had a 50% reduction in seizure frequency, but seizure-related injuries continued to occur. In the second case it was noted that seizure frequency was reduced by one-third, but seizures were milder and caused fewer injuries, thus improving the quality of life of this patient. STN DBS may hold significant future potential as a treatment for epilepsy; however, larger randomized, double-blind clinical trials are necessary.

Caudate Nucleus

The head of the caudate nucleus (HCN), thalamus, and neocortex communicate as a functional entity known as the "caudate loop."[57] Activation of HCN has been shown to correlate with hyperpolarization of cortical neurons, suggesting that suppression of epileptic activity may be a result of stimulation-induced inhibition on the cortex. Indeed, low-frequency stimulation (4 to 8 Hz) of the ventral part of HCN has been shown to suppress interictal epileptic activity, focal amygdalahippocampal discharges, and generalization of seizures[58,59]; however, clinical seizure data were not assessed. Thus, controlled clinical studies are necessary to further evaluate the caudate as a target for DBS in epilepsy.

Cerebellum

Cerebellar stimulation (CS) likely activates inhibitory Purkinje cells, which suppress the excitatory cerebellar output to the thalamus, decreasing the excitatory thalamocortical projection to motor cortex, resulting in a transient suppression of cortical excitability.[60] Cooper and colleagues were the first to report on CS for epilepsy in an open-label trial, demonstrating that 18 of the 34 patients experienced at least a 50% reduction in seizures.[61,62] A more recent uncontrolled study reported that 23 (85%) of 32 patients benefited overall from long-term CS[63]; however, controlled, double-blind trials demonstrated improvement in only 2 of (14%) 14 patients.[64,65] Recently, a double-blind trial of five patients showed a significant reduction in GTCSs and tonic seizures (TSs) at 2-year follow-up.[66] Improvement in GTCSs occurred sooner, however, and was more significant than that for TSs. Therefore, as suggested in animal studies, CS may act mainly at the supradiencephalic level.[67] Larger clinical trials are necessary to further assess the role of CS in epilepsy treatment.

Hippocampus

Enough evidence exists to suggest that temporal lobe seizures are initiated from and/or propagated through the hippocampal formation.[68,69] Furthermore, the hippocampus is an integral component of the circuit of Papez.[28-30] Subacute hippocampal stimulation (HS) using bilateral depth electrodes or unilateral electrode grids abolished complex partial and secondarily GTCs and significantly decreased the number of interictal EEG spikes at the focus in 7 of 10 patients with intractable temporal lobe seizures. A subsequent report by the same group of chronic HS in three patients demonstrated persistently blocked epileptogenesis with no negative effect on short-term memory.[70] As a follow-up, continuous high-frequency HS for about 2 weeks in 10 patients revealed a significant decrease in seizures and interictal paroxysmal activity.[71] A small, open series of three patients with complex partial seizures reported that DBS of the amygdalohippocampal region resulted in >50% reduction in seizure frequency at 5-month follow-up.[72] More recently, these investigators reported that at a mean follow up of 14 months, bilateral amygdalohippocampal DBS in seven patients resulted in one patient who was free of complex partial seizures.[73] Three other patients had >50% reduction in seizure frequency, whereas 2 of the 7 patients had a reduction of 25%. Only one patient had no change in seizure frequency. Controlled studies with larger sample sizes are mandatory to identify a potential treatment population for HS and optimal stimulation parameters.

Open Versus Closed-Loop Systems

Closed-loop systems are "intelligent" brain devices that can produce bursts of stimulation that react to and terminate physiological changes such as epileptiform activity.[9] These stimulators may provide comparable or even more effective seizure suppression than their "blind," "open-loop" counterparts (described above) that stimulate continuously or intermittently without reacting to any physiological changes. Penfield and Jasper were the first to apply focal electrical stimulation to a human's brain, and they successfully terminated spontaneous seizures detected by electrocorticography during resective surgery.[74] Closed-loop devices are more efficient and should be better tolerated than an open-loop modality because of lower daily doses of stimulation.[75] "Intelligent" detection may be less toxic than intermittent and continuous stimulation. A research group at the University of Pennsylvania, using EEG recordings in mesial temporal lobe epilepsy, identified a spontaneous progression of changes in brain activity that can lead to a full-blown convulsive seizure.[76] These changes can last up to 7 hours before the seizure, and, if detected, can be successfully suppressed by an implanted stimulator. Mapping cortical networks involved in seizure generation and determining the most effective time of stimulation relative to seizure onset still require further investigation.

A trial of four patients with refractory seizures treated with responsive cortical stimulation noted suppression of clinical seizures and resolution of electrographic seizure activity.[77] Recently, high-frequency stimulation was performed in eight patients with a closed-loop system, in which stimulation was delivered either to the epileptogenic cortex ($n = 4$) or ATN ($n = 4$) after automated seizure detection.[78] Three of the 4 patients in which stimulation was delivered to the cortex and 2 of 4 patients with ATN DBS responded with decreased seizure frequency. A multi-institutional clinical trial of a cranially implanted responsive neurostimulator (RNS™ System, NeuroPace, Inc., Mountain View, CA) is currently underway in patients with pharmacoresistant partial onset seizures. The RNS™ IPG continuously analyzes the patient's electrocortigram and triggers stimulation whenever the characteristics programmed by the clinician are indicative of seizures or epileptiform precursors. A feasibility study of this closed-loop device has already described about a 45% decrease in seizure frequency in the majority of patients at 9-month follow-up.[79]

Conclusions

There are a considerable amount of patients suffering from medically refractory epilepsy who are not candidates for resective brain surgery. Some of these patients may benefit from DBS. There are many potential targets for stimulation for epilepsy; however, evidence is limited to open-label pilot studies and very small double-blind clinical trials. Although there is an ongoing prospective double-blind randomized trial for ANT DBS (SANTE), it is difficult at this time to make any definitive judgments about the efficacy of targeting ANT with stimulation for epilepsy treatment. Further work is necessary to identify a potential patient population for whom this technique would be indicated, which target is most efficacious, optimal stimulation parameters, and the ideal mode of stimulation.

References

1. Sillanpaa M, Schmidt D. Natural history of treated childhood-onset epilepsy: prospective, long-term population-based study. Brain 2006; 129(Pt 3):617–624

2. Sander JW. Some aspects of prognosis in the epilepsies: a review. Epilepsia 1993;34(6):1007–1016

3. Juul-Jensen P. Epidemiology of intractable epilepsy. In: Schmidt D, Morselli P, eds. Intractable Epilepsy. New York: Raven Press 1986:5–11

4. Commission on Neurosurgery of Epilepsy. The International League Against Epilepsy. A global survey on epilepsy surgery, 1980–1990: a report by the Commission on Neurosurgery of Epilepsy, the International League Against Epilepsy. Epilepsia 1997;38(2):249–255

5. The Vagus Nerve Stimulation Study Group. A randomized controlled trial of chronic vagus nerve stimulation for treatment of medically intractable seizures. Neurology 1995;45(2):224–230

6. Krack P, Batir A, Van Blercom N, et al. Five-year follow-up of bilateral stimulation of the subthalamic nucleus in advanced Parkinson's disease. N Engl J Med 2003;349(20):1925–1934

7. Halpern C, Hurtig H, Jaggi J, et al. Deep brain stimulation in neurologic disorders. Parkinsonism Relat Disord 2007;13(1):1–16

8. Schuurman PR, Bosch DA, Bossuyt PM, et al. A comparison of continuous thalamic stimulation and thalamotomy for suppression of severe tremor. N Engl J Med 2000;342(7):461–468

9. Litt B. Evaluating devices for treating epilepsy. Epilepsia 2003;44 (Suppl 7):30–37

10. Litt B, Baltuch G. Brain stimulation for epilepsy. Epilepsy Behav 2001;2:S61–S67

11. Lee KH, Roberts DW, Kim U. Effect of high-frequency stimulation of the subthalamic nucleus on subthalamic neurons: an intracellular study. Stereotact Funct Neurosurg 2003;80(1–4):32–36

12. McIntyre CC, Savasta M, Kerkerian-Le Goff L, Vitek JL. Uncovering the mechanism(s) of action of deep brain stimulation: activation, inhibition, or both. Clin Neurophysiol 2004;115(6):1239–1248

13. Monnier M, Kalberer M, Krupp P. Functional antagonism between diffuse reticular and intralaminary recruiting projections in the medial thalamus. Exp Neurol 1960;2:271–289

14. Velasco M, Velasco F. State related brain stem regulation on cortical and motor excitability: effects on experimental focal motor seizures. Orlando: Academic Press, 1982.

15. Lado FA, Velisek L, Moshe SL. The effect of electrical stimulation of the subthalamic nucleus on seizures is frequency dependent. Epilepsia 2003;44(2):157–164

16. Vercueil L, Benazzouz A, Deransart C, et al. High-frequency stimulation of the subthalamic nucleus suppresses absence seizures in the rat: comparison with neurotoxic lesions. Epilepsy Res 1998;31(1):39–46

17. Shandra AA, Godlevsky LS. Antiepileptic effects of cerebellar nucleus dentatus electrical stimulation under different conditions of brain epileptisation. Indian J Exp Biol 1990;28(2):158–161

18. Mirski MA, McKeon AC, Ferrendelli JA. Anterior thalamus and substantia nigra: two distinct structures mediating experimental generalized seizures. Brain Res 1986;397(2):377–380

19. Bragin A, Wilson CL, Engel J Jr. Rate of interictal events and spontaneous seizures in epileptic rats after electrical stimulation of hippocampus and its afferents. Epilepsia 2002;43(Suppl 5):81–85

20. Mutani R. Experimental evidence for the existence of an extrarhinencephalic control of the activity of the cobalt rhinencephalic epileptogenic focus. Part 1. The role played by the caudate nucleus. Epilepsia 1969;10(3):337–350

21. Fisher R. SANTE (Stimulation of the Anterior Nucleus of Thalamus for Epilepsy) Interim Report. Presented at the American Epilepsy Society 60th Annual Meeting; 2006; San Diego, CA

22. Mirski MA, Ferrendelli JA. Interruption of the mammillothalamic tract prevents seizures in guinea pigs. Science 1984;226(4670):72–74

23. Mirski MA, Ferrendelli JA. Selective metabolic activation of the mammillary bodies and their connections during ethosuximide-induced suppression of pentylenetetrazol seizures. Epilepsia 1986;27(3):194–203

24. Mirski MA, Rossell LA, Terry JB, Fisher RS. Anticonvulsant effect of anterior thalamic high frequency electrical stimulation in the rat. Epilepsy Res 1997;28(2):89–100

25. Dempsey EW, Morrison RS. The production of rhythmically recurrent cortical potentials after localized thalamic stimulation. Am J Physiol 1941;135:293–300

26. Hamani C, Ewerton FI, Bonilha SM, et al. Bilateral anterior thalamic nucleus lesions and high-frequency stimulation are protective against pilocarpine-induced seizures and status epilepticus. Neurosurgery 2004;54(1):191–195, discussion 195–7

27. Lado FA. Chronic bilateral stimulation of the anterior thalamus of kainate-treated rats increases seizure frequency. Epilepsia 2006;47(1):27–32

28. Papez JW. A proposed mechanism of emotion. Arch Neur and Psych 1937;38:725–743

29. Carpenter MB. Core Text of Neuroanatomy. 4th ed. Baltimore: Williams & Wilkins; 1991

30. Oikawa H, Sasaki M, Tamakawa Y, Kamei A. The circuit of Papez in mesial temporal sclerosis: MRI. Neuroradiology 2001;43(3):205–210

31. Mullan S, Vailati G, Karasick J, Mailis M. Thalamic lesions for the control of epilepsy. A study of nine cases. Arch Neurol 1967;16(3):277–285

32. Lim SN, Lee ST, Tsai YT, et al. Electrical stimulation of the anterior nucleus of the thalamus for intractable epilepsy: a long-term follow-up study. Epilepsia 2007;48(2):342–347

33. Kerrigan JF, Litt B, Fisher RS, et al. Electrical stimulation of the anterior nucleus of the thalamus for the treatment of intractable epilepsy. Epilepsia 2004;45(4):346–354

34. Hodaie M, Wennberg RA, Dostrovsky JO, Lozano AM. Chronic anterior thalamus stimulation for intractable epilepsy. Epilepsia 2002;43(6):603–608

35. Osorio I, Overman J, Giftakis J, Wilkinson SB. High frequency thalamic stimulation for inoperable mesial temporal epilepsy. Epilepsia 2007;8(8):1561–1571

36. Samadani U, Baltuch GH. Anterior thalamic nucleus stimulation for epilepsy. Acta Neurochir Suppl (Wien) 2007;97:1–4

37. Andrade DM, Zumsteg D, Hamani C, et al. Long-term follow-up of patients with thalamic deep brain stimulation for epilepsy. Neurology 2006;66(10):1571–1573

38. Schaltenbrand G, Warren W. Atlas for Stereotaxy of the Human Brain. Stuttgart: Thieme; 1977

39. Upton AR, Amin I, Garnett S, et al. Evoked metabolic responses in the limbic-striate system produced by stimulation of anterior thalamic nucleus in man. Pacing Clin Electrophysiol 1987;10(1, Pt 2):217–225

40. Tasker RR. Deep brain stimulation is preferable to thalamotomy for tremor suppression. Surg Neurol 1998;49(2):145–153, discussion 153–4

41. Lang AE, Lozano AM. Parkinson's disease. Second of two parts. N Engl J Med 1998;339(16):1130–1143

42. Lee KJ, Jang KS, Shon YM. Chronic deep brain stimulation of subthalamic and anterior thalamic nuclei for controlling refractory partial epilepsy. Acta Neurochir Suppl (Wien) 2006;99:87–91

43. Penfield WB. The cerebral cortex in man, I: the cerebral cortex and consciousness (Harvey Lecture, 1936). Arch Neurol Psychiatry 1938;40:417

44. Velasco M, Velasco F, Velasco AL, et al. Acute and chronic electrical stimulation of the centromedian thalamic nucleus: modulation of reticulo-cortical systems and predictor factors for generalized seizure control. Arch Med Res 2000;31(3):304–315

45. Velasco AL, Velasco F, Jimenez F, et al. Neuromodulation of the centromedian thalamic nuclei in the treatment of generalized seizures and the improvement of the quality of life in patients with Lennox-Gastaut syndrome. Epilepsia 2006;47(7):1203–1212

46. Velasco F, Velasco M, Ogarrio C, Fanghanel G. Electrical stimulation of the centromedian thalamic nucleus in the treatment of convulsive seizures: a preliminary report. Epilepsia 1987;28(4):421–430

47. Velasco M, Velasco F, Velasco AL, et al. Effect of chronic electrical stimulation of the centromedian thalamic nuclei on various intractable seizure patterns, II: psychological performance and background EEG activity. Epilepsia 1993;34(6):1065–1074

48. Velasco F, Velasco M, Velasco AL, et al. Electrical stimulation of the centromedian thalamic nucleus in control of seizures: long-term studies. Epilepsia 1995;36(1):63–71

49. Velasco F, Velasco M, Jimenez F, et al. Stimulation of the central median thalamic nucleus for epilepsy. Stereotact Funct Neurosurg 2001;77(1–4):228–232

50. Fisher RS, Uematsu S, Krauss GL, et al. Placebo-controlled pilot study of centromedian thalamic stimulation in treatment of intractable seizures. Epilepsia 1992;33(5):841–851

51. Gale K. Role of the substantia nigra in GABA-mediated anticonvulsant actions. Adv Neurol 1986;44:343–364

52. Iadarola MJ, Gale K. Substantia nigra: site of anticonvulsant activity mediated by gamma-aminobutyric acid. Science 1982;218(4578):1237–1240

53. Benabid AL, Koudsie A, Benazzouz A, et al. Deep brain stimulation of the corpus luysi (subthalamic nucleus) and other targets in Parkinson's disease. Extension to new indications such as dystonia and epilepsy. J Neurol 2001;248(Suppl 3):III37–III47

54. Loddenkemper T, Pan A, Neme S, et al. Deep brain stimulation in epilepsy. J Clin Neurophysiol 2001;18(6):514–532

55. Chabardes S, Kahane P, Minotti L, et al. Deep brain stimulation in epilepsy with particular reference to the subthalamic nucleus. Epileptic Disord 2002;4(Suppl 3):S83–S93

56. Handforth A, DeSalles AA, Krahl SE. Deep brain stimulation of the subthalamic nucleus as adjunct treatment for refractory epilepsy. Epilepsia 2006;47(7):1239–1241

57. Heuser G, Buchwald NA, Wyers EJ. The "caudatespindle," II: facilitatory and inhibitory caudate-cortical pathways. Electroencephalogr Clin Neurophysiol 1961;13:519–524

58. Chkhenkeli SA, Sramka M, Lortkipanidze GS, et al. Electrophysiological effects and clinical results of direct brain stimulation for intractable epilepsy. Clin Neurol Neurosurg 2004;106(4):318–329

59. Chkhenkeli SA, Chkhenkeli IS. Effects of therapeutic stimulation of nucleus caudatus on epileptic electrical activity of brain in patients with intractable epilepsy. Stereotact Funct Neurosurg 1997;69(1–4, Pt 2):221–224

60. Molnar GF, Sailer A, Gunraj CA, et al. Thalamic deep brain stimulation activates the cerebellothalamocortical pathway. Neurology 2004; 63(5):907–909

61. Cooper IS, Amin I, Gilman S. The effect of chronic cerebellar stimulation upon epilepsy in man. Trans Am Neurol Assoc 1973;98:192–196

62. Cooper IS, Amin I, Riklan M, et al. Chronic cerebellar stimulation in epilepsy. Clinical and anatomical studies. Arch Neurol 1976;33(8):559–570

63. Davis R, Emmonds SE. Cerebellar stimulation for seizure control: 17-year study. Stereotact Funct Neurosurg 1992;58(1–4):200–208

64. Van Buren JM, Wood JH, Oakley J, Hambrecht F. Preliminary evaluation of cerebellar stimulation by double-blind stimulation and biological criteria in the treatment of epilepsy. J Neurosurg 1978;48(3):407–416

65. Wright GD, McLellan DL, Brice JG. A double-blind trial of chronic cerebellar stimulation in twelve patients with severe epilepsy. J Neurol Neurosurg Psychiatry 1984;47(8):769–774

66. Velasco F, Carrillo-Ruiz JD, Brito F, et al. Double-blind, randomized controlled pilot study of bilateral cerebellar stimulation for treatment of intractable motor seizures. Epilepsia 2005;46(7):1071–1081

67. Laxer KD, Robertson LT, Julien RM, Dow RS. Phenytoin: relationship between cerebellar function and epileptic discharges. Adv Neurol 1980; 27:415–427

68. Swanson TH. The pathophysiology of human mesial temporal lobe epilepsy. J Clin Neurophysiol 1995;12(1):2–22

69. Sperling MR, O'Connor MJ, Saykin AJ, et al. A noninvasive protocol for anterior temporal lobectomy. Neurology 1992;42(2):416–422

70. Velasco AL, Velasco M, Velasco F, et al. Subacute and chronic electrical stimulation of the hippocampus on intractable temporal lobe seizures: preliminary report. Arch Med Res 2000;31(3):316–328

71. Velasco F, Velasco M, Velasco AL, et al. Electrical stimulation for epilepsy: stimulation of hippocampal foci. Stereotact Funct Neurosurg 2001;77(1–4):223–227

72. Vonck K, Boon P, Achten E, et al. Long-term amygdalohippocampal stimulation for refractory temporal lobe epilepsy. Ann Neurol 2002; 52(5):556–565

73. Vonck K, Boon P, Claeys P, et al. Long-term deep brain stimulation for refractory temporal lobe epilepsy. Epilepsia 2005;46(Suppl 5):98–99

74. Penfield W, Jasper H. Epilepsy and the functional anatomy of the human brain. Boston: Little, Brown, 1954.

75. Osorio I, Frei MG, Manly BF, et al. An introduction to contingent (closed-loop) brain electrical stimulation for seizure blockage, to ultra-short-term clinical trials, and to multidimensional statistical analysis of therapeutic efficacy. J Clin Neurophysiol 2001;18(6):533–544

76. Litt B, Esteller R, Echauz J, et al. Epileptic seizures may begin hours in advance of clinical onset: a report of five patients. Neuron 2001; 30(1):51–64

77. Kossoff EH, Ritzl EK, Politsky JM, et al. Effect of an external responsive neurostimulator on seizures and electrographic discharges during subdural electrode monitoring. Epilepsia 2004;45(12):1560–1567

78. Osorio I, Frei MG, Sunderam S, et al. Automated seizure abatement in humans using electrical stimulation. Ann Neurol 2005;57(2):258–268

79. Fountas KN, Smith JR, Murro AM, et al. Implantation of a closed-loop stimulation in the management of medically refractory focal epilepsy: a technical note. Stereotact Funct Neurosurg 2005;83(4):153–158

19 Responsive (Closed-Loop) Stimulation

Robert E. Wharen Jr.

Partial epilepsy represents the most prevalent type of epilepsy, accounting for ~60% of cases overall and 90% of adult incident cases. Nearly 40% of these patients will be refractory to medications, resulting in more than 1 million patients in the US with medically refractory partial epilepsy.[1] A few of these patients will be lucky (i.e., a 34-year-old female with intractable complex partial seizures, a right temporal cavernous angioma on magnetic resonance imaging [MRI], and an electroencephalogram [EEG] with right temporal sharp waves who has resective surgery and achieves an Engel class I outcome). Most patients, however, will not be so fortunate (i.e., a 29-year-old with disabling complex partial seizures, bilateral medial temporal sclerosis on MRI, an EEG with independent sharp waves and bilateral independent seizures, and ictal asystole observed in the epilepsy monitoring unit). For these medically refractory patients a few options are available such as vagal nerve stimulation, ketogenic diet, and experimental medications. Most will have continued seizures and side effects from medications.

Given the significant need for improved therapeutics for patients with refractory seizures who are not candidates for resective surgery, there is considerable interest in device-based therapies. Vagal nerve stimulation, deep brain stimulation, and cortical stimulation are all being evaluated in clinical trials using open and closed-loop stimulation paradigms. The purpose of this chapter is to briefly review the use of neurostimulation for refractory epilepsy, and to describe in detail the use of responsive stimulation for the treatment of patients with medically refractory focal epilepsy using a cranially implanted responsive neurostimulator (RNS™ System, NeuroPace, Inc., Mountain View, CA).

Localization of Cortical Function

In 1870 two German physiologists, Gustav Fritch and Eduard Hitzig, examined localization of function by stimulating with electricity small regions of the exposed brain surfaces of awake dogs, providing evidence for localization of function in the cerebral cortex.[2] The work of Fritsch and Hitzig was considerably expanded by Sir David Ferrier, whose work on cerebral localization was considered a great advance in the physiology of the nervous system. He stimulated the cortex of animals and defined precise areas related to movement, and later demonstrated the loss of motor function following resection of the corresponding areas. Ferrier boldly predicted, with good accuracy, the application of these findings to the human brain, and he assisted Macewen in the localization and resection of a cortical lesion in a patient with unilateral paralysis of the fingers and forearm.[3] Penfield and Jasper greatly extended the use of electrical stimulation for localization of cortical function, and reported the first description of a seizure resulting from cortical stimulation.[4]

Deep Brain Stimulation for Epilepsy

Initial trials of electrical stimulation for epilepsy treatment by Cooper and colleagues targeted the cerebellum.[5–7] Although the subdural stimulation was well tolerated and was effective in small open trials, these results were not confirmed in later controlled trials[8,9] A double-blind, randomized controlled pilot study of supermedial cerebellar cortex in five patients with motor seizures found a significant reduction in tonic-clonic and tonic seizures over 6 months of stimulation, but further surgery was required in four of these patients.[10]

Over the past 20 years a variety of brain targets in addition to the cerebellum (centromedian thalamus,[11,12] anterior thalamus,[13–15] subthalamic nucleus,[16,17] hippocampus,[18] posterior hypothalamus,[19] and head of the caudate[20]) have been investigated for the capability of suppressing epileptic discharges using a variety of stimulation parameters. The potential use of brain stimulation to suppress seizures is based upon the premise that most forms of epilepsy result from an imbalance of excitatory and inhibitory processes due to debilitation of inhibitory processes,[21] and the potential existence of a control system responsible for seizure arrest.[22] The use of stimulation to artificially enhance the activity of such a control system can potentially suppress seizure activity. Experimental and clinical data have demonstrated that all of the above structures has some ability to exert inhibitory influences on both interictal and ictal epileptic electrical activity. Loddenkemper et al postulated a nigral control system capable of suppressing epilepsy via a dorsal midbrain anticonvulsant zone in the superior colliculi, and they suggested the potential interactions of the striatum, thalamus, and subthalamic nucleus, with the substantia nigra pars reticulata as the central part of the system that, when activated, inhibits seizure generation and propagation.[17]

Chronic anterior thalamic stimulation has been demonstrated in small, open-label clinical trials to reduce seizure frequency.[13,14] A multicenter prospective randomized trial evaluating the safety and efficacy of chronic bilateral anterior thalamic stimulation in adults with medically intractable partial onset seizures with or without secondary generalization has completed recruitment (SANTE trial, sponsored by Medtronic, Inc.).

Small, open-label trials have also reported seizure reduction in some patients treated with subthalamic stimulation.[16,17,23] A randomized, double-blind, placebo-controlled, crossover assignment trial to assess the safety and efficacy of subthalamic nucleus stimulation for adults with medically refractory epilepsy is currently recruiting patients in France (www.clinicaltrials.gov).

Cortical Stimulation for Epilepsy

Another approach to the treatment of refractory epilepsy involves attempting to interfere with the ictal onset zone. Preliminary experience with trials in animals and humans is promising and suggests efficacy with both continuous (open-loop) stimulation and with responsive intermittent (closed-loop) stimulation. In addition, clinical data thus far provide reassuring safety data for responsive stimulation.

Open-loop stimulation applied to mesial temporal structures reduced seizures in some patients with medically intractable temporal lobe epilepsy.[18] Scheduled stimulation with hippocampal electrodes for 2 to 3 weeks prior to epilepsy surgery reduced the seizure frequency in 7 of 10 patients.[24]

External Responsive Neurostimulation

An early clinical observation was that stimulation applied during functional cortical mapping was capable of disrupting induced afterdischarge potentials. The ability of applied cortical stimulation to successfully terminate spontaneous seizure activity in humans was explored in persons undergoing functional cortical mapping as part of an evaluation for epilepsy surgery. In several instances, a spontaneous electrographic seizure was recorded from the cortical electrodes. In some cases, delivery of a responsive stimulation (to the electrodes from which the electrographic event was recorded) appeared to stop the event (**Fig. 19.1**). Although this study was designed to explore safety and was not designed to demonstrate efficacy, one important observation in these early clinical evaluations was that stimulation was more likely to be effective if applied early in the electrographic event. Stimulation applied after electrographic seizure activity had become established did not appear to be effective in modifying or terminating the discharge (**Fig. 19.2**).

Safety of responsive stimulation was assessed in an early clinical study using an External Responsive Neurostimulation System. This external, nonminiaturized version of the RNS™ System duplicated the automatic seizure detection and stimulation of the implantable system. The external system was applied to patients with implanted electrodes who had completed prolonged EEG monitoring for possible resective surgery. The External Responsive Neurostimulator System feasibility study was designed to evaluate the safety of responsive cortical stimulation with a secondary intent of gathering preliminary evidence (not statistical proof) of efficacy. Results of this study on 129 patients revealed no unanticipated serious device-related adverse events. The study

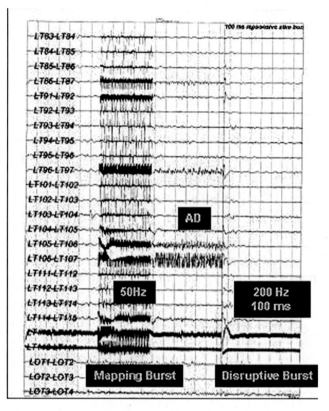

Fig. 19.1 Electrocorticography demonstrating that applied cortical stimulation disrupts afterdischarge potentials induced at surgery during functional cortical mapping. (Courtesy of Neuropace, Inc., Sunnyvale, CA. Reprinted with permission.)

also demonstrated that stimulation could be applied to multiple cortical areas without causing seizures, and that cortical stimulation at multiple frequencies and charge densities was well tolerated. Further observations were that stimulation applied early to an electrographic discharge could alter or terminate that discharge, that multiple electrodes in the vicinity of the seizure onset could be used for delivery of responsive stimulation, and that frequent responsive stimulation may be necessary to suppress clinical seizures.

The Implantable RNS™ System

System Components

The RNS™ System consists of an implantable pulse generator and two implantable leads (subdural and/or depth leads) a programmer comprising a laptop computer with a wand and telemetry box; and a data transmitter that is given to the patient, consisting of a laptop computer with a wand and telemetry box (**Figs. 19.3A and 19.3B**).

The neurostimulator continuously analyzes the patient's electrocorticogram (ECoG) and automatically triggers electrical stimulation when specific ECoG characteristics programmed by the clinician are detected that represent either seizure or preseizure epileptiform activity (**Fig. 19.4**). In addition, the implantable neurostimulator stores diagnostic

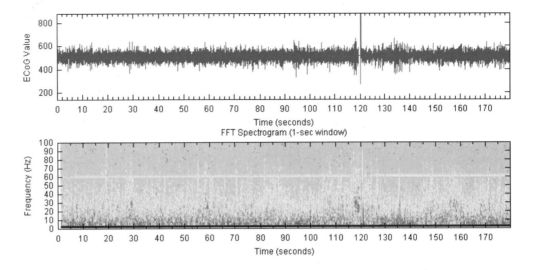

Stimulation appears to suppress the seizure

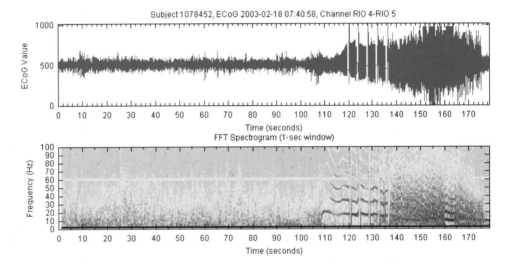

Stimulation is *too late* to suppress an ongoing seizure

Fig. 19.2 Electrocorticography and power spectral analysis of responsive stimulation demonstrating that stimulation must be applied early to effectively suppress seizure activity. (Courtesy of Neuropace, Inc., Sunnyvale, CA. Reprinted with permission.)

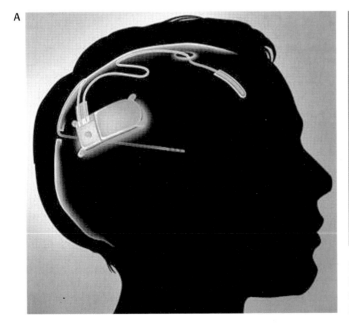

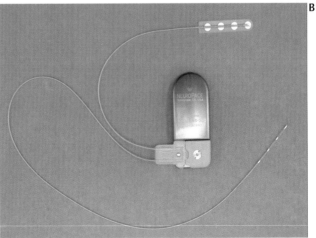

Fig. 19.3 Diagram **(A)** and photograph **(B)** of RNS™ System consisting of an implanted neurostimulator and two leads—one subdural and one depth electrode. (Courtesy of Neuropace, Inc., Sunnyvale, CA. Reprinted with permission.)

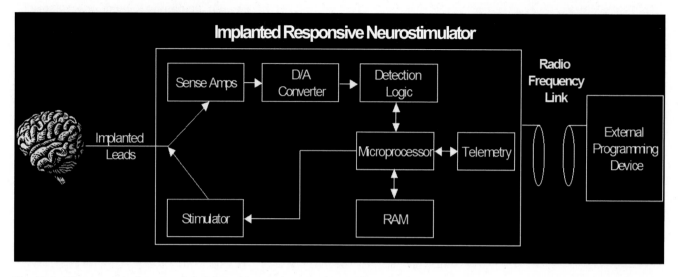

Fig. 19.4 Diagram of the functionality of the neurostimulator. (Courtesy of Neuropace, Inc., Sunnyvale, CA. Reprinted with permission.)

information including multichannel ECoGs and a detailed history of detections and stimulations. Using the data transmitter, the patient can upload this stored information to a secure Web site for analysis by the physician. Much of the technological basis of the RNS™ System builds on implanted defibrillator technology, in a sense creating an implantable brain defibrillator.

Responsive stimulation is a technology that is being initially investigated in persons with medically refractory epilepsy with partial onset seizures with or without secondary generalization. Early seizure detection and responsive stimulation necessitates that implanted electrodes be placed in or near the seizure foci.

Surgical Implantation

Implantation of the RNS™ System requires planning of a templated craniotomy for placement of the ferrule and neuro-

stimulator, which are designed to fit best in the contour of the parietooccipital skull. Placement of the neurostimulator must be coordinated with the implantation approach of the depth and/or subdural strip electrodes, which are to be applied to the site of the seizure focus. It is desirable to arrange the placement of the leads so that they do not traverse the incision. Additionally, prior surgeries and incisions must be considered so as not to compromise the vascularity of the scalp flap.

In this example, a patient with a left temporal lobe seizure focus who was not a candidate for resective surgery has the RNS™ System implanted with two stereotactically placed left temporal depth electrodes using an occipital approach. A horseshoe-shaped incision was planned in the left parieto-occipital region (**Fig. 19.5A and B**) and a single, left occipital bur hole was placed along with a templated craniotomy for the ferrule and pulse generator (**Fig. 19.6**). Next a bur hole base (Medtronic, Inc., Minneapolis, MN) and the RNS™ System ferrule were secured (**Fig. 19.7**). The depth electrodes

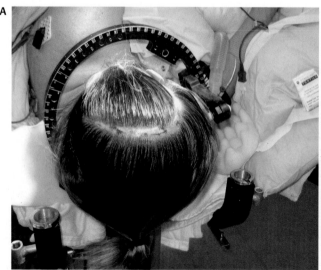
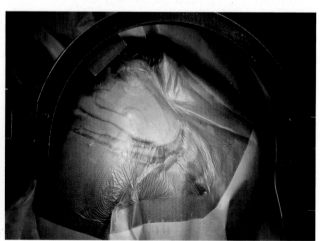

Fig. 19.5 Patient positioning and planning of the incision **(A)** and preparation **(B)** for implantation of an RNS™ System neurostimulator. (Courtesy of Neuropace, Inc., Sunnyvale, CA. Reprinted with permission.)

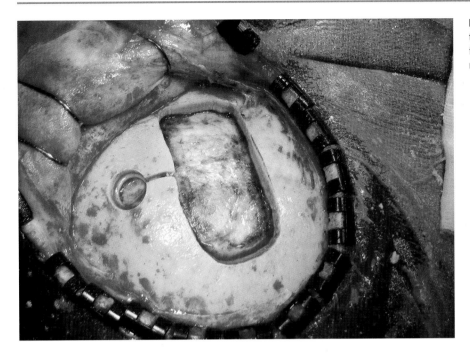

Fig. 19.6 Initial bur hole for depth electrode placement and template craniotomy for placement of RNS™ System ferrule and neurostimulator.

were then placed stereotactically (**Fig. 19.8**) and secured in the bur hole and the leads were connected to the neurostimulator, which is secured within the ferrule (**Fig. 19.9**).

Following implantation, detection algorithms were programmed to enable detection of the earliest possible onset of seizure activity for the patient. The detection algorithms are robust and include suggested algorithms for early detection based upon stored ECOGs.

Once detection parameters have been optimized, stimulation parameters can be programmed. Stimulation options are flexible and robust. Stimulation pathways can be any combination of nine possible contacts (eight electrode contacts plus the pulse generator housing), and parameters of frequency, duration of stimulation, pulse width, and current intensity can be varied. In addition, stimulation can be applied through various combinations of differing pulses or repetitive combinations of the same pulses. Achieving the most effective stimulation parameters for each individual patient remains one of the main challenges.

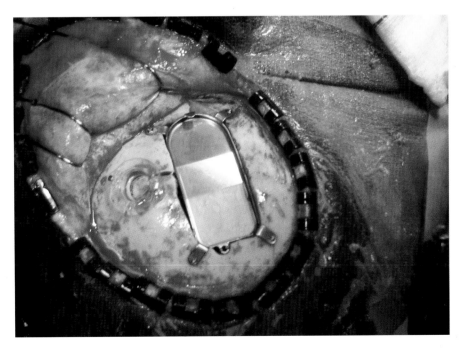

Fig. 19.7 Placement of RNS™ System ferrule into the template craniotomy.

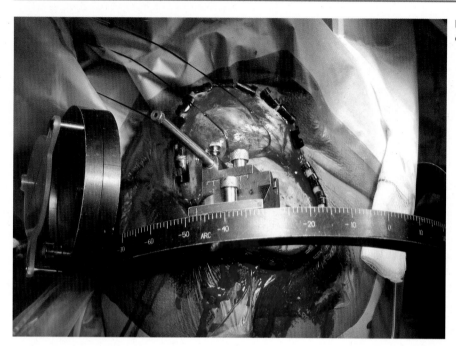

Fig. 19.8 Stereotactic placement of depth electrodes and RNS™ System neurostimulator.

Clinical Trials

Feasibility Clinical Trial

A feasibility investigation of the RNS™ System designed to assess safety with the secondary intent to gather seizure data for preliminary evidence of efficacy was completed in 2006. Patients were adults (18 to 65 years of age) with intractable partial onset seizures who had failed treatment with at least two antiepileptic drugs, and who had one or two localized epileptogenic onset zones and four or more seizures per month. Seizure frequency was assessed by a seizure diary and adverse events were monitored. The efficacy end point was defined as a 50% reduction in mean monthly seizure frequency. This was a multicenter design (12 sites) in which the first four subjects at each site entered an open-label protocol and subsequent subjects entered a double-blinded protocol. Following implantation there was a 28-day stabilization period during which detection parameters were optimized. A 3-month open-label or double-blinded efficacy evaluation was then completed followed by an open-label extension period to continue for 24 months after implant. Patients who completed the 24 months were eligible to enroll in a 5-year long-term treatment trial to assess ongoing safety and efficacy.

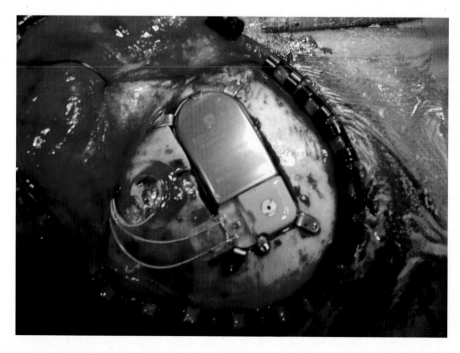

Fig. 19.9 Final placement of depth electrodes and RNS™ System neurostimulator.

Table 19.1 RNS™ System Feasibility Trial: Subject Demographics (*n* = 65)

Age (years)	31 (18–57)
Gender (female)	52%
Age at seizure onset (years)	14 (0–46)
Prior VNS	28%
Prior epilepsy surgery	37%
Intracranial monitoring	74%
Median baseline seizure rate	11/28 days

Data are current as of 12/31/2006; not completely verified.

Sixty-five subjects were implanted with the RNS™ System with a mean seizure frequency of 11 seizures per 28 days (**Table 19.1**). Thirty-seven percent had prior epilepsy surgery, and 28% had been previously treated with a vagus nerve stimulator (VNS). All 65 subjects completed the efficacy evaluation period with 50 subjects who received stimulation, 14 who were blinded off, and one open-label subject who did not receive stimulation during the efficacy evaluation period (**Table 19.2**). There were no unanticipated device-related serious adverse events. The study was not statistically powered to demonstrate efficacy. However, 32% of subjects demonstrated >50% reduction in seizures for complex partial seizures (CPS), 63% for generalized tonic-clonic seizures (GTCS), and 26% for simple partial motor, complex partial, and secondarily generalized tonic-clonic seizure combined (total disabling seizures [TDS]) (**Table 19.3**). In summary, the feasibility trial demonstrated that the RNS™ System device had an acceptable safety profile with no unanticipated serious device-related adverse events noted, and no unanticipated serious complications related to the surgical procedure. There was one death categorized by the data monitoring committee as probable sudden unexplained death in epilepsy (SUDEP). In addition there was preliminary evidence for efficacy with CPS and TDS. These data supported commencement of the long-term treatment trial and the start of a pivotal trial.

RNS™ System Pivotal Clinical Investigation in Epilepsy

The pivotal trial is a randomized, double-blinded, multicenter, sham-stimulation controlled clinical investigation designed to demonstrate safety and efficacy of the RNS™ System in reducing the frequency of disabling seizures in adults with medically intractable partial onset seizures. In this study, all patients will be randomized in a 1:1 fashion to sham stimulation or to active treatment. The plan is to enroll 240 patients at 28 sites. Inclusion criteria include age 18 to 70, with medically intractable partial epilepsy with seizure onset localized to one or two foci. Subjects must have an average of three or more disabling seizures for three consecutive 28-day periods and have failed at least two antiepileptic drugs. The trial design involves a baseline period in which subjects meet seizure frequency criteria, and a double-blinded efficacy analysis period followed by an open-label extension during which all subjects can receive stimulation (**Table 19.4**). All subjects will be followed for 2 years and then have the option of participating in the 5-year long-term treatment trial to assess ongoing safety and efficacy. This long-term treatment trial is currently in progress. Information regarding the pivotal trial and site information can be accessed at www.clinicaltrials.gov.

Case Examples

1. A 29-year-old man had intractable, simple and complex partial seizures with secondary generalization. Grid monitoring demonstrated a seizure focus in the left superior-posterior temporal lobe in the eloquent speech cortex near the area of a previous resection of an epidermoid cyst. The RNS™ System using two strip electrodes was implanted. Following optimization of detection algorithms, stimulation therapy was initiated using a pulse width of

Table 19.2 RNS™ System Feasibility Trial: Progress

- 65 subjects implanted with RNS™ System
  - All subjects completed efficacy evaluation period
    - 50 received stimulation
    - 1 never turned ON
    - 14 blinded OFF

- 127 patient years of experience (Feasibility & Long-term Treatment Trials)

- Subjects transitioning to long-term treatment trial
  - 23 subjects transitioned as of 12/31/2006

Table 19.3 RNS™ System Feasibility Trial: Efficacy Evaluation Period (*n* = 50)

- Subjects demonstrating >50% reduction in seizures
  - 32% (*n* = 44) for CPS
  - 63% (*n* = 16) for GTCS
  - 26% (*n* = 50) for total disabling seizures (SP motor, CPS, and GTCS combined)

Analysis excludes subjects who were blinded OFF.
Data not completely verified.

Table 19.4 RNS™ System Pivotal Trial: Timeline Schematic

	Enrollment / Implant Eligibility / Implant / Week 4	Week 8	Week 12	Week 20	Week 104
			Therapy ON Therapy OFF		(2 years postimplant)
	≤28 days				
Baseline Period (Min 12 weeks, Max 60 weeks)		Postop Stabilization and Stimulation Optimization Periods	Blinded Evaluation Period (12 weeks)		Open-Label Evaluation Period (84 weeks)
Assessment Protocol					
		Treatment Protocol			

200 microseconds, a pulse duration of 100 milliseconds, and a current of 8 mA. Since the initiation of therapy with the neurostimulator, the patient became seizure free and has remained so for 29 months (**Fig. 19.10**). He has obtained a driver's license and has full-time employment. His ECoGs and treatment log reveal that 40 to 400 stimulation treatments per day are administered following the detection of epileptogenic activity.

2. A 53-year-old woman had an 8-year history of complex partial seizures that began following an episode of viral encephalitis. EEG monitoring revealed independent bilateral temporal foci and MRI revealed bilateral mesial temporal sclerosis. Bilateral medial temporal depth elec-

trodes were implanted (**Fig. 19.11**). An example of the neurostimulator detection (**Fig. 19.11**) reveals a seizure of right temporal onset (**Fig. 19.12**). Effective stimulation parameters were found to suppress seizure activity in the right temporal lobe (**Fig. 19.13**). Application of similar stimulation parameters to the left temporal lobe seizure foci, however, was not effective (**Fig. 19.14**). Effective stimulation of the left temporal lobe seizure activity required different stimulation parameters (**Fig. 19.15**). The effectiveness of stimulation improved with increased duration of the stimulation (**Fig. 19.16**), and the patient became a consistent responder with >50% reduction in seizures only after 16 months of stimulation.

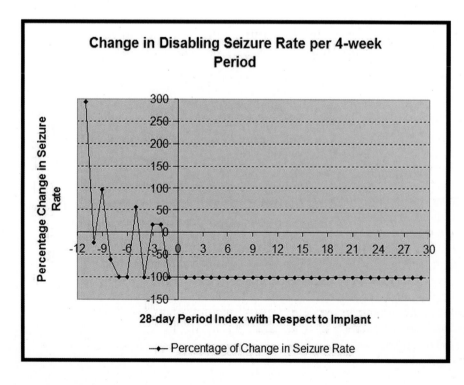

Fig. 19.10 Case 1. Changes in the rate of disabling seizures per 4-week period reveal no seizures since the activation of responsive neurostimulation therapy.

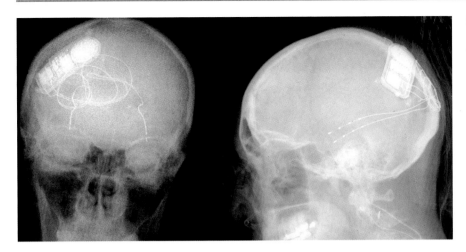

Q11

Fig. 19.11 Case 2. Anteroposterior and lateral skull x-rays of bilateral temporal depth electrodes and the RNS™ System neurostimulator.

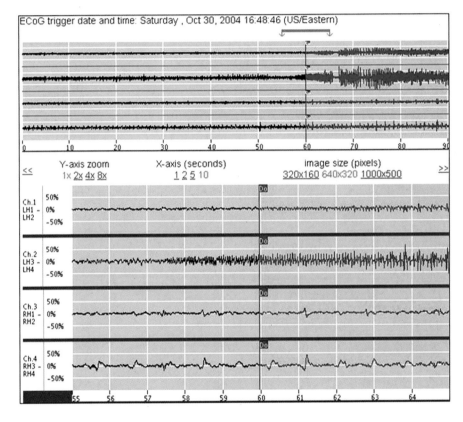

Fig. 19.12 Case 2. Example of stored ECoG demonstrating a seizure of left temporal origin.

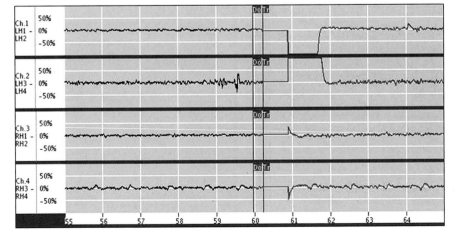

Fig. 19.13 Case 2. Example of left temporal detection and therapy using contacts 1 negative and 4 positive. Stimulation parameters are a frequency of 100 Hz, amplitude of 6 mA, pulse duration of 100 milliseconds, and a pulse width of 200 microseconds.

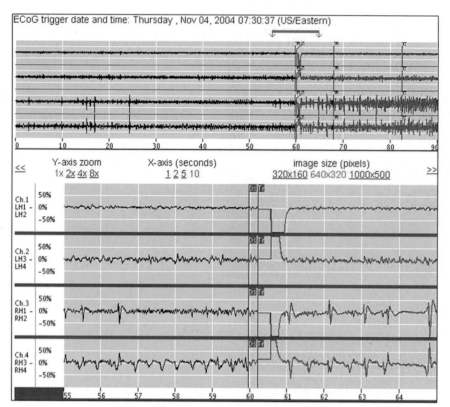

Fig. 19.14 Case 2. An example of ineffective stimulation of a seizure of right temporal lobe onset. Stimulation parameters are identical to those that were effective for left temporal seizure activity shown in **Fig. 19.13** and are a frequency of 100 Hz, amplitude of 6 mA, pulse duration of 100 milliseconds, and a pulse width of 200 microseconds.

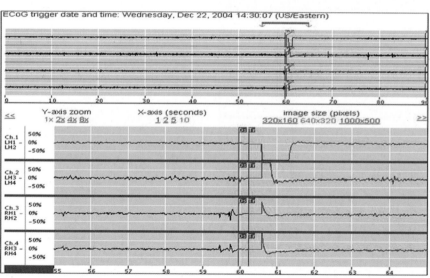

Fig. 19.15 Case 2. This figure demonstrates effective stimulation for suppression of right temporal lobe seizure-like activity. The parameters required (frequency 20 Hz, amplitude 10 mA, pulse width 200 microseconds, pulse duration 100 milliseconds) differed from stimulation parameters that were effective in the left temporal lobe.

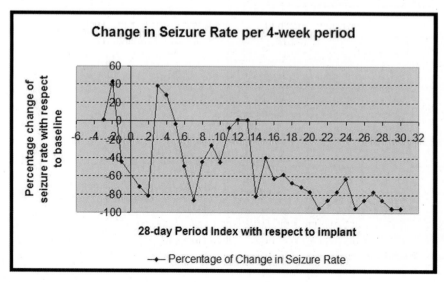

Fig. 19.16 Case 2. Seizure history reveals improved seizure control with increased duration of stimulation. The patient became a consistent responder only after 16 months of stimulation.

Conclusions

The RNS™ System has thus far demonstrated excellent safety. Responsive stimulation has been applied to all regions of the cortex. Preliminary evidence of efficacy was provided by the feasibility trial. Different electrographic onset patterns may require different stimulation programs, and the efficacy of stimulation may increase with the duration of the stimulation. This technology may ultimately provide an exciting new treatment option for a subgroup of patients with medically intractable epilepsy, but efficacy remains to be demonstrated by the ongoing pivotal trial.

References

1. Hauser WA, Annegers JF, Kurland LT. Prevalence of epilepsy in Rochester, Minnesota: 1940–1980. Epilepsia 1991;32(4):429–445
2. Frisch G, Hitzig E. Ueber die elektrische Erregbarkeit des Grosshirnes. Arch Anat Physiol (Leipzig) 1870;1:300–332
3. Pearce JM. Sir David Ferrier MD, FRS. J Neurol Neurosurg Psychiatry 2003;74(6):787
4. Penfield W, Jasper HH. Epilepsy and the Functional Anatomy of the Human Brain. 1st ed. Boston: Little; 1954
5. Cooper IS, Amin I, Gilman S. The effect of chronic cerebellar stimulation upon epilepsy in man. Trans Am Neurol Assoc 1973;98:192–196
6. Cooper IS, Amin I, Riklan M, Waltz JM, Poon TP. Chronic cerebellar stimulation in epilepsy. Clinical and anatomical studies. Arch Neurol 1976;33(8):559–570
7. Cooper IS, Amin I, Upton A, Riklan M, Watkins S, McLellan L. Safety and efficacy of chronic cerebellar stimulation. Appl Neurophysiol 1977;40(2–4):124–134
8. Van Buren JM, Wood JH, Oakley J, Hambrecht F. Preliminary evaluation of cerebellar stimulation by double-blind stimulation and biological criteria in the treatment of epilepsy. J Neurosurg 1978;48(3):407–416
9. Wright GD, McLellan DL, Brice JG. A double-blind trial of chronic cerebellar stimulation in twelve patients with severe epilepsy. J Neurol Neurosurg Psychiatry 1984;47(8):769–774
10. Velasco F, Carrillo-Ruiz JD, Brito F, et al. Double-blind, randomized controlled pilot study of bilateral cerebellar stimulation for treatment of intractable motor seizures. Epilepsia 2005;46(7):1071–1081
11. Fisher RS, Uematsu S, Krauss GL, et al. Placebo-controlled pilot study of centromedian thalamic stimulation in treatment of intractable seizures. Epilepsia 1992;33(5):841–851
12. Velasco F, Velasco M, Ogarrio C, Fanghanel G. Electrical stimulation of the centromedian thalamic nucleus in the treatment of convulsive seizures: a preliminary report. Epilepsia 1987;28(4):421–430
13. Hodaie M, Wennberg RA, Dostrovsky JO, Lozano AM. Chronic anterior thalamus stimulation for intractable epilepsy. Epilepsia 2002; 43(6):603–608
14. Kerrigan JF, Litt B, Fisher RS, et al. Electrical stimulation of the anterior nucleus of the thalamus for the treatment of intractable epilepsy. Epilepsia 2004;45(4):346–354
15. Upton AR, Cooper IS, Springman M, Amin I. Suppression of seizures and psychosis of limbic system origin by chronic stimulation of anterior nucleus of the thalamus. Int J Neurol 1985;19–20:223–230
16. Chabardes S, Kahane P, Minotti L, Koudsie A, Hirsch E, Benabid AL. Deep brain stimulation in epilepsy with particular reference to the subthalamic nucleus. Epileptic Disord 2002;4(Suppl 3):S83–S93
17. Loddenkemper T, Pan A, Neme S, et al. Deep brain stimulation in epilepsy. J Clin Neurophysiol 2001;18(6):514–532
18. Velasco M, Velasco F, Velasco AL, et al. Subacute electrical stimulation of the hippocampus blocks intractable temporal lobe seizures and paroxysmal EEG activities. Epilepsia 2000;41(2):158–169
19. Mirski MA, Fisher RS. Electrical stimulation of the mammillary nuclei increases seizure threshold to pentylenetetrazol in rats. Epilepsia 1994;35(6):1309–1316
20. Chkhenkeli SA, Chkhenkeli IS. Effects of therapeutic stimulation of nucleus caudatus on epileptic electrical activity of brain in patients with intractable epilepsy. Stereotact Funct Neurosurg 1997;69(1–4, Pt 2):221–224
21. Engel J Jr. Excitation and inhibition in epilepsy. Can J Neurol Sci 1996;23(3):167–174
22. Kreindler A. Active arrest mechanisms of epileptic seizures. Epilepsia 1962;3:329–337
23. Benabid AL, Minotti L, Koudsie A, de Saint Martin A, Hirsch E. Antiepileptic effect of high-frequency stimulation of the subthalamic nucleus (corpus luysi) in a case of medically intractable epilepsy caused by focal dysplasia: a 30-month follow-up: technical case report. Neurosurgery 2002;50(6):1385–1391, discussion 1391–1392
24. Vonck K, Boon P, Goossens L, et al. Neurostimulation for refractory epilepsy. Acta Neurol Belg 2003;103(4):213–217

V Radiosurgery

20 Radiosurgery

Jean Régis, Fabrice Bartolomei, and Patrick Chauvel

There is growing interest in the use of radiosurgery for treating medically intractable epilepsy. Our local clinical experience (122 patients), accumulated over the past 13 years, mainly includes treatment of temporal lobe epilepsy (56 patients), including 49 with pure mesial temporal lobe epilepsy (MTLE), 55 hypothalamic hamartomas (HHs), two callosotomies, and 11 other kind of epilepsies. The review of our cases, as well as other clinical and experimental data, suggests that the use of radiosurgery is beneficial only to those patients in whom a strict preoperative definition of the extent of the epileptogenic zone (or network) has been achieved, and where strict rules of dose planning have been followed. As soon as these principles are not observed, the risk of treatment failure and or side effects increases dramatically. Long-term outcome data are presently available for MTLE but not yet for other epilepsies.

Rationale

There are convincing arguments for investigating the potential role of radiosurgery for medically intractable seizures.

1. Radiosurgery (since its introduction in the 1950s) has been demonstrated to have advantages in terms of safety and efficacy, for the treatment of numerous small, deeply seated intracerebral lesions.
2. Radiosurgical treatment of small cortico-subcortical lesions associated with epilepsy has been demonstrated to lead to seizure cessation in a high percentage (58 to 80% in arteriovenous malformations [AVM]) of cases, long before the expected cure of the lesion and sometimes even in spite of radiosurgery's inability to totally eliminate the AVM.
3. Radiotherapeutic treatment of epilepsies with or without space-occupying lesions can lead to a reduction in seizure frequency and/or severity.
4. Experimental models of epilepsies treated with radiation therapy have demonstrated a dose-dependant positive effect of radiation on the frequency and severity of the seizures, and on the extent of discharge propagation.

Among 6102 Gamma Knife (GK) surgery procedures accomplished in our neurosurgical unit in a 14-year period (between July 1992 and December 2006), only 122 were performed in patients referred for epilepsy surgery (nine patients/year). The strategy of our treating team is to define the niche of patients in whom the safety/efficacy ratio makes radiosurgery advantageous or at least comparable to

craniotomy. Radiosurgery represents a small subset (15%) of patients in our overall epilepsy surgery series.

Lars Leksell conceived GK radiosurgery as a tool for functional neurosurgery.[1,2] Accordingly, he used GK in movement disorders, trigeminal neuralgia, and other pain syndromes, but not for epilepsy surgery.[3] The first radiosurgical treatments for epilepsy surgery were performed by Talairach in the fifties.[4] Unlike Leksell, he had specific expertise in epilepsy surgery and led one of the first large comprehensive programs for epilepsy surgery. As early as 1974, he reported on the use of radioactive Yttrium implants in patients with MTLE without space-occupying lesions, and he showed a high rate of seizure control in patients with epilepsies confined to the mesial structures of the temporal lobe.[4] In 1980, Elomaa,[5] promoted the idea of the use of focal irradiation for the treatment of temporal lobe epilepsy, based on the preliminary reports of Baudouin and Von Wieser.[6,7] Furthermore, clinical experience of the use of GK- and Linac-based radiosurgery in AVMs and cortico-subcortical tumors (mostly metastases and low-grade glial tumors) revealed an anticonvulsive effect of radiosurgery in absence of tissue necrosis.[8–10] A series of experimental studies in small animals confirmed this effect[11,12] and emphasized its relationship to the dose delivered.[13–16] Barcia Salorio et al, and later Lindquist et al, reported small and heterogenous groups of patients treated with the purpose of seizure cessation; their results, however, were poor.[17–20] Unfortunately, these results were never published in peer-reviewed articles.

The Department of Stereotactic and Functional Surgery at Timone University Hospital in Marseille is a major referral center for epilepsy surgery and radiosurgery. This expertise has facilitated the investigation and development of a potential role for GK radiosurgery in the treatment of intractable epilepsy. Since 1993, we have performed 122 cases of epilepsy surgery using GK radiosurgery. The majority of these patients presented with MTLE (56 patients) or HH (55 patients). The rest of the patients suffered from severe epilepsy associated with small benign lesions (11 patients), for which an epileptic zone was considered to be confined to the surrounding cortex.[21] In HH, GK radiosurgery offers very low morbidity, with similar efficacy when compared with microsurgical alternatives.[22,23] This has led us to consider radiosurgery systematically as the first-line treatment in patients with small HH of type I, II, III, and possibly type IV.[23] In MTLE, on the other hand, in spite of a good short- and middle-term safety-efficacy ratio,[24–26] the use of GK is still regarded as investigational,[25] given the well-established

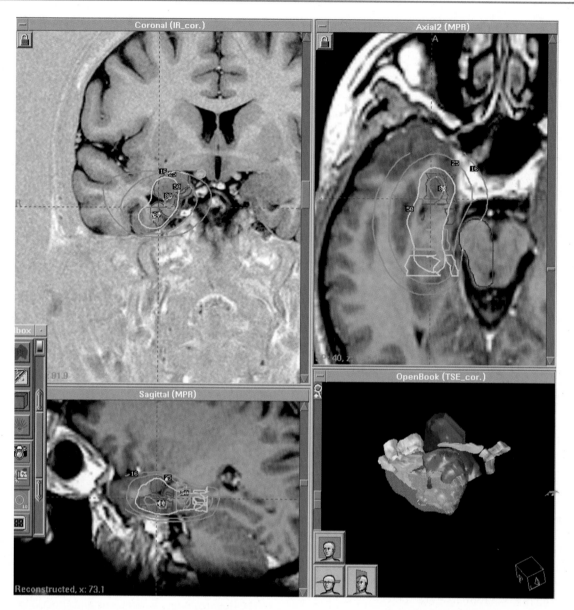

Fig. 20.1 Gamma Knife radiosurgery for a right MTLE. The dose is 24 Gy at the 50% isodose line (*yellow*). Doses to the brainstem are <12 Gy (25%), and the dose to the optic chiasm is <8 Gy (16%). Note the sparing of a large part of the amygdaloid complex and hippocampal head. Complete seizure cessation occurred 12 months after radiosurgery with no complication and no (even transient) side effects.

long-term safety and efficacy of the microsurgical resection in the temporal lobe. Since 1994, we have promoted the idea that seizure cessation may be generated by a specific neuromodulatory effect of radiosurgery, without induction of a significant amount of histological necrosis.[27–32] The selection of the appropriate technical parameters (dose, volume target, etc) allowing us to accurately obtain the desired functional effect without histological damage, remains an important challenge (**Fig. 20.1**).

Hypothalamic Hamartomas

HHs may be asymptomatic, associated with precocious puberty or with neurological disorders (including epilepsy, behavior disturbances, and cognitive impairment), or both. Usually, the seizures begin early in life and are often particularly drug-resistant from the outset. The natural history is unfavorable in the majority of the patients because of behavioral symptoms (particularly aggressive behavior) and mental decline, which occur as a direct effect of the seizures.[33] Interestingly, in our experience, the reversal of these behavioral symptoms after radiosurgery seems to begin even before complete cessation of the seizures and seems to be correlated to the improvement in background EEG activity. It is the authors' speculation that these continuous discharges lead to the disorganization of several systems, including the limbic system, and that their disappearance accounts for the improvement seen in attention, memory, cognitive performance, and impulsive behavior, etc. In these cases, radiosurgery's role in the reversal of the behavioral symptoms may be as or more important than its effect on decreasing seizures. Consequently, we consider that it is essential to operate on these young patients as early as possible, whatever the surgical approach considered (resection or radiosurgery).

The intrinsic epileptogenicity of HH has been demonstrated[34,35] even though the mechanisms of the epilepsy associated with HH are still debatable. The boundary of the target zone of treatment is that of the lesion visualized on magnetic resonance imaging (MRI). This contrasts greatly with cases of MTLE where there is no such clear delineation of an epileptogenic zone on the images used for planning radiosurgical intervention.

We retrospectively analyzed radiosurgery in a series of 10 patients collected from centers around the world.[22] The excellent safety-efficacy ratio (all improved, 50% cured and no adverse effects except one case of poikilothermia) led us to organize a prospective multicenter trial. Our series of 55 prospectively evaluated patients has been published in a preliminary report.[23] The number of patients operated by GK more than 3 years ago was 31, with a satisfactory follow-up being available for 27 patients. The preoperative cognitive deficits, behavioral disturbances, and investigated relationship of seizure severity and anatomical type to cognitive abilities were characterized.[36,37] The goal of the preoperative workup was to adequately select the candidates for inclusion and to evaluate the baseline neurological and endocrinological functions. All radiosurgical procedures were performed using the Leksell 201-source Cobalt 60 Gamma Knife (Elekta Instrument, Stockholm, Sweden). Consistently we developed multi-isocentric complex dose planning of high conformity and selectivity (**Fig. 20.2**). We used low peripheral doses to take into account the close relationship with the optic pathways and the hypothalamus (median 17 Gy; range 13 to 26 Gy). The lesions treated are generally small (median 9.5 mm; range 5 to 26 mm, **Fig. 20.2**). We pay special attention to the dose delivered to the mamillary body and to the fornix, and we always try to tailor the dose plan for each patient, based on the use of a single run of shots with the 4-mm collimator. Patients were evaluated with respect to seizures, cognition, behavior, and endocrine status 6, 12, 18, 24, and 36 months after radiosurgery and then every year. Among those, 10 are seizure free (37%), six are very much improved (22.2%) with a significant seizure reduction (usually only rare residual gelastic seizures) and with a dramatic behavioral and cognitive improvement. Overall an excellent result has been obtained in 60% of patients. Our strategy is to offer the patient and the family are offered a second radiosurgery in case of partial benefit when the lesion is anatomically small and well defined. Five patients (18.5%) with small hamartomas were only modestly improved and are being considered for two sessions of radiosurgery. Two have until

now reported no significant improvement. A microsurgical approach has been performed in four patients (14.8%) with quite large HHs and poor efficacy of radiosurgery. After this microsurgical approach, two are cured and two are failures. The radiosurgical treatment has been performed twice in nine patients.

Effect of Gamma Knife Surgery on Behavior and Cognitive Functions

The improvement was dramatic, in nine of these patients. All the patients with paroxystic aggressivity improved substantially. Increased alertness, elevated mood, and greater speech production were observed in some patients characterized by excessive behavioral inhibition. A positive effect on sleep was frequently reported by the parents, mainly in the younger patients. Finally, dramatic developmental acceleration was observed in three young patients.

Topological Classification

Topological classification of the lesion based on good high-resolution MRI is a key feature in the decision-making process.[23] Previous classification has been based on anatomical[38-40] or surgical[41] considerations. These classifications do not describe the large diversity of these lesions and their therapeutic consequences. As underlined by Palmini and coworkers, the exact location of the lesion in relation to the interpeduncular fossa and the walls of the third ventricle correlates with the extent of excision, seizure control, and complication rate.[42] On this basis, we classify the HH according to their topology based on our original classification.[23,43] In our experience this classification correlates with the clinical semiology and severity and is especially critical for surgical strategy selection. Type I HHs (small HH located inside the hypothalamus extending more or less into the third ventricle) are certainly the best candidates for GK surgery. In this population the morbidity of microsurgical removal is likely to be potentially high.

In type II (when the lesion is small and mainly in the third ventricle) radiosurgery is certainly a safer alternative. Even though the endoscopic and transcallosal interforniceal approach has been well described (see Chapter 9), the risks of short-term memory worsening, endocrinological disturbance (hyperphagia with obesity, low tyroxine, sodium metabolism disturbance), and thalamic or thalamocapsular infarcts have been reported even in the hands of highly skilled and experienced neurosurgeons. In exceptional cases of recurrent status epilepticus we recommend open surgery through either a transcallosal interforniceal approach or an endoscopic approach (depending on the width of the third ventricle). If the lesion is small and the third ventricle large, an endoscopic approach is chosen.

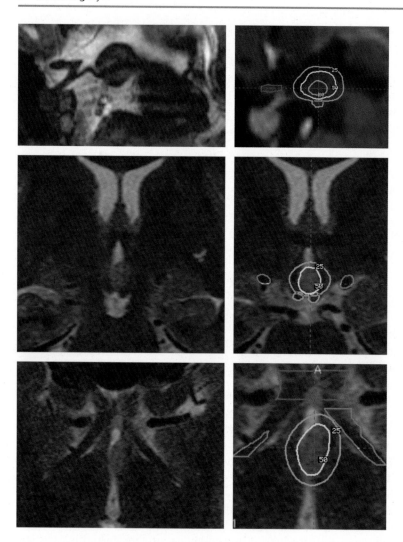

Fig. 20.2 Typical good indication of radiosurgery in hypothalamic hamartoma type II according to our original classification (ref). The dose at the margin was 17 Gy.[23,43] The volume of the target is 268,2 mm³. The average number of seizures prior to radiosurgery was 300 per month. Five months after radiosurgery seizures have disappeared completely.

In type III (lesion located essentially in the floor) with the extremely close relationship between the mammilary body, the fornix, and the lesion, we prefer GK surgery. We speculate that sessile HHs have always more or less of an "extension" into the hypothalamus close to the mammilary body. Thus when a lesion is classified as a type II, that means that the lesion appears on the MRI as being located in the third ventricle but is likely to have a "root" in the hypothalamus. The same assumption is made for type III.

In type IV (the lesion sessile in the cistern) a disconnection can be discussed (pterional approach with or without orbitozygomatic osteotomy). However, if the lesion is small, GK surgery can be recommended due to its safety and to its ability to simultaneously treat the small associated part of the lesion in the hypothalamus itself, frequently visible on the high-resolution MRI. In Delalande's experience only two patients among 14 are seizure free after a single disconnection through a pterional approach.[41] Consequently, we only recommend this approach in cases of lesions too large for GK surgery as a first step of a staged approach. In most circumstances, the patient is improved but not seizure free after

the first surgical step, and GKS is organized at 3 months as a second step in the treatment.

Type V HHs (pediculate) are rarely epileptic and can be easily cured by radiosurgery or disconnection through a pterional approach. In cases of severe epilepsy the second therapeutic modality will result in a more rapid cessation of seizures. However, a distant extension of the HH in the hypothalamus close to the mammillary bodies must be cautiously searched for on high-resolution MRI, and its discovery will eventually lead to the recommendation of GK surgery, allowing for treatment of both parts of the lesion, especially in cases in which the cisternal component is small.

Type VI (giant) are not good candidates for up-front radiosurgery, and in nearly all the cases, a combination of several therapeutic modalities should be utilized (**Fig. 20.3**). Even if GK surgery does not seem to be suitable when the lesion is large, "radiosurgical" disconnection can been be envisaged. Radiosurgically targetting only the superior part in the hypothalamus and/or the third ventricle leaving untreated all of the lesion lower than the floor has been uniformly

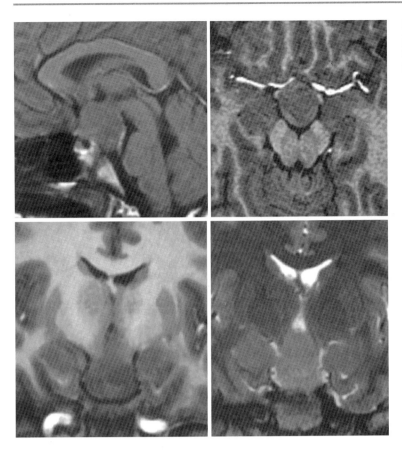

Fig. 20.3 Typical good indication for a combined approach. Our proposal in this case is a disconnection by a pterional approach and then a radiosurgery on the residual.

disappointing. In our opinion, this strategy in children may result in a loss of precious developmental time in which a child could be treated effectively. Consequently, we do not advocate such a strategy. When microsurgical resection has left a small remnant in the third ventricle and the patient is not seizure free, we recommend GK surgery.

Limits and Strengths of Radiosurgery in Hypothalamic Hamartoma

Two major questions remain. First, we know that complete treatment or resection of the lesion is not always necessary for control,[44-46] but we do not know how to predict in an individual patient the amount (and mapping) of the HH that must be treated to obtain a complete antiepileptic effect. Second, we know that these patients frequently present with an electroclinical semiology suggesting involvement of the temporal or frontal lobe and which can mimic a secondary epileptogenesis phenomenon.[35,47] In our experience, some of these patients can be completely cured by the isolated treatment of the HH, whereas in others, a partial result is obtained, with residual seizures despite a significant overall psychiatric and cognitive improvement. In this second group, it is tempting to propose that such a secondary epileptogenic area accounts for the partial failure.

Our initial results indicate that GK surgery is as effective as microsurgical resection with reduced morbidity. GK sur-

gery also avoids the vascular risk related to radiofrequency lesioning or stimulation. The disadvantage of radiosurgery is its delayed action. Longer follow-up is mandatory for proper evaluation of the role of GK surgery. Results are faster and more complete in patients with smaller lesions inside the third ventricle (stage II). The early effect on subclinical EEG discharges appears to play a major role in the dramatic benefit to sleep quality, behavior, and cognitive-developmental improvement. GK surgery can safely lead to the reversal of the epileptic encephalopathy.

Due to the poor clinical prognosis of a majority of patients with HH and the invasiveness of microsurgical resection, GK can be now be considered a first-line intervention for small- to middle-sized HH associated with epilepsy, as it can lead to dramatic improvements in these unfortunate young patients. The role of secondary epileptogenesis or of widespread cortical dysgenesis in these patients needs to be further evaluated and understood, to optimize patient selection and define the best treatment strategy.

Mesial Temporal Lobe Epilepsy

The first GK surgery operations for MTLE were performed in Marseille in March 1993. As far as no similar experience was available at that time in the literature, we were obliged to base our technical choices on the experience of radiosurgery for other pathological conditions. Four patients were treated with different technical strategies (dose, volume, target definition). The delayed, huge radiological changes observed some months after radiosurgery[30] led us to stop such treatment and follow these first four patients. Due to the clinical safety of the procedure in these patients and the gradual disappearance of the acute changes shown on the MR after some months, we treated several new series of patients under strict prospective controlled trial conditions (with ethical committee approval). The treatment for the following 17 patients was based upon that of the first patient who had a successful outcome (as opposed to the three others who had partial or no effect). This "classic planning" (**Fig. 20.1**) was based on the use of two 18-mm shots, covering a volume of around 7 cc at the 50% isodose (24 Gy), and has turned out to produce a high rate of seizure cessation.[24,26]

To decrease morbidity, the targeting was centered on the parahippocampal cortex and spared a significant part of the amygdaloid complex and hippocampus. The refinement of the GK surgery technique, and the desire to find a dose which would create less transient acute changes shown on the MR, led us to reduce the dose from 24 Gy to 20 Gy, and 18 Gy at the margin. However, this brought about a significant decrease in the rate of seizure cessation. We have recently reviewed the long-term follow-up of our first 15 patients operated by GK surgery for MTLE at the state of the art (24 Gy). The mean follow-up was 8 years, and at the last follow-up, 73% were seizure free. These long-term results compare favorably with open surgery. No permanent neurological deficit was reported out of a visual field deficit in nine patients.[48]

The timetable of events after radiosurgery and the follow-up is quite standardized. Patients are informed that delayed efficacy of radiosurgery is its main drawback. Typically, the frequency of the seizures is not modified significantly for the first few months. Thereafter, there is a rapid and dramatic increase in auras for some days or weeks, and then the seizures disappear. Usually the peak in seizure cessation is observed around the eighth to 18th month with a clear variability in the delay in onset. In one patient, this occurred 26 months after GK radiosurgery. We usually consider a delay of 2 years as a minimum for postradiosurgery follow-up. In the absence of initial radiological changes or clinical benefit, the recommendation is to wait for the onset of the MRI changes and their subsequent disappearance. All our patients had the same pattern of MR changes whatever marginal dose (18 to 24 Gy) and volume of treatment (5 to 8.5 cc) were used. However, the degree of these changes and their delay of onset varied according to the dose delivered to the margin, the volume treated, and the individual patient. To allow an optimal evaluation, we recommend that subsequent microsurgery not be considered before the third year after radiosurgery. Similarly, we believe that a patient who undergoes a craniotomy before the onset of the MR changes has occurred cannot be assumed to have failed radiosurgical treatment. Before considering any further surgery, the reason for the treatment failure needs to be addressed. After reviewing files of patients treated for MTLE with radiosur-

gery, it was sometimes possible to identify likely causes of failure, such as:

1. Poor patient selection (e.g., patients with epilepsy involving more than the MTL structures)
2. Patients with the diagnosis of "treatment failure" (<3 years) who had been operated upon too early after radiosurgery[11]
3. Targeting of the amygdala and hippocampus (which is not in our opinion the optimal target in term of safety and efficacy) instead of the parahippocampal cortex[49]
4. Insufficient dosage[50,51]

Our current strategy of treatment is based on our first series of MTLE patients who were strictly selected and treated systematically with a very simple but very reproducible dose-planning strategy.[26,32] The identification of putative improvements in the methodology requires a systematic analysis of the influence of the technical data from our experience and from the literature on the outcome of those patients.

Technical Questions

The Dose Issue

The first targets used in functional GK radiosurgery (capsulotomy, thalamotomy of ventral intermedius (VIM) or the centromedianum, pallidotomy) were treated using high doses (300 to 150 Gy) delivered in very small volumes (3 to 5 mm in diameter).[3] The goal was to ablate a predefined, very small anatomical structure with stereotactic precision. Significant variability in the delay and amplitude of the MR changes has been reported with defined doses.[52,53]

Barcia Salorio et al have documented a small and heterogeneous group of patients treated with different types of radiosurgical techniques and variable patient-to-patient dosimetry.[54] Some of these patients had no expanding lesion and were treated with very large volumes and very low doses (around 10 Gy). Based on this experience, several teams have suggested that very low doses, as low as 10 to 20 Gy at the margin, should be as effective as the 24 Gy protocol (at the margin) that we used for our first series of patients with MTLE.[26]

A careful review of the last Congress proceeding of Barcia Salorio et al pools patient data on the margin dose, and the volume and topography of the epileptogenic zone. Moreover, among the 11 patients reported, the real rate of seizure cessation is apparently only 36% (4/11), which is much lower than what we would expect with resection in MTLE.[2] In a heterogeneous group of 176 patients, Yang et al confirmed that only a very low rate of seizure control is achieved when low doses (from 9 to 13 Gy at the margin) are used.[51]

The experience of the radiosurgical treatment of HH indicates that 18 Gy at the margin appears to be a threshold in terms of probability of seizure cessation.[22] In this group of patients (36 cases), only one showed MR changes. The majority of the AVM case patients with worsening seizures were treated with a range of doses between 15 and 18 Gy. Similarly, poor results have been reported by Cmelak et al in one case patient with MTLE treated with Linac-based radiosurgery, with 15 Gy at the 60% isodose line, who underwent surgical resection 1 year later. In this case, the authors first observed a slight improvement followed by an obvious worsening.[50] A desescalation study has allowed us to demonstrate poorer results in patients receiving doses of 18 or 20 Gy at the margin as compared with 24 Gy.[55,56] Due to the rate of seizure cessation that is achievable by conventional resection, a radiosurgical strategy associated with a much lower rate of seizure cessation appears unacceptable. Fractionated stereotactically guided radiotherapy has been demonstrated to fail systematically in controlling seizures. Among 12 patients treated by Grabenbauer et al, none have achieved seizure cessation; only seizure reduction was obtained in this series.[57,58]

Experimental studies on small animals have demonstrated the antiepileptic effect of radiosurgery,[13,15,59] the dose dependence of this effect,[13–15,60] and the possibility of obtaining clear antiepileptic effect without macroscopic necrosis using certain doses.[14] Although the rat model of epilepsy is not an ideal model of human MTLE, it is intriguing to notice that similar to our clinical experience in humans, a similar maximum dose range of 40 to 50 Gy is currently the dose range that provides the optimal safety-efficacy ratio.

Target Definition

When the target is a lesion that is precisely defined radiologically, the question of the selection of the marginal dose can be quite easily addressed by correlating safety-efficacy individual outcome to the marginal dose. This can be refined based upon stratification according to volume, location, age, etc. However, in patients presenting with MTLE, this process is invalid for two reasons. First, there is no consensus regarding the requirement for the extent of mesial temporal lobe resection. Second, the concept of MTLE syndrome with a stable extent of the epileptogenic zone and surgical target is increasingly a topic of debate.[61,62]

The volume (in association with marginal dose) is well known to be a major determinant of the tissue effect, as shown in integrated risk/dose volume formulae.[63] In the first series of patients that we treated, this marginal isodose volume (or prescription isodose volume) was ~7 cc (range 5 to 8,5 cc).

An attempt to correlate dose/volume and the effect on seizures and on the MR changes (as evaluated by volume of the contrast enhancement ring, extent of the high T2 signal, and the importance of the mass effect) has been published.[55] In this study, we found, not surprisingly, that the higher the dose and the volume, the higher the risk of having more severe MR changes, but also the higher the chance of achieving seizure cessation. However, these data may have limited value. Hence, more precise identification of those structures

of the mesial temporal lobe that need to be "covered" by the radiosurgical treatment may allow more selective, but just as efficacious, dose-planning strategies, in spite of smaller prescription isodose volumes.

There is growing evidence to support the organization of the epileptogenic zone in networks, meaning that several different and possibly distant structures are discharging simultaneously at the onset of the electroclinical seizure. This kind of organization explains why the risk of failure is so high when a simple topectomy (without preoperative investigations) is performed in severe drug-resistant epilepsies associated with a benign lesion.[64] This has been also reported in MTLE.[61,62] Certain nuclei of the amygdaloid complex of the head, body, tail of the hippocampus, of the perirhinal, entorhinal (EC), and parahippocampal cortices may be associated with genesis of the seizures. The role of the EC cortex in epilepsy is supported by experimental studies in animals.[65,66] The EC is considered to be the amplifier of the "amygdalohippocampal epileptic system." The pattern of the associated structures, including that of the structure playing the lead role, can vary significantly from one patient to another.[61,62] There is a subgroup of patients who have clonic discharges and the involvement of the EC, amygdale, and head of the hippocampus, with a clear lead role of the EC. Wieser et al have analyzed the postoperative MR images of patients operated by Yasargil (amygdalohippocampectomy) and was able to correlate the quality of the resection of each substructure of the mesial temporal lobe area and the outcome with respect to seizures.[67] Only the quality of the removal of the anterior parahippocampal cortex was correlated strongly with a higher chance of seizure cessation.[67] We tried to perform a similar study in patients treated with GK radiosurgery.[55] We defined and manually drew the limits of subregions on the stereotactic images of all these patients. The amygdala, the head, the body, and the tail of the hippocampus were first delineated. The white matter, the parahippocampal cortex, and the cortex of the anterior wall of the collateral fissure were then separately drawn and divided into four sectors in the rostrocaudal axis, corresponding to the amygdala, the head, the body, and the tail of the hippocampus.[55]

Patient Selection

Whang et al treated patients with epilepsy associated with slowly growing lesions and observed seizure cessation in only 38% (12/31) of the patients[68] This kind of observation emphasizes the importance of preoperative definition of the extent of the epileptic zone and of its relationship with the lesion.[64,69] In our institution, the philosophy is to adapt the investigations for each individual case. In some patients, the electroclinical data, the structural and functional imaging, and the neuropsychological examination are sufficiently concordant for surgery of the temporal lobe to be proposed without depth electrode recording. In other cases, the level of evidence for MTLE is judged insufficient, and a stereoelectroencephalographic (SEEG) study is performed. The strategy of SEEG implantation is based on the primary hypothesis (mesial epileptogenic zone) and alternative hypotheses (early involvement of the temporal pole, lateral cortex, basal cortex, insular cortex, or other cortical areas). The goal of these studies is to record the patient's habitual seizures, to establish the temporospatial pattern of involvement of the cortical structures during these seizures. Clearly, in these patients, the high resolution of depth electrode recording allows fine tailoring of surgical resection, according to the precise temporospatial course of the seizures. The main limitation of radiosurgery is that of size of the target (prescription isodose volume). The radiosurgical treatment of MTLE is certainly the most selective surgical therapy for this group of patients. The requirements for precision and accuracy in the definition of the epileptogenic zone is consequently higher. Furthermore, if depth electrode investigation enables demonstration of a particular subtype of MTLE, this can lead to tailoring of the treatment volume and frequently allows this to be reduced.

Potential Concerns

The risk of long-term complications must always be cautiously scrutinized in functional neurosurgery. Radiotherapy is most frequently used in the brain for short-term life-threatening pathologies. The use of radiotherapy in young patients with benign disease such as pituitary adenomas or craniopharyngiomas has been associated with a significant rate of cognitive decline[70,71] and tumor genesis[72] including some carcinogenesis.[73] If the risk of radiation-induced tumor was similar with radiosurgery, we should have by now already observed numerous cases. However, such reported cases[74–76] are extremely rare and frequently fail to meet the classic criteria by which tumors are deemed to be "radiation-induced."[77] If this risk exists, it is likely to be around 1/10 000, which is far lower than the mortality risk associated with temporal lobectomy.[78–82]

Epilepsy is a life-threatening condition. The risk of sudden unexplained death in epileptic patients (SUDEP) is higher than in the general population.[83,84] This risk is higher in patients treated with more than two antiepileptic drugs and IQ lower than 70 (as independent factors). Because seizure cessation after surgery reduces the mortality risk to that of the general population,[84] microsurgical resection of the epileptogenic zone may confer a benefit in terms of the possibility of immediate seizure cessation and therefore reduced mortality risk, as compared with the more delayed benefits of radiosurgical treatment. Our patients are systematically informed about this disadvantage of radiosurgery.

Current Indications

We still consider the use of radiosurgery for MTLE to be investigational. The demonstrated advantages of radiosurgery are the comfort of the procedure, the absence of general anesthesia, the absence of surgical complications and mortality, the very short hospital stay, and the immediate return to the previous level of functioning and employment. Potential sparing of memory function is still a matter of debate and needs to be established using comparative studies. There is also a requirement for further demonstration of long-term efficacy and safety of radiosurgery. Worldwide, microsurgical craniotomies for MTLE are proving to be very satisfactory due to the rarity of surgical complications and a high rate of seizure freedom. In our experience, the most important selection parameters are the demonstration of the purely mesial location of the epileptogenic zone, as well as a clear understanding by the patient of the advantages, disadvantages, and limitations. One other very good indication in our experience is that of patients with proven MTLE but previous failure of open surgery, supposedly due to insufficient extent (usually posteriorly) of resection. The best candidates are young patients, with middle severity epilepsy (working, socially well adapted), a high level of functioning (able to understand well the limits and constraints of radiosurgery), a quite high risk of memory deficit with open surgery (MTLE on the dominant side with little hippocampal atrophy, small deficits in verbal memory preoperatively), and potentially huge social and professional consequences in case of a postoperative memory deficit.

Conclusions

The field of epilepsy surgery is a new and promising one for radiosurgery. However, determination of the extent of the epileptogenic zone requires specific expertise, which is crucial to achieve a reasonable rate of seizure cessation. In addition, the huge impact of fine technical detail on the efficacy and eventual toxicity of the procedure means that, at present, its use for these indications remains under investigation, and further prospective work is necessary.

References

1. Leksell L. The stereotaxic method and radiosurgery of the brain. Acta Chir Scand 1951;102:316–319
2. Leksell L. Sterotaxic radiosurgery in trigeminal neuralgia. Acta Chir Scand 1971;137:311–314
3. Lindquist C, Kihlstrom L, Hellstrand E. Functional neurosurgery–a future for the gamma knife? Stereotact Funct Neurosurg 1991;57:72–81
4. Talairach J, Bancaud J, Szikla G, et al. Approche nouvelle de la neurochirurgie de l'epilepsie. Méthodologie stéréotaxique et résultats thérapeutiques. Neurochirurgie 1974;20:92–98
5. Elomaa E. Focal irradiation of the brain: an alternative to temporal lobe resection in intractable focal epilepsy? Med Hypotheses 1980; 6:501–503

6. Baudouin M, Stuhl L, Perrard A. Un cas d'épilepsie focale traité par la radiothérapie. Rev Neurol 1951;84:60–63

7. Von Wieser W. Die Roentgentherapie der traumatischen Epilepsie. Monatsschr Psychiatr Neurol 1939;101:422–424

8. Heikkinen ER, Konnov B, Melnikow L. Relief of epilepsy by radiosurgery of cerebral arteriovenous malformations. Stereotact Funct Neurosurg 1989;53:157–166

9. Rogers LR, Morris H, Lupica K. Effect of cranial irradiation on seizure frequency in adults with low-grade astrocytoma and medically intractable epilepsy. Neurology 1993;43:1599–1601

10. Rossi GF, Scerrati M, Roselli R. Epileptogenic cerebral low grade tumors: effect of interstital stereotactic irradiation on seizures. Appl Neurophysiol 1985;48:127–132

11. Barcia Salorio JL, Roldan P, Hernandez G, et al. Radiosurgery treatment of epilepsy. Appl Neurophysiol 1985;48:400–403

12. Gaffey CT, Monotoya V, Lyman J, et al. Restriction of the spread of epileptic discharges in cats by mean of Bragg Peak intracranial irradiation. Int J Appl Radiat Isot 1981;32:779–787

13. Chen ZF, Kamiryo T, Henson SL, et al. Anticonvulsant effects of gamma surgery in a model of chronic spontaneous limbic epilepsy in rats. J Neurosurg 2001;94:270–280

14. Maesawa S, Kondziolka D, Dixon C, et al. Subnecrotic stereotactic radiosurgery controlling epilepsy produced by kainic acid injection in rats. J Neurosurg 2000;93:1033–1040

15. Mori Y, Kondziolka D, Balzer J, et al. Effects of stereotactic radiosurgery on an animal model of hippocampal epilepsy. Neurosurgery 2000; 46:157–165

16. Ronne-Engström E, Kihlström L, Flink R, et al. Gamma Knife surgery in epilepsy: an experimental model in the rat, in European Society for Stereotactic and Functional Neurosurgery, Acta Neurochirurgica, 1993

17. Barcia Salorio JL, Garcia JA, Hernandez G, et al. Radiosurgery of epilepsy: long-term results, in European Society for Stereotactic and Functional Neurosurgery, Acta Neurochirurgica, 1993

18. Lindquist C. Gamma knife surgery in focal epilepsy. 1 year follow-up in 4 cases. Unpublished, 1992

19. Lindquist C, Hellstrand E, Kilström L, et al. Stereotactic localisation of epileptic foci by magnetoencephalography and MRI followed by gamma surgery, in International Stereotactic Radiosurgery Symposium, 1991

20. Lindquist C, Kihlström L, Hellstrand E, et al. Stereotactic radiosurgery instead of conventional epilepsy surgery, in European Society for Stereotactic and Functional Neurosurgery, 1993

21. Régis J, Bartolomei F, Hayashi M, et al. The role of gamma knife surgery in the treatment of severe epilepsies. Epileptic Disord 2000;2: 113–122

22. Régis J, Bartolomei F, de Toffol B, et al. Gamma knife surgery for epilepsy related to hypothalamic hamartomas. Neurosurgery 2000; 47:1343–1351

23. Régis J, Hayashi M, Eupierre LP, et al. Gamma knife surgery for epilepsy related to hypothalamic hamartomas. Acta Neurochir Suppl (Wien) 2004;91:33–50

24. Régis J, Bartolomei F, Rey M, et al. Gamma knife surgery for mesial temporal lobe epilepsy. J Neurosurg 2000;93(Suppl 3):141–146

25. Régis J, Rey M, Bartolomei F, et al. Gamma knife surgery in mesial temporal lobe epilepsy: a prospective multicenter study. Epilepsia 2004;45:504–515

26. Régis J, Bartolomei F, Rey M, et al. Gamma knife surgery for mesial temporal lobe epilepsy. Epilepsia 1999;40:1551–1556

27. Régis J, Bartolomei F, Hayashi M, et al. Gamma Knife surgery, a neuromodulation therapy in epilepsy surgery! Acta Neurochir Suppl (Wien) 2002;84:37–47

28. Régis J, Levivier M. M H: Radiosurgery for intractable epilepsy. Tech Neurosurg 2003;9:191–203

29. Régis Y, Roberts D. Gamma Knife radiosurgery relative to microsurgery: epilepsy. Stereotact Funct Neurosurg 1999;72(Suppl 1):11–21

30. Régis J, Semah F, Bryan R, et al. Early and delayed MR and PET changes after selective temporomesial radiosurgery in mesial temporal lobe epilepsy. AJNR Am J Neuroradiol 1999;20:213–216

31. Régis J, Kerkerian-Legoff L, Rey M, et al. First biochemical evidence of differential functional effects following gamma knife surgery. Stereotact Funct Neurosurg 1996;66:29–38

32. Régis J, Peragut JC, Rey M, et al. First selective amygdalohippocampic radiosurgery for mesial temporal lobe epilepsy. Stereotact Funct Neurosurg 1995;64:193–201

33. Deonna T, Ziegler AL. Hypothalamic hamartoma, precocious puberty and gelastic seizures: a special model of "epileptic" developmental disorder. Epileptic Disord 2000;2:33–37

34. Kuzniecky R, Guthrie B, Mountz J, et al. Intrinsic epileptogenesis of hypothalamic hamartomas in gelastic epilepsy. Ann Neurol 1997;42:60–67

35. Munari C, Kahane P, Francione S, et al. Role of the hypothalamic hamartoma in the genesis of gelastic fits (a video-stereo-EEG study). Electroencephalogr Clin Neurophysiol 1995;95:154–160

36. Frattali CM, Liow K, Craig GH, et al. Cognitive deficits in children with gelastic seizures and hypothalamic hamartoma. Neurology 2001; 57:43–46

37. Weissenberger AA, Dell ML, Liow K, et al. Aggression and psychiatric comorbidity in children with hypothalamic hamartomas and their unaffected siblings. J Am Acad Child Adolesc Psychiatry 2001;40: 696–703

38. Arita K, Ikawa F, Kurisu K, et al. The relationship between magnetic resonance imaging findings and clinical manifestations of hypothalamic hamartoma. J Neurosurg 1999;91:212–220

39. Debeneix C, Bourgeois M, Trivin C, et al. Hypothalamic hamartoma: comparison of clinical presentation and magnetic resonance images. Horm Res 2001;56:12–18

40. Valdueza JM, Cristante L, Dammann O, et al. Hypothalamic hamartomas: with special reference to gelastic epilepsy and surgery. Neurosurgery 1994;34:949–958

41. Delalande O, Fohlen M. Disconnecting surgical treatment of hypothalamic hamartoma in children and adults with refractory epilepsy and proposal of a new classification. Neurol Med Chir (Tokyo) 2003;43:61–68

42. Palmini A, Chandler C, Andermann F, et al. Resection of the lesion in patients with hypothalamic hamartomas and catastrophic epilepsy. Neurology 2002;58:1338–1347

43. Regis J, Scavarda D, Tamura M, et al. Epilepsy related to hypothalamic hamartomas: surgical management with special reference to gamma knife surgery. Childs Nerv Syst 2006;22:881–895

44. Pascual-Castroviejo I, Moneo JH, Viano J, et al. [Hypothalamic hamartomas: control of seizures after partial removal in one case.] Rev Neurol 2000;31:119–122

45. Rosenfeld JV, Harvey AS, Wrennall J, et al. Transcallosal resection of hypothalamic hamartomas, with control of seizures, in children with gelastic epilepsy. Neurosurgery 2001;48:108–118

46. Watanabe T, Enomoto T, Uemura K, et al. [Gelastic seizures treated by partial resection of a hypothalamic hamartoma] No Shinkei Geka 1998;26:923–928

47. Cascino GD, Andermann F, Berkovic SF, et al. Gelastic seizures and hypothalamic hamartomas: evaluation of patients undergoing chronic intracranial EEG monitoring and outcome of surgical treatment. Neurology 1993;43:747–750

48. Bartolomei F, Hayashi M, Tamura M, Rey M, Fischer C, Chauvel P, Regis J. Long term efficacy of Gamma Knife radiosurgery in mesial temporal lobe epilepsy. Neurology, 2008;70:1658–1663

49. Kawai K, Suzuki I, Kurita H, et al. Failure of low-dose radiosurgery to control temporal lobe epilepsy. J Neurosurg 2001;95:883–887

50. Cmelak AJ, Abou-Khalil B, Konrad PE, et al. Low-dose stereotactic radiosurgery is inadequate for medically intractable mesial temporal lobe epilepsy: a case report. Seizure 2001;10:442–446

51. Yang KJ, Wang KW, Wu HP, et al. Radiosurgical treatment of intractable epilepsy with low radiation dose. Di Yi Jun Yi Da Xue Xue Bao 2002;22:645–647

52. Kihlstrom L, Hindmarsh T, Lax I, et al. Radiosurgical lesions in the normal human brain 17 years after gamma knife capsulotomy. Neurosurgery 1997;41:396–401

53. Kihlström L, Guo WY, Lindquist C, et al. Radiobiology of radiosurgery for refractory anxiety disorders. Neurosurgery 1995;36:294–302

54. Barcia-Salorio JL, Barcia JA, Hernandez G, et al. Radiosurgery of epilepsy. Long-term results. Acta Neurochir Suppl (Wien) 1994;62:111–113

55. Hayashi M, Bartolomei F, Rey M, et al. MR changes after Gamma Knife radiosurgery for mesial temporal lobe epilepsy: an evidence for the efficacy of subnecrotic doses. In Kondziolka D, ed. Radiosurgery. Vol 4. Basel: Karger; 2002:192–202

56. Hayashi M, Regis J, Hori T. [Current treatment strategy with gamma knife surgery for mesial temporal lobe epilepsy.] No Shinkei Geka 2003;31:141–155

57. Grabenbauer GG, Reinhold C, Kerling F, et al. Frationated stereotactically guided radiotherapy of pharmacoresistant temporal lobe epilepsy. Acta Neurochir Suppl (Wien) 2002;84:65–70

58. Stefan H, Hummel C, Grabenbauer GG, et al. Successful treatment of focal epilepsy by fractionated stereotactic radiotherapy. Eur Neurol 1998;39:248–250

59. Barcia Salorio JL, Vanaclocha V, Cerda M, et al. Focus irradiation in epilepsy. Experimental study in the cat. Appl Neurophysiol 1985;48:152–154

60. Maesawa S, Kondziolka D, Balzer J, et al. The behavioral and electro-encephalographic effects of stereotactic radiosurgery for the treatment of epilepsy evaluated in the rat kainic acid model. Stereotact Funct Neurosurg 1999;73:115

61. Bartolomei F, Wendling F, Bellanger JJ, et al. Neural networks involving the medial temporal structures in temporal lobe epilepsy. Clin Neurophysiol 2001;112:1746–1760

62. Spencer SS, Spencer D. Entorhinal-hippocampal interactions in medial temporal lobe epilepsy. Epilepsia 1994;35:721–727

63. Flickinger JC. An integrated logistic formula for prediction of complications from radiosurgery. Int J Radiat Oncol Biol Phys 1989;17:879–885

64. Régis J, Bartolomei F, Kida Y, et al. Radiosurgery of epilepsy associated with cavernous malformation: retrospective study in 49 patients. Neurosurgery 2000;47:1091–1097

65. Jones R, Heinemann U, Lambert J. The entorhinal cortex and generation of seizure activity: studies of normal synaptic transmission and epileptogenesis in vitro In: Avanzini G, Engel J, Fariello R, et al, eds. Neurotransmitters in Epilepsy. Amsterdam: Elsevier Science; 1992:173–180

66. Wilson WA, Swartzwelder HS, Anderson WW, et al. Seizure activity in vitro: a dual focus model. Epilepsy Res 1988;2:289–293

67. Wieser HG, Siegel AM, Yasargil GM. The Zurich amygdalo-hippocampectomy series: a short up-date. Acta Neurochir Suppl (Wien) 1990;50:122–127

68. Whang CJ, Kwon Y. Long-term follow-up of stereotactic Gamma Knife radiosurgery in epilepsy. Stereotact Funct Neurosurg 1996;66 (Suppl 1):349–356

69. Kitchen N. Experimental and clinical studies on the putative therapeutic efficacy of cerebral irradiation (radiotherapy) in epilepsy. Epilepsy Res 1995;20:1–10

70. Glosser G, McManus P, Munzenrider J, et al. Neuropsychological function in adults after high dose fractionated radiation therapy of skull base tumors. Int J Radiat Oncol Biol Phys 1997;38:231–239

71. McCord MW, Buatti JM, Fennell EM, et al. Radiotherapy for pituitary adenoma: long-term outcome and sequelae. Int J Radiat Oncol Biol Phys 1997;39:437–444

72. Strasnick B, Glasscock ME, Haynes D. The natural history of untreated acoustic neuromas. Laryngoscope 1994;104:1115–1119

73. Simmons NE, Laws E. Gliomas Occurence after sellar Irradiation: case report and review. Neurosurgery 1998;42:172–178

74. Kaido T, Hoshida T, Uranishi R, et al. Radiosurgery-induced brain tumor. Case report. J Neurosurg 2001;95:710–713

75. Shamisa A, Bance M, Nag S, et al. Glioblastoma multiforme occurring in a patient treated with gamma knife surgery. Case report and review of the literature. J Neurosurg 2001;94:816–821

76. Yu JS, Yong WH, Wilson D, et al. Glioblastoma induction after radiosurgery for meningioma. Lancet 2000;356:1576–1577

77. Cahan W, Woodard H, Highinbotham N, et al. Sarcoma arising in irradiated bone: report of eleven cases. Cancer 1948;1:3–29

78. Ganz JC. Gamma knife radiosurgery and its possible relationship to malignancy: a review. J Neurosurg 2002;97:644–652

79. Loeffler JS, Niemierko A, Chapman PH. Second tumors after radiosurgery: tip of the iceberg or a bump in the road? Neurosurgery 2003;52:1436–1440

80. Lunsford LD, Niranjan A, Flickinger JC, et al. Radiosurgery of vestibular schwannomas: summary of experience in 829 cases. J Neurosurg 2005;102(Suppl):195–199

81. Muracciole X, Cowen D, Regis J. [Radiosurgery and brain radio-induced carcinogenesis: update.] Neurochirurgie 2004;50:414–420

82. Rowe J, Grainger A, Walton L, et al. Risk of malignancy after gamma knife stereotactic radiosurgery. Neurosurgery 2007;60:60–65

83. Ficker DM, So EL, Shen WK, et al. Population-based study of the incidence of sudden unexplained death in epilepsy. Neurology 1998;51:1270–1274

84. Sperling MR, Feldman H, Kinman J, et al. Seizure control and mortality in epilepsy. Ann Neurol 1999;46:45–50

Index

Note: Page numbers followed by *f* and *t* indicate figures and tables, respectively.

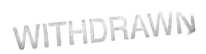